OXFORD MEDICAL PUBLICATIONS

Oxford Handbook of
Critical Care

KU-214-783

Oxford Handbook of Critical Care

M. SINGER
and
A. R. WEBB

Oxford New York Tokyo
OXFORD UNIVERSITY PRESS
1997

Oxford University Press, Walton Street, Oxford OX2 6DP

Oxford New York
Athens Auckland Bangkok Bombay Bogota
Buenos Aires Calcutta Cape Town Dar es Salaam
Delhi Florence Hong Kong Istanbul Karachi
Kuala Lumpur Madras Madrid Melbourne
Mexico City Nairobi Paris Singapore
Taipei Tokyo Toronto

and associated companies in
Berlin Ibadan

Oxford is a trade mark of Oxford University Press

Published in the United States
by Oxford University Press Inc., New York
© M. Singer and A. R. Webb, 1997

A catalogue record for this book is available from the British Library

Library of Congress Cataloging in Publication Data
Singer, Mervyn.
Oxford handbook of critical care / M. Singer and A. R. Webb.
p. cm.
1. Critical care medicine—Handbooks, manuals, etc.
I. Webb, A.R. (Andrew Roy) II. Title.
RC86.8.S595 1997 616'.028—dc20 96-20157
ISBN 0 19 262542 X

Typeset by Joshua Associates Ltd, Oxford
Printed in Great Britain by
The Bath Press Ltd, Bath.

Preface

Of all the medical specialties, few if any are as exacting and complex as critical care medicine. The required knowledge of physiology, pathophysiology, biochemistry, technology and pharmacology; the unpredictability; the need to act and react decisively; the ability to communicate clearly with colleagues, patients and relatives, often in stressful situations; the importance of working cohesively within an expanded team drawn from different backgrounds; and the regular occurrences of ethical and life-and-death dilemmas all place heavy demands on the intensive care staff member.

This book does not aim to be a panacea; many areas of uncertainty in diagnosis and management remain. However, current best practice (at least as practised by us!) is described in succinct, concise, clinically orientated sections covering therapeutic and monitoring, drugs and fluids, specific organ system disorders and complications, and general management philosophies. Ample space is provided to append or amend sections to suit your particular practice.

It will hopefully serve the consultant, junior doctor, nurse or other paramedical staff as a reference book, aide mémoire and handy pocket book providing rationales and solutions to most of the problems encountered.

1996   Mervyn Singer
                                                             Andrew Webb

Acknowledgements

We would like to thank all our colleagues from whom we have sought advice during the preparation of this book. In particular, we acknowledge the assistance of Dr E Ahmed for providing helpful criticism and Drs G Ridgway and P Wilson for microbiological advice.

Respiratory Therapy Techniques

Oxygen therapy

All critically ill patients should receive additional inspired oxygen on a 'more not less is best' philosophy.

Principles

High flow, high concentration oxygen should be given to any acutely dyspnoeic or hypoxaemic patient until accurate titration can be performed using arterial blood gas analysis.

Generally maintain SaO_2 > 90% though preferably > 95%. Compromises may need to be made during (i) severe ARDS/acute respiratory failure or (ii) acute on chronic hypoxaemic respiratory failure when target values > 80–85% may be sufficient provided tissue oxygen delivery is maintained.

All patients placed on mechanical ventilation should initially receive a high FIO_2 until accurate titration is performed using arterial blood gas analysis.

Apart from patients receiving hyperbaric O_2 therapy (e.g. carbon monoxide poisoning, diving accidents), there is no need to maintain very high levels of PaO_2.

Cautions

A *small* proportion of patients in chronic Type II (hypoxaemic, hypercapnic) respiratory failure will develop apnoea if their central hypoxic drive is removed by supplemental oxygen. However, this is seldom (if ever) abrupt and a period of deterioration and increasing drowsiness will alert medical and nursing staff to consider either (i) FIO_2 reduction if overall condition allows (ii) mechanical ventilation if fatiguing or (iii) use of respiratory stimulants such as doxepram. The corollary is that close supervision and monitoring is necessary in all critically ill patients.

A normal pulse oximetry reading may obscure deteriorating gas exchange and progressive hypercapnia.

Oxygen toxicity is described in animal models and normal volunteers will become symptomatic after several hours of breathing pure oxygen. Furthermore, washout of nitrogen may lead to microatelectasis. However, the relevance and relative importance of oxygen toxicity compared to other forms of ventilator trauma in critically ill patients is still far from clear. Efforts should nevertheless be made to minimise FIO_2 whenever possible. Debate continues as to whether FIO_2 or other ventilator settings (e.g. PEEP, V_T, inspiratory pressures) should be reduced first. The authors' present view is to minimise the risks of ventilator trauma first, using as high an FIO_2 as necessary.

Monitoring

An oxygen analyser in the inspiratory limb of the ventilator or CPAP circuit confirms the patient is receiving a known FIO_2. Some ventilators have a built-in calibration device.

Adequacy and changes in arterial oxygen saturation can be continuously monitored by pulse oximetry and intermittent or continuous invasive blood gas analysis.

Techniques

- Hudson-type masks or nasal 'spectacles' give an imprecise FIO_2 and should only be used when hypoxaemia is not a major concern. Hudson-type masks do allow delivery of humidified gas (e.g. via an 'Aquapak'). Valves fitted to the Aquapak system do not deliver an accurate FIO_2.
- Masks fitted with a Venturi valve deliver a reasonably accurate FIO_2 (0.24, 0.28, 0.35, 0.40, 0.60) except in patients with very high inspiratory flow rates. These masks do not allow delivery of humidified gas but are preferable in the short-term for dyspnoeic patients as they enable more precise monitoring of PaO_2 /FIO_2 ratios.
- Tight-fitting anaesthetic mask and reservoir bag—allows 100% oxygen to be delivered.

See also:
Ventilatory support—indications, 5; Continuous positive airway pressure, 23;
Basic resuscitation, 259; Respiratory failure, 271

Ventilatory support—indications

Acute ventilatory insufficiency

Defined by an acute rise in $PaCO_2$ and respiratory acidosis (pH < 7.2). $PaCO_2$ is directly proportional to the body's CO_2 production and inversely proportional to alveolar ventilation (minute ventilation minus dead space ventilation). May be caused by:

- Respiratory centre depression, e.g. by depressant drugs or intracranial pathology
- Peripheral neuromuscular disease, e.g. Guillain–Barré syndrome, myasthenia gravis or spinal cord pathology
- Therapeutic muscle paralysis, e.g. as part of balanced anaesthesia, tetanus or status epilepticus
- Loss of chest wall integrity, e.g. chest trauma, diaphragmatic rupture
- High CO_2 production, e.g. burns, sepsis or severe agitation
- Reduced alveolar ventilation, e.g. airways obstruction (asthma, acute bronchitis, foreign body), atelectasis, pneumonia, pulmonary oedema (ARDS, cardiac failure), pleural pathology, fibrotic lung disease, obesity
- Pulmonary vascular disease (pulmonary embolus, cardiac failure, ARDS)

Oxygenation failure

Hypoxaemia is defined by $PaO_2 < 11kPa$ on $FIO_2 \geqslant 0.4$. May be due to:

- Ventilation / perfusion mismatching (reduced ventilation in or preferential perfusion of some lung areas), e.g. pneumonia, pulmonary oedema, pulmonary vascular disease, extremely high cardiac output
- Shunt (normal perfusion but absent ventilation in some lung zones), e.g. pneumonia, pulmonary oedema
- Diffusion limitation (reduced alveolar surface area with normal ventilation, e.g. emphysema; reduced inspired oxygen tension, e.g. altitude, suffocation
- Acute ventilatory insufficiency (as above)

To reduce intracranial pressure

Reduction of $PaCO_2$ to approximately 4kPa causes cerebral vasoconstriction and therefore reduces intracranial pressure after brain injury. Recent studies suggest this effect is transient and may impair an already critical cerebral blood flow.

To reduce work of breathing

Controlled ventilation ± sedation and muscle relaxation reduces respiratory muscle activity and therefore work of breathing. In cardiac failure or non-cardiogenic pulmonary oedema the resulting reduction in myocardial oxygen demand is easier matched to oxygen supply.

Indications for ventilatory support

Ventilatory support should be considered if:

Respiratory rate $> 30/\text{min}$
Vital capacity $< 10\text{--}15\,\text{ml/min}$
$PaO_2 < 11\,\text{kPa}$ on $FIO_2 \geqslant 0.4$
$PaCO_2$ high with respiratory acidosis (pH < 7.2)
$V_D/V_T > 60\%$
$Q_S/Q_T > 15\text{--}20\%$
Exhaustion
Confusion
Severe shock
Severe LVF
Raised ICP

See also:

IPPV—description of ventilators

Classification of mechanical ventilators

Mechanical ventilators may be classified according to the method of cycling from inspiration to expiration. This may be when a pre-set time has elapsed (time-cycled), when a pre-set pressure has been reached (pressure-cycled) or when a pre-set volume has been delivered (volume-cycled). Although the method of cycling is classified according to a single constant, modern ventilators allow a greater degree of control. In volume-cycled mode with pressure limit the upper pressure alarm limit is set or the maximum inspiratory pressure is controlled. The ventilator delivers a pre-set tidal volume (V_T) unless lungs are non-compliant or airway resistance is high. This is useful to avoid high peak airway pressures. In volume-cycled mode with time limit inspiratory flow is reduced; the ventilator delivers the pre-set V_T unless impossible at the set respiratory rate. If pressure limitation is not available this is useful to limit peak airway pressures. In time-cycled mode with pressure control, pre-set pressure is delivered throughout inspiration (unlike pressure-cycled ventilation), cycling being determined by time. V_T is dependent on respiratory compliance and airway resistance and high peak airway pressures can be avoided.

Setting up the mechanical ventilator

Tidal volume
Normally 7–10ml/kg but may require 10–12ml/kg in acute respiratory failure. In severe airflow limitation (e.g. asthma, acute bronchitis) smaller V_T and minute volume may be needed to allow prolonged expiration.

Respiratory rate
Usually set in accordance with V_T to provide minute ventilation of 85–100ml/kg/min. In time-cycled or time-limited modes the set respiratory rate determines the timing of ventilator cycles.

Inspiratory flow
Usually set between 40–80L/min. A higher flow rate is more comfortable for alert patients and also allows for longer expiration in patients with severe airflow limitation. However, it is also associated with higher peak airway pressures. In addition, the flow pattern may be adjusted on most ventilators. A square wave is common but decelerating flow, by reducing the average flow rate at a set peak flow rate, may reduce peak airway pressure.

I:E ratio
A function of respiratory rate, V_T, inspiratory flow and inspiratory time. Prolonged expiration is useful in severe airflow limitation and a prolonged inspiratory time is used in ARDS to allow slow reacting alveoli time to fill. Alert patients are more comfortable with shorter inspiratory times and high inspiratory flow rates.

FIO_2
Set according to arterial blood gases. Usual to start at $FIO_2 = 0.6–1$.

Airway pressure
In pressure controlled or pressure limited modes the peak airway pressure (circuit rather than alveolar pressure) can be set (usually $\leqslant 40cmH_2O$). PEEP can be used to maintain FRC when respiratory compliance is low.

Initial ventilator set-up

Check for leaks
Check oxygen on
FIO_2 0.6–1
V_T 7–12ml/kg
Rate 10–15/min
I:E ratio 1:2
Peak pressure $\leqslant$40cmH_2O
PEEP 0–5cmH_2O

Ventilator adjustments in response to blood gas measurements

Low PaO_2
Increase FIO_2
Increase PEEP (may increase peak airway pressure or reduce CO)
Increase I:E ratio
Review V_T and respiratory rate
Consider CMV, increased sedation $\pm$ muscle relaxants

High PaO_2
Decrease PEEP (usually to 5cmH_2O before reducing FIO_2)
Decrease FIO_2
Decrease I:E ratio

High $PaCO_2$
Increase V_T (if peak airway pressure will allow)
Increase respiratory rate
Consider reducing respiratory rate if too high (to reduce intrinsic PEEP)
Consider reducing dead space
Consider CMV, increased sedation $\pm$ muscle relaxants
Consider tolerating (permissive hypercapnia)

Low $PaCO_2$
Decrease respiratory rate (to 10–12/min)
Decrease V_T (to < 7ml/kg)

IPPV—modes of ventilation

Controlled mechanical ventilation (CMV)

A pre-set number of breaths are delivered to supply all the patient's ventilatory requirements. These breaths may be at a pre-set V_T (volume controlled) or at a pre-set inspiratory pressure (pressure controlled).

Assist—control mechanical ventilation (ACMV)

Patients can trigger the ventilator to determine the respiratory rate but, as with CMV, a pre-set number of breaths are delivered if the spontaneous respiratory rate falls below the pre-set level.

Intermittent mandatory ventilation (IMV)

A pre-set mandatory rate is set but patients are free to breathe spontaneously between set ventilator breaths. Mandatory breaths may be synchronised with a patient's spontaneous efforts (SIMV) to avoid mandatory breaths occurring during a spontaneous breath. This effect, known as 'stacking' may lead to excessive tidal volumes, high airway pressure, incomplete exhalation and air trapping. Pressure support may be added to spontaneous breaths to overcome the work of breathing associated with opening the ventilator demand valve.

Pressure support ventilation (PSV)

A pre-set inspiratory pressure is added to the ventilator circuit during inspiration in spontaneously breathing patients. The pre-set pressure should be adjusted to ensure adequate V_T.

Choosing the appropriate mode

Pressure controlled ventilation avoids the dangers associated with high peak airway pressures, although it may result in marked changes in V_T if compliance alters. Allowing the patient to make some spontaneous respiratory effort may reduce sedation requirements, re-train respiratory muscles and reduce mean airway pressures.

Apnoeic patient
Use of IMV or ACMV in patients who are totally apnoeic provides the total minute volume requirement if the pre-set rate is high enough (this is effectively CMV) but allows spontaneous respiratory effort on recovery.

Patient taking limited spontaneous breaths
A guaranteed minimum minute volume is assured with both ACMV and IMV depending on the pre-set rate. The work of spontaneous breathing is reduced by supplying the pre-set V_T for spontaneously triggered breaths with ACMV, or by adding pressure support to spontaneous breaths with IMV. With ACMV the spontaneous tidal volume is guaranteed whereas with IMV and pressure support spontaneous tidal volume depends on lung compliance and may be less than pre-set tidal volume. The advantage of IMV and pressure support is that gradual reduction of pre-set rate, as spontaneous effort increases, allows a smooth transition to pressure support ventilation. Subsequent weaning is by reduction of pressure support level.

IPPV—failure to tolerate ventilation

Agitation or 'fighting the ventilator' may occur at any time.

Poor tolerance during initial phase of ventilation

Immediately after initiating mechanical ventilation the most likely cause is a failure to match ventilator settings to the patient's requirements. Careful adjustment of V_T, respiratory rate, inspiratory flow and trigger sensitivity may resolve the problem; alternatively, additional sedation $\pm$ muscle relaxation may be required.

Poor tolerance after previous good tolerance

If agitation occurs in a patient who has previously tolerated mechanical ventilation, either the patient's condition has deteriorated (e.g. tension pneumothorax) or there is a problem in the ventilator circuit (including artificial airway) or the ventilator itself.

- The patient should be removed from the ventilator and placed on manual ventilation while the problem is resolved. Resorting to increased sedation $\pm$ muscle relaxation in this circumstance is dangerous until the cause is resolved.
- Check patency of the endotracheal tube (e.g. with a suction catheter) and re-intubate if in doubt.
- Consider malposition of the endotracheal tube (e.g. cuff above vocal cords, tube tip at carina, tube in main bronchus)
- Where patients are making spontaneous respiratory efforts it is often better to allow this with IMV and pressure support or, if ventilatory drive is adequate, with PSV alone, rather than increasing sedation.
- If patients fail to synchronise with IMV by stacking spontaneous and mandatory breaths, increasing pressure support and reducing mandatory rate may help; alternatively, the use of PSV may be appropriate.

IPPV—complications of ventilation

Haemodynamic complications

Venous return is dependent on passive flow from central veins to right atrium. As right atrial pressure increases secondary to the transmitted increase in intrathoracic pressure across compliant lungs there is a reduction in venous return. This is less of a problem if lungs are stiff (e.g. ARDS) although will be exacerbated by the use of inverse I:E ratio. As lung volume is increased by IPPV the pulmonary vasculature is constricted, thus increasing pulmonary vascular resistance. This increases the diastolic volume of the right ventricle and, by septal shift, impedes filling of the left ventricle. These effects all contribute to a reduced stroke volume. This reduction can be minimised by reducing airway pressures, avoiding prolonged inspiratory times and maintaining blood volume.

Ventilator trauma

The term barotrauma relates to gas escape into cavities and interstitial tissues occurring during IPPV. The complication is a misnomer since it is probably the distending volume which is responsible rather than the pressure. It is most likely to occur with high V_T and high PEEP. It also occurs in IPPV and conditions associated with overinflation of the lungs (e.g. asthma). Tension pneumothorax is life threatening and should be suspected in any patient on IPPV who becomes suddenly agitated, tachycardic, hypotensive or exhibits sudden deterioration in their blood gases. An immediate chest drainage tube should be inserted if tension pneumothorax develops. Prevention of ventilator trauma relies on avoidance of high V_T, high PEEP and high airway pressures.

Nosocomial infection

Endotracheal intubation bypasses normal defence mechanisms. Ciliary activity and cellular morphology in the tracheobronchial tree are altered. The requirement for endotracheal suction further increases susceptibility to infection. In addition, the normal heat and moisture exchanging mechanisms are bypassed requiring artificial humidification of inspired gases. Failure to provide adequate humidification increases the risk of sputum retention and infection.

Acid–base disturbance

Ventilating patients with chronic respiratory failure or hyperventilation may, by rapid correction of hypercapnia, cause respiratory alkalosis. This reduces pulmonary blood flow and may contribute to hypoxaemia. A respiratory acidosis due to hypercapnia may be due to inappropriate ventilator settings or may be desired in an attempt to avoid high V_T and ventilator trauma.

Water retention

Vasopressin released from the anterior pituitary is increased due to a reduction in intrathoracic blood volume and psychological stress. Reduced urine flow thus contributes to water retention. In addition, the use of PEEP reduces lymphatic flow with consequent peripheral oedema, especially affecting the upper body.

Respiratory muscle wasting

Prolonged ventilation may lead to disuse atrophy of the respiratory muscles.

IPPV—weaning techniques

Patients may require all or part of their respiratory support to be provided by a mechanical ventilator. Weaning from mechanical ventilation may follow several patterns. In patients ventilated for a short period (less than a few days), it is common to allow 20–30min breathing on a 'T' piece before removing the endotracheal tube. For patients who have received longer term ventilation it is unlikely that mechanical support can be withdrawn suddenly; several methods are commonly used to wean mechanical ventilation from these patients. There is, however, no evidence that any technique is superior in terms of weaning success or speed of weaning.

Intermittent 'T' piece or continuous positive airway pressure (CPAP)

Spontaneous breathing is allowed for increasingly prolonged periods with a rest on mechanical ventilation in between. The use of a 'T' piece for longer than 30min may lead to basal atelectasis since the endotracheal tube bypasses the physiological PEEP effect of the larynx. It is therefore common to use 5cmH$_2$O CPAP as spontaneous breathing periods get longer. With these techniques mechanical ventilation is continued at night to encourage sleep and respiratory muscle rest. Once unaided spontaneous breathing continues throughout the day it is likely that it will continue successfully through the night.

Intermittent mandatory ventilation (IMV)

The set mandatory rate is gradually reduced as the spontaneous rate increases. Spontaneous breaths are usually pressure supported to overcome circuit and ventilator valve resistance. With this technique it is important that the patient's required minute ventilation is provided by the combination of mandatory breaths and spontaneous breaths without an excessive spontaneous rate. The reduction in mandatory rate should be slow enough to maintain adequate minute ventilation. It is also important that the patient can synchronise his own respiratory efforts with mandatory ventilator breaths; many cannot, particularly where there are frequent spontaneous breaths, some of which may 'stack' with mandatory breaths causing hyperinflation.

Pressure support ventilation

All respiratory efforts are spontaneous but positive pressure is added to each breath, the level being chosen to maintain an appropriate tidal volume. Weaning continues with a gradual reduction of the pressure support level while the respiratory rate is < 30/min. The patient is extubated or allowed to breathe with 5cmH$_2$O CPAP when pressure support is only overcoming the resistance of the ventilator circuit and valves (< 10–15cmH$_2$O with modern ventilators) .

Choice of ventilator

Modern ventilators have enhancements to aid weaning; however, weaning most patients from ventilation is possible with a basic ventilator and the intermittent 'T' piece technique, provided an adequate fresh gas flow is provided. If IMV and/or pressure support are used the ventilator should provide the features listed in the table opposite.

Key features in the choice of ventilator

15

Ventilator must allow patient triggering (i.e. not a minute volume divider)

Fresh gas flow must be greater than spontaneous peak inspiratory flow

Minimum circuit resistance (short, wide bore, smooth internal lumen)

Low resistance ventilator valves

Sensitive pressure or flow trigger (ideally monitored close to the ET tube)

Synchronised IMV (avoids 'stacking' mandatory on spontaneous breaths)

See also:
IPPV—assessment of weaning, 16

IPPV—assessment of weaning

Assessment prior to weaning

Prior to weaning it is important that the cause of respiratory failure and any complications arising from respiratory failure have been corrected. Sepsis should be eradicated as should other factors that increase oxygen demand. Attention is required to nutritional status and fluid and electrolyte balance. The diaphragm should be allowed to contract unhindered by choosing the optimum position for breathing (sitting up unless quadriplegic) and ensuring that intra-abdominal pressure is not high. Adequate analgesia must be provided but sedatives should have been withdrawn unless the patient has a raised intracranial pressure. Weaning should start when staffing is at its best (i.e. not at night) and only after adequate explanation has been given to the patient. Factors predicting weaning success are detailed in the table opposite. Spontaneous (pressure supported) breathing should start as soon as possible to allow reduction in sedation levels, and maintain respiratory muscle function. However, weaning with the intention of removing mechanical ventilatory support is unlikely to be successful while $FIO_2 > 0.4$.

Assessment during weaning

Continuous pulse oximetry and regular clinical review are essential during weaning. Arterial blood gases should be taken after 20–30min spontaneous breathing and, after short term ventilation, extubation should follow if arterial gases and respiratory pattern are satisfactory, the cough reflex is adequate and the patient can clear any sputum. Patients who are being weaned from longer term ventilation should be allowed to breathe spontaneously for at least 24h before extubation.

Indications for reventilation

If spontaneous respiration is discoordinate or the patient is exhausted, agitated or clammy the ventilator should be reconnected. However, clinical monitoring should avoid exhaustion. Successful weaning is more easily accomplished if excessive tiredness is not allowed to set in. Tachypnoea (>30/min), tachycardia (>110/min), respiratory acidosis ($pH < 7.2$), rising $PaCO_2$ and hypoxaemia ($SaO_2 < 90\%$) should all prompt reconnection of the ventilator.

Factors associated with weaning failure

Failure to wean is associated with:
- Increased oxygen cost of breathing
- Muscle fatigue (hypophosphataemia, hypomagnesaemia, hypokalaemia, hypothyroidism, malnutrition, peripheral neuropathy, myopathy and drugs, e.g. muscle relaxants, aminoglycosides,)
- Inadequate respiratory drive (alkalosis, opiates, sedatives, malnutrition, hypothyroidism, cerebrovascular accident, coma)
- Inadequate cardiac reserve and heart failure.

In the latter case cardiac output should be monitored during spontaneous breathing periods. Any deterioration in cardiac function should be treated aggressively (e.g. optimal fluid therapy, vasodilators, inotropes)

Factors predicting weaning success

$PaO_2 > 11kPa$ on $FIO_2 = 0.4$ (PaO_2/FIO_2 ratio $> 27.5kPa$)
Minute volume $< 12L/min$
Vital capacity $> 10ml/kg$
Maximum inspiratory force (PI_{max}) $> 20cmH_2O$
Respiratory rate / tidal volume < 100
$Q_S/Q_T < 15\%$
Dead space / tidal volume $< 60\%$
Haemodynamic stability

See also:
IPPV—weaning techniques, 14

High frequency jet ventilation

A high pressure jet of gas entrains further fresh gas which is directed by the jet towards the lungs.

- Respiratory rates of 100–300/min ensure minute volumes of about 20L/min although tidal volume may be lower than dead space volume.
- CO_2 elimination is usually more efficient than on conventional IPPV.
- The method of gas exchange is not fully elucidated but includes turbulent gas mixing and convection.
- Oxygenation is dependent on mean airway pressure.
- Peak airway pressures are lower than with conventional mechanical ventilation but auto-PEEP and mean airway pressures are maintained.

There is often a reduction in SaO_2 when patients start on high frequency jet ventilation (HFJV), although this usually improves with time.

The high gas flow rates employed require additional humidification to be provided, usually nebulised with the jet.

Indications

Bronchopleural fistula is the only definite indication in the ICU but HFJV has been used to help wean patients from mechanical ventilation and for respiratory support in ARDS. In weaning patients the open circuit allows spontaneous breaths without the drawbacks of demand valves. The HFJV ensures adequate ventilation if the patient fails to breathe adequately. In ARDS conventional ventilation can lead to ventilator trauma if high V_T is used. HFJV avoids the problems associated with high V_T but does not provide adequate ventilation for all patients.

Setting up HFJV

- A jet must be provided either by using a modified endotracheal tube or modified catheter mount. Entrainment gas is provided via a T-piece.
- Tidal volume cannot be set during HFJV. A display of V_T or minute volume is calculated according to jet size, I:E ratio, driving pressure and respiratory rate via an in-built algorithm.
- Respiratory rate is usually set between 100–200/min. As respiratory rate increases at constant driving pressure CO_2 may increase since increasing auto-PEEP increases the effective physiological dead space.
- I:E ratio is usually set between 1:3 and 1:2. V_T is determined by airway pressure and I:E ratio.
- Driving pressure is usually set between 1–2 bar. Note these pressures are extremely high compared to the 60–100cmH$_2$O used in conventional ventilation. Jet ventilators are designed to cut out on occlusion.
- Auto-PEEP is related to the driving pressure, I:E ratio and respiratory rate. External PEEP can be added to increase mean airway pressure should this be necessary to improve oxygenation.

Weaning HFJV

If HFJV is used with an open breathing circuit the patient may take conventional breaths. Reducing the driving pressure and increasing the respiratory rate may facilitate weaning.

Combined HFJV and conventional CMV

May be useful in ARDS where HFJV alone cannot provide adequate gas exchange. Low frequency pressure limited ventilation with PEEP provides an adequate mean airway pressure to ensure oxygenation whilst CO_2 clearance is effected by HFJV. Care must be taken to avoid excessive peak airway pressures when HFJV breaths stack on CMV breaths.

Adjusting HFJV according to blood gases

Increasing PaO_2
Increase FIO_2
Increase I:E ratio
Increase driving pressure
Add external PEEP
Consider reducing respiratory rate

Decreasing $PaCO_2$
Increase driving pressure
Decrease respiratory rate

See also:
Ventilatory support—indications, 4; Positive end expiratory pressure, 20; Adult respiratory distress syndrome 1, 280; Adult respiratory distress syndrome 2, 282

Positive end expiratory pressure

Positive end-expiratory pressure (PEEP) is a modality used in positive pressure ventilation to prevent the alveoli returning to atmospheric pressure during expiration. An integral setting in all modern positive pressure ventilators, it can also be obtained by adding a valve (or underwater seal of measured depth) to the expiratory limb of the ventilator circuit. It is usually set $\leqslant 10cmH_2O$ and rarely $> 20cmH_2O$ to avoid cardiorespiratory complications (see below). It does not prevent nor attenuate ARDS, reduce capillary leak or lung water, nor hasten lung recovery.

Respiratory effects

PEEP improves oxygenation by recruiting collapsed alveoli, re-distributing lung water, decreasing A-V mismatch and increasing FRC.

Haemodynamics

PEEP usually lowers both left and right ventricular preload and increases RV afterload. Though PEEP may increase cardiac output in left heart failure and fluid overload states by preload reduction, in most other cases cardiac output falls, even at PEEP levels as low as $5cmH_2O$. PEEP may also compromise a poorly functioning right ventricle. An improved PaO_2 resulting from decreased venous admixture may sometimes arise solely from reductions in cardiac output.

Physiological PEEP

A small degree of PEEP (2–$3cmH_2O$) is usually provided physiologically by a closed larynx. It is lost when the patient is intubated or tracheostomised and breathing spontaneously on a T-piece with no CPAP valve.

Intrinsic PEEP (auto-PEEP, air-trapping, PEEPi)

Increased level of PEEP due to insufficient time for expiration, leading to 'air trapping', CO_2 retention, increased airway pressures and increased FRC. Seen in pathological conditions of increased airflow resistance (e.g. asthma, emphysema) and when insufficient expiratory time is set on the ventilator. Used clinically in inverse ratio ventilation to increase oxygenation and decrease peak airway pressures. High levels of PEEPi can however slow weaning by increased work of breathing; use of extrinsic PEEP may overcome this. PEEPi can be measured by temporarily occluding the expiratory outlet of the ventilator at end-expiration for a few seconds to allow equilibration of pressure between upper and lower airway and then reading ventilator pressure gauge (or print-out).

'Best' PEEP

Initially described as the level of PEEP producing the lowest shunt value. Now generally considered to be the lowest level of PEEP that achieves $SaO_2 \geqslant 90\%$ allowing, wherever possible, lowering of FIO_2 (ideally $\leqslant 0.6$) though not at the expense of peak airway pressures $> 40cm\ H_2O$ or significant reductions in DO_2.

Adjusting PEEP

1 Measure blood gases and monitored haemodynamic variables.
2 If indicated, alter level of PEEP by 3–5cmH$_2$O increments.
3 Re-measure gases and haemodynamic variables after 15–20min.
4 Consider further changes as necessary (including additional changes in PEEP, fluid challenge or vasoactive drugs)

Indications

- Hypoxaemia requiring high FIO$_2$.
- Hypoxaemia secondary to left heart failure.
- Improvement of cardiac output in left heart failure.
- Reduced work of breathing during weaning in patients with high PEEPi

Complications

- Reduced cardiac output. May need additional fluid loading or even inotropes. This should generally be avoided unless higher PEEP is necessary to maintain adequate arterial oxygenation. Caution should be exercised in patients with myocardial ischaemia.
- Increased airway pressure (and potential risk of ventilator trauma).
- Overinflation leading to air-trapping and raised PaCO$_2$. Use with caution in patients with chronic airflow limitation or asthma.
- High levels will decrease venous return, raise intracranial pressure and increase hepatic congestion.
- PEEP may change the area of lung in which a pulmonary artery catheter tip is positioned from West Zone III to non-Zone III. This is suggested by a rise in wedge pressure of at least half the increase in PEEP and requires re-siting of the PA catheter.

Continuous positive airway pressure

Continuous positive airway pressure (CPAP) is the addition of positive pressure to the expiratory side of the breathing circuit of a spontaneously ventilating patient who may or may not be intubated. This sets the baseline upper airway pressure above atmospheric pressure, prevents alveolar collapse and possibly recruits already collapsed alveoli. It is usually administered in increments of $2.5cmH_2O$ to a maximum of $10cmH_2O$ and applied via either a tight-fitting face mask (face CPAP), nasal mask (nasal CPAP) or expiratory limb of a T-piece breathing circuit. A high-flow (i.e. > peak inspiratory flow) inspired air-oxygen supply, or a large reservoir bag in the inspiratory circuit, is necessary to keep the valve open. CPAP improves oxygenation and may reduce the work of breathing by reducing the alveolar-to-mouth pressure gradient in patients with high levels of intrinsic PEEP.

Indications
- Hypoxaemia requiring high respiratory rate, effort, and FIO_2.
- Left heart failure to improve hypoxaemia and cardiac output.
- Weaning modality.
- Reducing work of breathing in patients with high PEEPi (e.g. asthma, chronic airflow limitation) NB use with caution and monitor closely.

Complications
- With mask CPAP there is an increased risk of aspiration as gastric dilatation may occur from swallowed air. Insert a nasogastric tube, especially if consciousness is impaired or gastric motility is reduced.
- Reduced cardiac output due to reduced venous return 2° to raised intra-thoracic pressure). May need additional fluid loading or even inotropes.
- Overinflation leading to air-trapping and high $PaCO_2$. Caution is urged in patients with chronic airflow limitation or asthma.
- High levels will reduce venous return and increase intracranial pressure.
- Occasional poor patient compliance with tight-fitting face mask due to feelings of constriction, claustrophobia and discomfort on bridge of nose.
- Inspissated secretions due to high flow, dry gas.

Management

1 Measure blood gases, monitor haemodynamic variables and respiratory rate.

2 Prepare T-piece circuit with a 5cmH$_2$O CPAP valve on the expiratory limb. Connect inspiratory limb to flow generator/Large volume reservoir bag. Adjust air–oxygen mix to obtain desired FIO$_2$ (measured by oxygen analyser in circuit). Use a heat–moisture exchanger to humidify the inhaled gas. If not intubated, consider either nasal or face CPAP. Attach mask to face by appropriate harness and attach T-piece to mask. Ensure no air leak around the mask. If using a nasal mask, encourage patient to keep his mouth closed as much as possible.

3 Measure gases, respiratory rate, and haemodynamics after 15–20min.

4 Consider further changes in CPAP (by 2.5cmH$_2$O increments)

5 Consider need for (i) fluid challenge (or vasoactive drugs) if circulatory compromise and (ii) a nasogastric tube if gastric atony is present.

See also:
Positive end expiratory pressure, 20; Inotropes, 184; Fluid challenge, 262

Non-invasive respiratory support

Devices of varying sophistication are available to augment spontaneous breathing in the compliant patient by either assisting inspiration (inspiratory support) and/or providing CPAP. Non-invasive support is usually delivered by face or nasal mask though inspiratory support can also be delivered by mouthpiece. Some devices allow connection to an endotracheal tube for the intubated but spontaneously breathing patient.

Indications

- Hypoxaemia requiring high respiratory rate, effort, and FIO_2.
- Weaning modality
- To avoid endotracheal intubation where possible (e.g. severe chronic airflow limitation, immunosuppressed)
- Reducing work of breathing in patients with high PEEPi (e.g. asthma, chronic airflow limitation). Use with caution and monitor closely.
- Physiotherapy technique for improving FRC.
- Sleep apnoea

Inspiratory support (IS)

A pre-set inspiratory pressure is given which is triggered by the patient's breath. This trigger can be adjusted according to the degree of patient effort. Some devices will deliver breaths automatically at adjustable rates and the I:E ratio may also be adjustable.

The tidal volume delivered for a given level of inspiratory support will vary according to the patient's respiratory compliance. An example of an IS device is the Bird ventilator commonly used by physiotherapists for improving FRC and expanding lung bases.

BiPAP

This device delivers inspiratory pressure support and/or CPAP depending on clinical and patient preference.

Management

1 Select type and delivery mode of ventilatory support.
2 Connect patient as per device instructions.
3 For IS, a delivered pressure of 10–15cmH$_2$O is a usual starting point which can be adjusted according to patient response (rate, degree of fatigue, comfort, blood gases...).
4 Patients in respiratory distress may have initial difficulty in coping with these devices. Constant attention and encouragement help to accustom the patient to the device while different levels of support, I:E ratios etc. are being experimented with to find the optimal setting. Cautious administration of low dose subcutaneous opiate injections (e.g. diamorphine 2.5mg) may help to calm the patient without depressing respiratory drive.

Non-ventilatory respiratory support

Several techniques are available to support gas exchange when severe lung failure ensues. These include extracorporeal respiratory support (ECCO$_2$R and ECMO) and intravenous oxygenation (IVOX).

ECCO$_2$R

An extracorporeal veno-venous circulation is used to allow CO$_2$ clearance via a gas exchange membrane. Blood flows of 25–33% cardiac output are typically used which only allow for partial oxygenation support. A technique of low frequency (4–5/min) positive pressure ventilation (LFPPV) is usually used with ECCO$_2$R with continuous oxygenation throughout inspiration and expiration. The lungs are 'held open' with high PEEP (20–25cmH$_2$O), limited peak airway pressures (40–45cmH$_2$O) and a continuous fresh gas supply. Thus oxygenation is effected with lung rest to aid recovery. Oxygenating the pulmonary blood provides pulmonary vasodilatation which helps to overcome the pulmonary hypertension associated with ARDS. Anticoagulation of the extracorporeal circulation can now be achieved with heparin bonded circuits and membranes. Survival of 50–60% has been achieved with this technique in ARDS but superiority to conventional ventilation has not been demonstrated in controlled studies.

ECMO

An extracorporeal veno-arterial circulation is used with high blood flows (approaching cardiac output). It is possible to supply the whole of the body's gas exchange requirement via a membrane, although it is more usual to support gas exchange supplied with conventional CMV. The main disadvantages of ECMO compared to ECCO$_2$R are the need for large bore arterial puncture with its consequent risks and the high extracorporeal blood flows with the potential for cell damage. Furthermore, there is no oxygenation of the pulmonary blood.

IVOX

The device consists of multiple hollow fibres which are placed in the vena cavae and right atrium via a femoral venotomy. Gas exchange support is partial across the hollow fibres and is limited by the surface area which can be provided. Oxygenation of pulmonary blood flow is provided but full ventilatory support is usually required. Full systemic anticoagulation is also required.

Indications

Failure of maximum intensive therapy and ventilatory support to sustain adequate gas exchange as evidenced by the criteria opposite.

Contraindications

- Chronic systemic disease involving any major organ system (e.g. irreversible chronic CNS disease, chronic lung disease with $FEV_1 < 1L$, $FEV_1/FVC < 0.3$ of predicted, chronic $PaCO_2 > 6.0$kPa, emphysema or previous admission for chronic respiratory insufficiency, incurable or rapidly fatal malignancy, chronic left heart failure, chronic renal failure, chronic liver failure, HIV related disease)
- Lung failure for > 14 days (although treatment with extracorporeal respiratory support may persist for longer than 14 days)
- Burns ($> 40\%$ of body surface)
- More than 3 organ failures in addition to lung failure

Criteria for non-ventilatory respiratory support

i) Rapid failure of ventilatory support prompting the immediate use of these techniques should be considered for those meeting the following gas exchange criteria for a period of > 2h despite maximum intensive therapy:

PaO_2	< 6.7kPa
FIO_2	1.0
PEEP	> 5cmH$_2$O

ii) Slow failure of ventilatory support should be considered after 48h maximum intensive therapy for those meeting the following gas exchange and mechanical pulmonary function criteria for a period > 12h:

PaO_2	< 6.7kPa
FIO_2	> 0.6
PaO_2/FIO_2	< 11.2kPa
PEEP	> 5cmH$_2$O
Q_S/Q_T	$> 30\%$ on $FIO_2 = 1.0$
TSLC	< 30ml/cmH$_2$O at 10ml/kg inflation

See also:
Adult respiratory distress syndrome 1, 280; Adult respiratory distress syndrome 2, 282

Endotracheal intubation

Indications

An artificial airway is necessary in the following circumstances:
- Apnoea—The provision of mechanical ventilation, e.g. unconsciousness, severe respiratory muscle weakness, self-poisoning
- Respiratory failure—The provision of mechanical ventilation, e.g. ARDS, pneumonia
- Airway protection—Unconsciousness, trauma, aspiration risk, poisoning
- Airway obstruction—To maintain airway patency, e.g. trauma, laryngeal oedema, tumour, burns
- Haemodynamic instability—To facilitate mechanical ventilation, e.g. shock, cardiac arrest

Choice of endotracheal tube

Most adults require a standard high volume, low pressure cuffed endotracheal tube. The average sized adult will require a size 9.0mm id tube (size 8.0mm id for females) cut to a length of 23cm (21cm for females). Obviously, different sized patients may require changes to these sizes and particular problems with the upper airway, e.g. trauma, oedema, may require a smaller tube. In specific situations non-standard tubes may be used, e.g. jet ventilation, armoured tubes (where head mobility is expected or for patients who are to be positioned prone), double lumen tubes to isolate the right or left lung.

Route of intubation

The usual routes of intubation are oro-tracheal and naso-tracheal. Oro-tracheal intubation is preferred. The naso-tracheal route has the advantages of increased patient comfort and the possibility of easier blind placement; it is also easier to secure the tube. However, there are several disadvantages. The tube is usually smaller, there is a risk of sinusitis and otitis media and the route is contraindicated in coagulopathy, CSF leak and nasal fractures.

Difficult intubation

If a difficult intubation is predicted it should not be attempted by an inexperienced operator. Difficulty may be predicted in the patient with a small mouth, high arched palate, large upper incisors, hypognathia, large tongue, anterior larynx, short neck, immobile temporomandibular joints, immobile cervical joints or morbid obesity. If a difficult intubation presents unexpectedly the use of a stylet, a straight bladed laryngoscope or a fibreoptic laryngoscope may help. It is important not to persist for too long; revert to bag and mask ventilation to ensure adequate oxygenation.

Complications of intubation

Early complications
- Trauma, e.g. haemorrhage, mediastinal perforation
- Haemodynamic collapse, e.g. positive pressure ventilation, vasodilatation, arrhythmias or rapid correction of hypercapnia
- Tube malposition, e.g. failed or endobronchial intubation.

Later complications
- Infection including maxillary sinusitis if nasally intubated
- Cuff pressure trauma (maintain cuff pressure $< 25cmH_2O$)
- Mouth/Lip trauma

Equipment required

Suction (Yankauer tip)
Oxygen, rebreathing bag and mask
Laryngoscope (two curved blades and straight blade)
Stylet / bougie
Endotracheal tubes (preferred size and smaller)
Magill forceps
Drugs (Induction agent, muscle relaxant, sedative, anticholinergic)
Syringe for cuff inflation
Tape to secure tube

See also:

Tracheostomy

Indications

To provide an artificial airway where oro- or naso-tracheal intubation is to be avoided. This may be to provide better patient comfort, to avoid mouth or nasal trauma or, in an emergency, where there is acute upper airway obstruction. Converting an oro- or naso-tracheal tube to a tracheostomy should be considered early in cases of difficult intubation to avoid the risks of repeat intubation, or later in cases of prolonged intubation to avoid laryngeal trauma. The exact time that one should consider performing a tracheostomy in cases of prolonged intubation is not known although current practice is at about 10–16 days. High volume, low pressure cuffs on modern endotracheal tubes do not cause more tracheal damage than the equivalent cuffs of a tracheostomy tube, but avoiding the risks of laryngeal and vocal cord damage may provide some advantage for a tracheostomy. The reduced need for sedation is a definite advantage.

Percutaneous tracheostomy

A more rapid procedure with less tissue trauma and scarring than the standard open surgical technique. Can be performed in the intensive care unit avoiding the need to transfer patients to theatre. The technique involves infiltration of the subcutaneous tissues with lignocaine and adrenaline. A 1–1.5cm skin crease incision is made in the midline. Subcutaneous tissue is blunt dissected to the anterior tracheal wall. The trachea is punctured with a 14G needle between the 1st and 2nd tracheal cartilages and a guide wire is inserted into the trachea. The stoma is created either by progressive dilatation to 36Fr (Ciaglia technique) or by use of a single stage guided dilating tool (Schachner-Ovill technique). In the former case the tracheostomy tube is introduced over an appropriate sized dilator and in the latter through the open dilating tool.

Complications

The main early complication is haemorrhage, either from trauma to the thyroid isthmus or aberrant superior thyroid vessels. Although most early haemorrhage is easily controlled, coagulation disorder in critically ill patients may create additional problems. Tracheal stenosis is related to creation of the tracheal stoma and subsequent low grade infection. This is thought to be a greater problem with open surgical tracheostomies than percutaneous tracheostomies. The presence of a foreign body in the trachea, bypassing the normal upper airway defence mechanisms, together with an open neck wound, presents an obvious infection risk. Subglottic infection is more likely after trans-laryngeal intubation. Tracheo-oesophageal fistula is a rare complication due to trauma or pressure necrosis of the posterior wall of the trachea.

Maintenance of a tracheostomy

Since the upper air passages have been bypassed artificial humidification is required. Cough is less effective without a functioning larynx so regular tracheal suction will be necessary. Furthermore, the larynx provides a small amount of natural PEEP which is lost with a tracheostomy. The risk of basal atelectasis can be overcome with CPAP or attention to respiratory exercises which promote deep breathing. A safe fistula forms within 3 days allowing replacement of the tracheostomy tube.

Tracheostomy tubes

Standard high volume, low pressure cuff

Fenestrated with or without cuff
Useful where airway protection is not a primary concern. May be closed during normal breathing while providing intermittent suction access.

Fenestrated with inner tube
As above but with an inner tube to facilitate closure of the fenestration during intermittent mechanical ventilation.

Fenestrated with speaking valve
Inspiration allowed through the tracheostomy to reduce dead space and inspiratory resistance. Expiration through the larynx, via the fenestration, allowing speech and the advantages of laryngeal PEEP.

Adjustable flange
Accommodates extreme variations in skin to trachea depth while ensuring the cuff remains central in the trachea.

Pitt speaking tube
A non-fenestrated, cuffed tube for continuous mechanical ventilation and airway protection with a port to direct airflow above the cuff to the larynx. When airflow is directed through the larynx some patients are able to vocalise.

Silver tube
An uncuffed tube which is used occasionally in ENT practice to maintain a tracheostomy fistula.

Minitracheotomy

A 4mm diameter uncuffed plastic tube inserted through the cricothyroid membrane under local anaesthetic.

Indications

- Removal of retained secretions, usually when the patient's cough is weak
- Emergency access to lower airway if upper airway obstructed

Contraindications / cautions

- Coagulopathy
- Non-compliant, agitated patient (unless sedated)

Technique

Some commercial kits rely on blind insertion of a blunt introducer; others use a Seldinger technique where a guidewire is inserted via the cricothyroid membrane into the trachea. An introducer passed over the wire dilates the track allowing easy passage of the tube.

1 Use aseptic technique. Cleanse site with antiseptic. Locate cricothyroid membrane (midline 'spongy' area between cricoid and thyroid cartilages)

2 Infiltrate local skin and subcutaneous tissues with 1% lignocaine ± adrenaline. Advance needle into deeper tissues, aspirating to confirm absence of blood then infiltrating with lignocaine until cricothyroid membrane is pierced and air can be easily aspirated.

3 (If using Seldinger technique insert guidewire through membrane into trachea). Tether thyroid cartilage with one hand, incise skin and tissues vertically in midline (alongside wire) with short-bladed guarded scalpel provided with pack. Insert scalpel to blade guard level to make adequate hole through cricothyroid membrane. Remove scalpel.

4 Insert blunt introducer through incision site into trachea (or over guidewire). Angle caudally. Relatively light resistance will be felt during correct passage—do not force introducer if resistance proves excessive.

5 Lubricate plastic tube with gel. Slide tube over introducer into trachea.

6 Remove introducer (+ wire), leaving plastic tube in situ.

7 Confirm correct position by placing own hand over tube and feeling airflow during breathing. Suction down tube to aspirate intratracheal contents (check pH if in doubt). Cap opening of tube. Suture to skin.

8 Perform CXR (unless very smooth insertion and no change in cardiorespiratory variables).

9 O_2 can be entrained through the tube, or an appropriate connector (provided in pack) placed to allow bagging, use of the Bird ventilator and/or short-term assisted ventilation.

Complications

- Puncture of blood vessel at cricothyroid membrane may cause significant intratracheal or external bleeding. Apply local pressure if this occurs after blade incision. If bleeding continues, insert minitracheotomy tube for a tamponading effect. If bleeding persists, insert deep sutures either side of minitracheotomy; if this fails, contact surgeon for assistance.
- Perforation of oesophagus
- Mediastinitis (rare)
- Pneumothorax

33

Chest drain insertion

Indications

Drainage of air (pneumothorax), fluid (effusion), blood (hae-mothorax) or pus (empyema) from the pleural space.

Contraindications / Cautions

Coagulopathy (unless emergency).

Subsequent management

- Drains should not be clamped prior to removal or transport of patient.
- Drains may be removed in spontaneously breathing patients when the lung has re-expanded and there is no air leak (no respiratory swing in fluid level or air leak on coughing).
- Drains inserted for haemothorax/empyema/effusion may be removed during IPPV if there is no air leak and the lung has re-expanded.
- Unless long-term ventilation is necessary, a drain inserted for a pneumothorax should usually be left *in situ* during IPPV.
- Remove drain at end-expiration. Cover hole with thick gauze and elastoplast; a purse-string suture is not usually necessary. Repeat chest X-ray if indicated by deteriorating clinical signs or blood gas analysis.

Complications

Morbidity associated with chest drainage may be up to 10%.

- Puncture of intercostal vessel. This may cause significant bleeding. Consider (i) correcting any coagulopathy, (ii) placing deep tension sutures around drain or (iii) removing drain, inserting Foley catheter through hole, inflating balloon and applying traction on catheter to tamponade bleeding vessel. If these measures fail, contact (thoracic) surgeon.
- Puncture of lung tissue causing bronchopleural fistula. If chest drain suction (up to 15–20cmH$_2$O) fails, consider (i) pleurodesis (e.g. with tetracycline), (ii) high frequency jet ventilation ± double-lumen endo-bronchial tube, or (iii) surgery.
- Perforation of major vessel (often fatal). Clamp but do not remove drain. Resuscitate with blood. Contact surgeon. Consider placing double-lumen endotracheal tube.
- Infection. Take cultures; antibiotics (staphylococcal ± anaerobic cover); consider removing/resiting drain.
- Local discomfort/pain from pleural irritation. Coughing may be impaired. Consider (unless contraindicated) either subcutaneous lignocaine, instilling local anaesthetic into pleural space, intercostal block, thoracic epidural, non-steroidal analgesia, etc.
- Drain dislodgement. If needed, replace/resite new drain, depending on cleanliness of original site. Don't advance old drain (infection risk).
- Lung entrapment/infarction. Avoid milking chest drain in pneumothorax.

Insertion technique

1 Use 28Fr drain (or larger) for haemothorax or empyema; 20Fr will suffice for a pure pneumothorax. Usually inserted through 5th intercostal space in the mid-axillary line, first anaesthetising skin and pleura with 1% plain lignocaine. Ensure that air/fluid/blood/pus is aspirated.

2 Make a 1–1.5cm skin crease incision and create a track with gloved finger (or artery forceps) to separate muscle fibres and to open pleura.

3 Insert drain through open pleura with trochar withdrawn to ensure tip is blunt to avoid lung damage. Angle and insert drain to correct position (towards lung apex for a pneumothorax and lung base for a haemothorax). Connect drain to underwater seal. CT scan or ultrasound may be useful for directing placement for focal/small collections.

4 Secure drain to chest wall by properly placed sutures.

5 Perform chest X-ray to ensure correct siting and lung reinflation.

6 Place on 5–10cmH$_2$O (0.5–1.3 kPa) negative pressure (low pressure wall suction) if lung has not fully expanded.

See also:
IPPV—complications of ventilation, 12; High frequency jet ventilation, 18; Pleural aspiration, 36; Basic resuscitation, 258; Pneumothorax, 288; Haemothorax, 290

Pleural aspiration

Drainage of fluid from the pleural space using either a needle, cannula or flexible small-bore drain. Increasingly being performed under ultrasound guidance. Blood/pus usually requires large-bore drain insertion.

Indications
- Improvement of blood gases.
- Symptomatic improvement of dyspnoea.
- Diagnostic 'tap'.

Contraindications / Cautions
- Coagulopathy.

Complications
- Puncture of lung or subdiaphragmatic viscera.
- Bleeding.

Fluid protein level

Protein > 30g/L—exudate—causes: inflammatory e.g. pneumonia, pulmonary embolus, neoplasm, collagen vascular diseases

Protein < 30g/L—transudate— causes: (i) increased venous pressure (e.g. heart failure, fluid overload), (ii) decreased colloid osmotic pressure (e.g. critical illness leading to reduced [plasma protein] from capillary leak and hepatic dysfunction, hepatic failure, nephrotic syndrome).

Technique

1 Confirm presence of effusion by CXR or ultrasound.
2 Select drainage site either by maximum area of stony dullness under percussion or under ultrasound guidance.
3 Use aseptic technique. Clean area with antiseptic and infiltrate local skin and subcutaneous tissues with 1% lignocaine. Advance into deeper tissues, aspirating to confirm absence of blood then infiltrating with local anaesthetic until pleura is pierced and fluid can be aspirated.
4 Advance drainage needle/cannula/drain slowly, applying gentle suction, through chest wall and intercostal space (above upper border of rib to avoid neurovascular bundle) until fluid can be aspirated.
5 Withdraw 50ml for microbiological (M,C&S, TB stain), biochemical (protein, glucose, rheumatoid factor, etc.) and cytological (malignant cells) analysis as indicated
6 Either leave drain in situ connected to drainage bag or connect needle/cannula by three-way tap to drainage apparatus.
7 Continue aspiration/drainage until no further fluid can be withdrawn or patient becomes symptomatic (pain/dyspnoea). Dyspnoea or haemodynamic changes may occasionally be due to removal of large volumes of fluid (> 1–2L) and subsequent fluid shifts; if this is considered to be a possibility, remove no more than one litre at a time either by clamping/declamping drain or repeating needle aspiration after an equilibration interval (e.g. 4–6h).
8 Remove needle/drain. Cover puncture site with firmly applied gauze dressing.

Bronchoscopy

Flexible fibre-optic bronchoscopy is performed for diagnostic and/or therapeutic reasons. Because of the risks involved in ICU patients, it should be performed by an experienced operator. As patients are often intubated, care must be taken to not damage the instrument on insertion through the tight-fitting port of the endotracheal tube catheter mount. An assistant should support the endotracheal tube during the procedure to minimise trauma to both trachea and scope. Rigid bronchoscopy may be indicated for removal of large foreign bodies.

Indications

Diagnostic
- Collection of microbiological ± cytological specimens (by broncho-alveolar lavage, protected brush specimen, biopsy) from affected areas.
- Cause of full/partial lung/Lobar obstruction (e.g. blood clot, foreign body, neoplasm).
- Extent of inhalation injury.
- Diagnosis of ruptured trachea/bronchus.

Therapeutic
- Clearance of secretions, inhaled vomitus, etc.
- Removal of lumen-obstructing matter (e.g. mucus plug, blood clot, food, tooth).
- Cleansing—removing soot and other toxic materials, irrigation with saline
- Directed physiotherapy ± saline to loosen secretions.
- Directed placement of balloon catheter to arrest pulmonary bleeding.

Contraindications / cautions
- Coagulopathy.
- Severe hypoxaemia.

Complications
- Hypoxaemia—from suction, loss of PEEP, partial obstruction of endotracheal tube and non-delivery of tidal volume.
- Haemodynamic disturbances including hypertension and tachycardia (related to hypoxaemia, agitation, tracheal stimulation, etc.)
- Bleeding.
- Perforation (unusual though more common if biopsy taken).

General

It is difficult to perform flexible bronchoscopy in a nasally intubated patient. A narrow lumen scope can be used but this may impair suctioning abilities. Orotracheal intubation may be necessary, with a size 8.0 tube. Bronchoalveolar lavage is performed by instillation of at least 60ml of (preferably warm) isotonic saline into affected area of lung with suction tubing removed/temporarily obstructed. Reconnect suction and aspirate into sterile catheter trap for microbiological investigation. All bronchoscopic samples should be sent promptly to the laboratory.

Proximal obstruction rather than consolidation is suggested by the radiological appearance of a collapsed lung/Lobe & no air bronchogram.

Soot should be promptly and thoroughly removed. Irrigate lungs until clean with copious amounts of isotonic saline. Rigid bronchoscopy requires removal of the endotracheal tube and gas exchange performed by a Sanders injector.

Procedure

1 Pre-oxygenate with FIO_2 1.0. Monitor throughout with pulse oximetry.
2 Increase pressure alarm limit on ventilator.
3 Lubricate scope with lubricant gel/saline.
4 If unintubated, apply lignocaine gel to nares ± spray to pharynx.
5 Consider short-term IV sedation ± paralysis ± ventilator adjustments.
6 Insert scope nasally (in unintubated patient) or through catheter mount port in an intubated patient.
7 Inject 2% lignocaine into trachea to prevent coughing and haemodynamic effects from tracheal/carinal stimulation.
8 Perform thorough inspection and any necessary procedures. If $SpO_2 \leqslant 85\%$ or haemodynamic disturbance occurs, remove scope from patient and allow patient to re-oxygenate before continuing.
9 After procedure, reset ventilator as appropriate.

See also:
Endotracheal intubation, 28; Chest physiotherapy, 40; Atelectasis and pulmonary collapse, 272; Haemoptysis, 292; Inhalation injury, 294

Chest physiotherapy

This encompasses a variety of techniques aimed at expanding collapsed alveoli, mobilising chest secretions and, occasionally, re-inflating collapsed lung, lobe or lobar segments. Though sufficient anecdotal experience suggests benefit, no scientific validation of its effectiveness has been reported other than prevention of post-suctioning hypoxaemia.

Techniques

Hyperinflation
Hyperinflating to 50% above ventilator-delivered V_T, aiming to expand collapsed alveoli and mobilise secretions. V_T is rarely measured, so either excessive or inadequate hyperinflations may be given depending on lung compliance and operator technique. Pressure-limiting devices ('blow-off valves') or manometers can avoid excessive airway pressures. Usually performed with a manual resuscitation bag, a recommended technique is slow inspiration, a 1–2 second plateau phase and then rapid release of the bag to simulate a 'huff' and mobilise secretions. Though the FIO_2 is 1.0, preoxygenation may be needed as PEEP may be lost and the delivered V_T may be inadequate. Cardiac output often falls in relation to the generated V_T with variable blood pressure and heart rate responses. Sedation may be required to blunt the haemodynamic response. Allow full expiration to prevent air trapping.

Suction
Removing secretions from trachea and main bronchi (usually right). A cough reflex may be stimulated to mobilise secretions further. Tenacious secretions may be loosened by instillation of 2–5ml 0.9% saline. Falls in SaO_2 and cardiovascular disturbances may be prevented by pre-oxygenation.

Percussion and vibration
Drumming and shaking actions over chest wall to mobilise secretions.

Inspiratory pressure support (Bird ventilator)
Delivery of inspiratory pressure support to increase FRC and expand collapsed alveoli.

Postural drainage
Patient positioning to assist drainage-depends on affected area(s) of lung.

Complications
- Hypoxaemia—from suction, loss of PEEP, etc.
- Haemodynamic disturbances affecting cardiac output, heart rate and blood pressure which may be related to supranormal tidal volumes and airway pressures, hypoxaemia, agitation, tracheal stimulation, etc..
- Direct trauma from suction.
- Barotrauma/volutrauma including pneumothorax.

General
Adequate hydration and lung humidification prevents development of tenacious secretions and mucus plugs. Pain relief is important to encourage good chest excursion and coughing. Mobilisation of patient (into chair) and encouragement to take deep breaths (e.g. using incentive spirometry) are important facets of both rehabilitation and prophylaxis against infection.

Indications

- Mobilisation of secretions.
- Re-expansion of collapsed lung/Lobes.
- Prophylaxis against alveolar collapse and secondary infection.

Contraindications / cautions

- Aggressive hyperinflation in patients with already hyperinflated lungs e.g. asthma, emphysema—though can be very useful in removing mucus plugs.
- Undrained pneumothorax.
- Raised intracranial pressure.

When to request urgent physiotherapy

- Collapsed lung/Lobe with no air bronchogram visible i.e. suggesting proximal obstruction rather than consolidation
- Mucus plugging causing subsegmental collapse e.g. asthma

When not to request urgent physiotherapy

- Clinical signs of chest infection with no secretions being produced.
- Radiological consolidation with air bronchogram but no secretions present.

See also:
Ventilatory support—indications, 4; Bronchoscopy, 38

Cardiovascular Therapy Techniques

Defibrillation

Electrical conversion of a tachyarrhythmia to restore normal sinus rhythm. This may be an emergency procedure (when the circulation is absent or severely compromised), semi-elective (when the circulation is compromised to a lesser degree), or elective (when synchronised cardioversion is performed to restore sinus rhythm for a non-compromising supra-ventricular tachycardia). Synchronisation requires initial connection of ECG leads from the patient to the defibrillator so that the shock is delivered on the R wave to minimise the risk of ventricular fibrillation.

Indications
- Compromised circulation, e.g. VF, VT
- Restoration of sinus rhythm and more effective cardiac output
- Lessens risk of cardiac thrombus formation

Contraindications / cautions
- Aware patient
- Severe coagulopathy
- Caution with recent thrombolysis
- Digoxin levels in toxic range

Complications
- Surface burn
- Pericardial tamponade
- Electrocution of bystanders

Technique
(see algorithm opposite).
- The chances of maintaining sinus rhythm are increased in elective cardioversion if $K^+ > 4.5$mmol/L and plasma Mg^{2+} levels are normal.
- Prior to defibrillation, ensure self and onlookers are not in contact with patient or bed frame.
- To reduce the risk of superficial burns, replace gel/gelled pads after every 3shocks.
- Consider resiting paddle position (e.g. antero-posterior) if defibrillation fails.
- The risk of intractable VF following defibrillation in a patient receiving digoxin is small unless the plasma digoxin levels are in the toxic range or the patient is hypovolaemic.

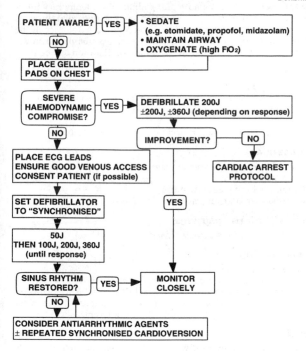

45

See also:
Cardiac arrest, 260; Tachyarrhythmias, 304

Temporary internal pacing

When the heart's intrinsic pacemaking ability fails, temporary internal pacing can be instituted. Electrodes can be endocardial (inserted via a central vein) or epicardial (placed on the external surface of the heart at thoracotomy). The endocardial wire may be placed under fluoroscopic control or 'blind' using a balloon flotation catheter.

Indications
- Third-degree heart block
- Mobitz Type II second-degree heart block when the circulation is compromised or an operation is planned
- Overpacing (rarely)
- Asystole (although external pacing is more useful initially)

Complications
- As for central venous catheter insertion
- Arrhythmias
- Infection (including endocarditis)
- Myocardial perforation (rare)

Contraindications / cautions
- As for central venous catheter insertion

Troubleshooting
Failure to pace may be due to:
1 No pacemaker output (no spikes seen)—check connections, battery
2 No capture (pacing spikes seen but no QRS complex following)—poor positioning/dislodgement of wire. Temporarily increase output as this may regain capture. Reposition/replace wire.

General
1 Check threshold daily as it will rise slowly over 48–96h, probably due to fibrosis occurring around the electrodes.
2 Overpacing is occasionally indicated for a tachycardia not responding to antiarrhythmic therapy or cardioversion. For SVT, pacing is usually attempted with the wire sited in the right atrium. Pace at rate 20–30 bpm above patient's heart rate for 10–15sec then either decrease rate immediately to 80 bpm or slowly, by 20 bpm every 5–10sec.
3 If overpacing fails, underpacing may be attempted with the wire situated in either atrium (for SVT) or, usually, ventricle (for either SVT or VT). A paced rate of 80–100 bpm may produce a refractory period sufficient to suppress the intrinsic tachycardia.
4 Epicardial pacing performed during cardiac surgery requires siting of either two epicardial electrodes or one epicardial and one skin electrode (usually a hypodermic needle). The pacing threshold of epicardial wires rises quickly and may become ineffective after 1–2 days.

Technique (for endocardial electrode placement)

1 If using fluoroscopy, move patient to X-ray suite or place lead shields around bed area. Place patient on 'screening table'. Staff should wear lead aprons. **47**

2 Use aseptic technique throughout. Insert 6Fr sheath in internal jugular or subclavian vein. Suture in position.

3 Connect pacing wire electrodes to pacing box (black = negative polarity = distal, red = positive polarity = proximal). Set pacemaker to demand. Check box is working and battery charge adequate. Turn pacing rate to ⩾30 bpm above patient's intrinsic rhythm. Set voltage to 4V.

4 Insert pacing wire through sheath into central vein. If using balloon catheter, insert to 15–20cm depth then inflate balloon. Advance catheter, viewing ECG monitor for change in ECG morphology and capture of pacing rate. If using screening, direct wire toward the apex of the right ventricle. Approximate insertion depth from a neck vein is 35–40cm.

5 If pacing impulses not captured, (deflate balloon), withdraw wire to 15cm insertion depth then repeat step 4.

6 Once pacing captured, decrease voltage by decrements to determine threshold at which pacing is no longer captured. Ideal position determined by a threshold ⩽0.4V. If not achieved, re-position wire.

7 If possible, ask patient to cough to check that the wire does not dislodge.

8 Set voltage at 3 × threshold and set desired heart rate on 'demand' mode. Tape wire securely to patient to prevent dislodgement.

See also:
External pacing, 49; Central venous catheter—use, 109; Central venous catheter—insertion, 111; Tachyarrhythmias, 305; Bradyarrhythmias, 307

External pacing

External pacing can be rapidly performed by placement of two electrodes on the front and rear chest wall when asystole or third degree heart block has produced acute haemodynamic compromise. It is often used as a bridge to temporary internal pacing. It can also be used as a prophylactic measure e.g. for Mobitz Type II second-degree heart block.

Indications
- Asystole (in conjunction with cardiopulmonary resuscitation)
- Third-degree heart block
- Prophylactic

Complications
- Discomfort

Technique
1 Connect pacing wire gelled electrodes to pacemaker. Place black (= negative polarity) electrode on the anterior chest wall to the left of the lower sternum and red (= positive polarity) electrode to the corresponding position on the posterior hemithorax.
2 Connect ECG electrodes from ECG monitor to external pacemaker and another set of electrodes from pacemaker to patient.
3 Set pacemaker to demand. Turn pacing rate to ≥30 bpm above patient's intrinsic rhythm. Set current to 70mA.
4 Start pacing. Increase current (by 5mA increments) until pacing rate captured on monitor.
5 If pacing rate not captured at current of 120–130mA, re-site electrodes and repeat steps 3–4.
6 Once pacing captured, set current at 5–10mA above threshold.

General
- In asystole, even though an electrical rhythm is produced by the external pacing, this does not guarantee an adequate output is being generated.
- Although the patient may complain of discomfort, external chest wall pacing is better tolerated and more reliable than other forms of external pacing e.g. oesophageal.

See also:
Temporary internal pacing, 46; Cardiac arrest, 260; Bradyarrhythmias, 306

Intra-aortic balloon counterpulsation

Principle

A 40cm^3 balloon is placed in the descending aorta. The balloon is inflated with helium during diastole thus increasing diastolic blood pressure above the balloon. This serves to increase coronary and cerebral perfusion. The balloon is deflated during systole thus decreasing peripheral resistance and increasing stroke volume. No pharmacological technique exists which can increase coronary blood flow while reducing peripheral resistance. Intra-aortic balloon counterpulsation may improve cardiac performance in situations where drugs are ineffective.

Indications

The most obvious indication is to support the circulation where a structural cardiac defect is to be repaired surgically. However, it may be used in acute circulatory failure in any situation where resolution of the cause of cardiac dysfunction is expected. In acute myocardial infarction resolution of peri-infarct oedema may allow spontaneous improvement in myocardial function; the use of intra-aortic balloon counterpulsation may provide temporary circulatory support and promote myocardial healing by improving myocardial blood flow. Other indications include acute myocarditis and poisoning with myocardial depressants. Intra-aortic balloon counterpulsation should not be used in aortic regurgitation since the increase in diastolic blood pressure would increase regurgitant flow.

Insertion of the balloon

The usual route is via a femoral artery. Percutaneous Seldinger catheterisation (with or without an introducer sheath) provides a rapid and safe technique with minimal arterial trauma and bleeding. Open surgical catheterisation may be necessary in elderly patients with atheromatous disease. The balloon position should be checked on a chest X-ray to ensure that the radio-opaque tip is at the level of the 2nd intercostal space.

Anticoagulation

The presence of a large foreign body in the aorta requires systemic anticoagulation to prevent thrombosis. The balloon should not be left deflated for longer than a minute while in situ otherwise thrombosis may occur despite anticoagulation.

Control of balloon inflation and deflation

Helium is used to inflate the balloon, its low density facilitating rapid transfer from pump to balloon. Inflation is commonly timed to the 'R' wave of the ECG, although timing may be taken from an arterial pressure waveform. Minor adjustment may be made to the timing to ensure that inflation occurs immediately after closure of the aortic valve (after the dicrotic notch of the arterial pressure waveform) and deflation occurs at the end of diastole. The filling volume of the balloon can be varied up to the maximum balloon volume. The greater the filling volume the greater the circulatory augmentation. The rate at which balloon inflation occurs may coincide with every cardiac beat or every 2nd or 3rd cardiac beat. Slower rates are necessary in tachyarrhythmias. Weaning of intra-aortic balloon counterpulsation may be achieved by reducing augmentation or the rate of inflation.

Renal Therapy Techniques

Haemo(dia)filtration 1

These are alternatives to dialysis which requires a pressurised, purified water supply, more expensive equipment and operator expertise, and a greater risk of haemodynamic instability due to rapid fluid and osmotic shifts. Haemo(dia)filtration can be arterio-venous, using the patient's blood pressure to drive blood through the haemofilter or pumped veno-venous. The latter is advantageous in that it is not dependent on the patient's BP and the pump system incorporates alarms and safety features. Veno-venous haemo(dia)filtration is increasingly the technique of choice. Blood is usually drawn and returned via a 10–12Fr double lumen central venous catheter.

Indications

- Azotaemia (uraemia)
- Hyperkalaemia
- Anuria/oliguria; to make space for nutrition
- Severe metabolic acidosis of non-tissue hypoperfusion origin
- Fluid overload
- Drug removal
- Hypothermia/hyperthermia

Techniques

Numerous including haemofiltration, haemodiafiltration, ultrafiltration, continuous ultrafiltration with intermittent dialysis (CUPID). [See Figure].

Filtrate is usually removed at 1–2Litres/h and fluid balance adjusted by varying the fluid replacement rate.

Creatinine and potassium clearances are higher with diafiltration though filtration alone is usually sufficient provided an adequate ultrafiltrate volume is achieved. (1000ml/h = creatinine clearance of 16ml/min).

Anticoagulation

Anticoagulation of the circuit is with either heparin (200–1000IU/h), a prostanoid (epoprostenol or PGE_1) at 2–10 ng/kg/min, or a combination of the two.

No anticoagulant may be needed if the patient is auto-anti-coagulated.

No major advantage is gained by using low molecular weight heparin instead of unfractionated heparin though may be considered if heparin-induced thrombocytopenia is a concern.

Premature clotting may be due to insufficient anticoagulation, inadequate blood flow rates, mechanical kinking/obstruction of the circuit or to lack of endogenous anticoagulants (antithrombin III, heparin cofactor II).

Usual filter lifespan should be at least two days but is often decreased in septic patients due to decreased endogenous anticoagulant levels.

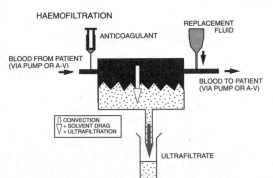

HAEMOFILTRATION

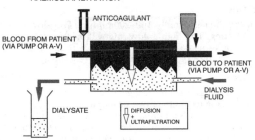

HAEMODIAFILTRATION

Haemo(dia)filtration 2

Membranes
Usually polyacrylonitrile, polyamide or polysulphone. May be hollow fibre or flat-plate in design. Surface area usually $0.6-1m^2$.

Replacement fluid
A buffered balanced electrolyte solution is given to replace losses and achieve desired fluid balance. Buffers include lactate (metabolised by liver to bicarbonate), acetate (metabolised by muscle), and bicarbonate. Acetate causes most haemodynamically instability, bicarbonate is the most complex to administer (requires separate infusions of calcium, magnesium, etc.), while lactate may not be metabolised in liver failure. An increasing metabolic alkalosis may be due to excessive buffer. Potassium can be added if necessary to maintain normokalaemia. Having 20mmol KCl in a 4.5Litre bag provides a concentration of 4.44mmol/L. Clearance is increased by decreasing the concentration within the replacement fluid or the dialysate.

Filter blood flow
Flow through the filter is usually 100–200ml/min. Too slow a flow rate promotes clotting. Too high a flow rate will increase transmembrane pressures and decrease filter lifespan without significant improvement in clearance of 'middle molecules' (e.g. urea).

Complications
- Disconnection leading to haemorrhage
- Infection risk (sterile technique must be employed)
- Electrolyte, acid–base or fluid imbalance (excess input or removal)
- Haemorrhage (vascular access sites, peptic ulcers) related to anticoagulation therapy or consumption coagulopathy. Heparin-induced thrombocytopenia may rarely occur

Cautions
- Haemodynamic instability related to hypovolaemia (especially at start)
- Vasoactive drug removal by the filter (e.g. catecholamines)
- Membrane biocompatibility problems (especially with cuprophane)
- Drug dosages may need to be revised (consult pharmacist)
- Amino acid losses through the filter
- Heat loss leading to hypothermia
- Masking of pyrexia

See also:
Haemo(dia)filtration 1, 54

Peritoneal dialysis

A slow form of dialysis, utilising the peritoneum as the dialysis membrane. Slow correction of fluid and electrolyte disturbance may be better tolerated by critically ill patients and the technique does not require complex equipment. However, treatment is labour intensive and there is considerable risk of peritoneal infection. It has been largely superseded by haemofiltration in most intensive care units.

Peritoneal access

For acute peritoneal dialysis a trochar and cannula are inserted through a small skin incision under local anaesthetic. The skin is prepared and draped as for any sterile procedure. The commonest approach is through a small midline incision 1cm below the umbilicus. The subcutaneous tissues and peritoneum are punctured by the trocar which is withdrawn slightly before the cannula is advanced towards the pouch of Douglas. In order to avoid damage to intra-abdominal structures 1–2L warmed peritoneal dialysate may be infused into the peritoneum by a standard, short intravascular cannula prior to placement of the trocar and cannula system. If the midline access site is not available an alternative is to use a lateral approach, lateral to a line joining the umbilicus and the anterior superior iliac spine (avoiding the inferior epigastric vessels).

Dialysis technique

Warmed peritoneal dialysate is infused into the peritoneum in a volume of 1–2L at a time. During the acute phase fluid is flushed in and drained continuously (i.e. with no dwell time). Once biochemical control is achieved it is usual to leave fluid in the peritoneal cavity for 4–6h before draining. Heparin (500IU/L) may be added to the first 6 cycles to prevent fibrin catheter blockage. Thereafter it is only necessary if there is blood or cloudiness in the drainage fluid.

Peritoneal dialysate

The dialysate is a sterile balanced electrolyte solution with glucose at 75mmol/L for a standard fluid or 311mmol/L for a hypertonic fluid (used for greater fluid removal). The fluid is usually potassium free since potassium exchanges slowly in peritoneal dialysis although potassium may be added if necessary.

Complications

- Fluid leak   Poor drainage
  Steroid therapy
  Obese or elderly patient
- Catheter blockage   Bleeding
  Omental encasement
- Infection   White cells > 50/ml, cloudy drainage fluid
- Hyperglycaemia   Absorption of hyperosmotic glucose
- Diaphragm splinting

Treatment of infection

It is possible to sterilise the peritoneum and catheter by adding appropriate antibiotics to the dialysate. Suitable regimens include:
Cefuroxime 500mg/L for 2 cycles then 200mg/L for 10 days
Gentamicin 8mg/L for 1 cycle daily

Plasma exchange

Indications

Plasma exchange may be used to remove circulating toxins or to replace missing plasma factors. It may be used in sepsis (particularly meningococcaemia). In patients with immune-mediated disease plasma exchange is usually a temporary measure while systemic immunosuppression takes effect. There are, however, some immune mediated diseases (e.g. Guillain–Barré syndrome) where an isolated rather than a continuous antibody-antigen reaction can be treated with early plasma exchange and no follow-up immunosuppression. Most diseases require a daily 3–4L plasma exchange repeated for at least 4 further occasions over 10 days.

Techniques

Cell separation by centrifugation
Blood is separated into components in a centrifuge. Plasma (or other specific blood components) are discarded and a plasma replacement fluid is infused in equal volume. Centrifugation may be continuous where blood is withdrawn and returned by separate needles or intermittent where blood is withdrawn, separated and then returned via the same needle.

Membrane filtration
Plasma is continuously filtered through a large pore filter (molecular weight cut-off typically 1 000 000 daltons). The plasma is discarded and replaced by infusion of an equal volume of replacement fluid. The technique is similar to haemofiltration and uses the same equipment.

Replacement fluid
Most patients will tolerate replacement with a plasma substitute. The authors' preference is to replace plasma loss with equal volumes of 6% hydroxyethyl starch and 5% albumin. However, some use partial crystalloid replacement and others use all albumin replacement. Some fresh frozen plasma will be necessary after the exchange to replace coagulation factors. The only indication to replace plasma loss with all fresh frozen plasma is where plasma exchange is being performed to replace missing plasma factors.

Complications

- Circulatory instability — intravascular volume changes
  removal of circulating catecholamines
  hypocalcaemia
- Reduced intravascular COP — if replacement is crystalloid
- Infection — reduced plasma opsonisation
- Bleeding — removal of coagulation factors

Indications

Autoimmune disease
Goodpasture's syndrome
Guillain–Barré syndrome
Myasthenia gravis
Pemphigus
Rapidly progressive glomerulonephritis
SLE
Thrombotic thrombocytopenic purpura

Immunoproliferative disease
Cryoglobulinaemia
Multiple myeloma
Waldenstrom's macroglobulinaemia

Poisoning
Paraquat

Others
Meningococcal septicaemia (possible benefit)
Sepsis syndrome (possible benefit)
Reye's syndrome

See also:
   Coagulation monitoring, 146; Anticoagulants, 236; Guillain–Barré syndrome,
370; Myasthenia gravis, 372; Poisoning—general principles, 438; Systemic
inflammatory response, 488; Vasculitides, 508

Gastrointestinal Therapy Techniques

Sengstaken-type tube

Used in the management of oesophageal variceal haemorrhage that continues despite pharmacological ± per-endoscopic therapy. The device (Sengstaken-Blakemore or similar) is a large-bore rubber tube usually containing two balloons (oesophageal and gastric) and two further lumens (oesophageal and gastric) that open above and below the balloons. This device works usually by the gastric balloon alone compressing the varices at the cardia. Inflation of the oesophageal balloon is only rarely necessary.

Insertion technique

The tubes are usually kept in the fridge to provide added stiffness for easier insertion.

1 The patient often requires judicious sedation or mechanical ventilation (as warranted by conscious state/level of agitation) prior to insertion.
2 Check balloons inflate properly beforehand. Lubricate end of tube.
3 Insert via mouth. Place to depth of 55–60cm, i.e. to ensure gastric balloon is in stomach prior to inflation.
4 Inflate gastric balloon with water ± small amount of radio-opaque contrast to volume instructed by manufacturer (usually 200ml). Negligible resistance to inflation should be felt. Clamp gastric balloon lumen.
5 Pull tube back until resistance is felt, i.e. gastric balloon is at cardia. Fix tube in place by applying counter-traction at the mouth. Old-fashioned methods, such as attaching the tube to a free-hanging litre bag of saline, have been superseded by more manageable techniques. For example, two wooden tongue depressors, 'thickened' by having Elastoplast wound around them, are placed either side of the tube at the mouth and then attached to each other at both ends by more Elastoplast. The tube remains gripped at the mouth/cheek by the attached tongue depressors but can be retracted until adequate but not excessive traction is being applied.
6 Perform X-ray to check satisfactory position of gastric balloon.
7 If bleeding continues (continued large aspirates from gastric or oesophageal lumens), inflate oesophageal balloon (to approx. 50ml).

Subsequent management

1 The gastric balloon is usually kept inflated for 12–24h and deflated prior to endoscopy ± sclerotherapy. The traction on the tube should be tested hourly by the nursing staff. The oesophageal lumen should be placed on continuous drainage while enteral nutrition and administration of drugs can be given via the gastric lumen
2 If the oesophageal balloon is used, deflate for 5–10min every 1–2h to reduce the risk of oesophageal pressure necrosis. Do not leave oesophageal balloon inflated for longer than 12h after sclerotherapy.
3 The tube may need to stay *in situ* for 2–3 days though periods of deflation should then be allowed.

Indications
- Oesophageal variceal haemorrhage

Complications
- Aspiration
- Perforation
- Ulceration
- Oesophageal necrosis

See also:
Bleeding varices, 334

Upper gastrointestinal endoscopy

Oesophago-gastro-duodenoscopy is identical in ventilated and non-ventilated patients though a protected airway ± sedation usually facilitates the procedure.

Indications

- Investigation of upper G-I signs/symptoms. e.g. bleeding, pain, mass, obstruction
- Therapeutic—e.g. sclerotherapy for varices, local adrenaline injection for discrete bleeding points, e.g. in an ulcer base
- Placement of nasojejunal tube (when gastric atony prevents enteral feeding) or percutaneous gastrostomy (PEG).
- ERCP—unusual in the ICU patient

Complications

- Local trauma causing haemorrhage or perforation.
- Abdominal distension compromising respiratory function.

Contraindications / cautions

- Any coagulopathy should ideally be corrected.

Procedure

Upper G-I endoscopy should be performed by an experienced operator to minimise the duration and trauma of the procedure and G-I tract gaseous distension.

1 The patient is usually placed in a lateral position though can be supine if intubated.
2 Increase FIO_2 and ventilator pressure alarm settings. Consider increasing sedation and adjusting ventilator mode.
3 Monitor ECG, SpO_2, airway pressures and haemodynamic variables throughout. If patient is on pressure support or pressure control ventilatory modes also monitor tidal volumes. The operator should cease the procedure, at least temporarily, if the patient becomes compromised.
4 At the end of the procedure the operator should aspirate as much air as possible out of the G-I tract to decompress the abdomen.

See also:
Pulse oximetry, 86; Upper gastrointestinal haemorrhage, 332; Bleeding varices, 334

Nutrition

Nutrition—use and indications

Malnutrition leads to poor wound healing, post-operative complications and sepsis. Adequate nutritional support is important for critically ill patients and should be provided early during the illness. Evidence for improved outcome from early nutritional support exists for patients with trauma and burns. Enteral nutrition is indicated when swallowing is inadequate or impossible but gastrointestinal function is otherwise intact. Parenteral nutrition is indicated where the gastrointestinal tract cannot be used to provide adequate nutritional support, e.g. obstruction, ileus, high small bowel fistula or malabsorption. Parenteral nutrition may be used to supplement enteral nutrition where gastrointestinal function allows partial nutritional support.

Consequences of malnutrition

Underfeeding	*Overfeeding*
Loss of muscle mass	Increased VO_2
Reduced respiratory function	Increased VCO_2
Reduced immune function	Hyperglycaemia
Poor wound healing	Fatty infiltration of liver
Gut mucosal atrophy	
Reduced protein synthesis	

Calorie requirements

Various formulae exist to calculate the patient's basal metabolic rate but they are often misleading in critical illness. Metabolic rate can be measured at the bedside by indirect calorimetry but most patients will require 2000–2700Cal/day or less if starved or underweight.

Nitrogen requirements

Nitrogen excretion can be calculated in the absence of renal failure according to the 24h urea excretion.

Nitrogen (g/24h) = 2 + Urinary urea (mmol/24h) × 0.028

However, as with most formulae, this method lacks accuracy. Most patients require 7–14g/day.

Other requirements

The normal requirements of substrates, vitamins and trace elements are tabled opposite. Most critically ill patients require folic acid and vitamin supplementation during nutritional support, e.g. Solvito. Trace elements are usually supplemented in parenteral formulae but should not be required during enteral nutrition.

Normal daily requirements (for a 70kg adult)

Water	2100ml
Energy	2000–2700Cal
Nitrogen	7–14g
Glucose	210g
Lipid	140g
Sodium	70–140mmol
Potassium	50–120mmol
Calcium	5–10mmol
Magnesium	5–10mmol
Phosphate	10–20mmol
Vitamins	
Thiamine	16–19mg
Riboflavin	3–8mg
Niacin	33–34mg
Pyridoxine	5–10mg
Folate	0.3–0.5mg
Vitamin C	250–450mg
Vitamin A	2800–3300iu
Vitamin D	280–330iu
Vitamin E	1.4–1.7iu
Vitamin K	0.7mg
Trace elements	
Iron	1–2mg
Copper	0.5–1.0mg
Manganese	1–2µg
Zinc	2–4mg
Iodide	70–140µg
Fluoride	1–2mg

Additional requirements are needed to satisfy excess loss of increased metabolic activity

Enteral nutrition

Routes include naso-gastric, naso-duodenal, gastrostomy and jeju-nostomy. Nasal tube feeding should be via a soft fine bore tube to aid patient comfort and avoid ulceration of the nose or oesophagus. Prolonged enteral feeding may be accomplished via a percutaneous gastrostomy. Enteral feeding provides a more complete diet than parenteral nutrition, maintains structural integrity of the gut, improves bowel adaptation after resection and reduces infection risk.

Feed composition

Most patients tolerate an iso-osmolar, non-lactose feed. Carbohydrates are provided as sucrose or glucose polymers (other than lactose). Protein may be as whole protein or oligopeptides. There is evidence that oligopeptides are better absorbed than free amino acids in 'elemental' feeds. Fats may be provided as medium chain or long chain triglycerides. Medium chain triglycerides are better absorbed. A standard feed will be formulated at 1Cal/ml. Special feeds are available for special purposes, e.g. high protein, fat or carbohydrate requirements, restricted salt, concentrated (1.5 or 2Cal/ml) for fluid restriction, or glutamine enriched. Impact® is a formula supplemented with arginine, nucleotides and fish oil; it may reduce hospital stay and infectious complications in critically ill patients.

Management of enteral nutrition

Once a decision is made to start enteral nutrition 30ml/h full strength standard feed may be started immediately. Starter regimens incorporating dilute feed are not necessary. After 4h at 30ml/h the feed should be stopped for 30min prior to aspiration of the stomach. Since gastric juice production is increased by the presence of a nasogastric tube, it is reasonable to accept an aspirate of < 200ml as evidence of gastric emptying and therefore to increase the infusion rate to 60ml/h. This process is repeated until the target feed rate is achieved. Thereafter aspiration of the stomach can be reduced to 8hrly. If the gastric aspirate volume is > 200ml the infusion rate is not increased (the feed is continued). If aspirates remain at high volume despite measures to promote gastric emptying (e.g. metoclopramide, erythromycin or cisapride) then nasoduodenal / nasojejunal feeding or parenteral nutrition should be considered.

Complications

- Tube placement: tracheobronchial intubation, nasopharyngeal perforation, intracranial penetration (basal skull fracture), oesophageal perforation
- Reflux
- Pulmonary aspiration
- Nausea and vomiting
- Diarrhoea: large volume, bolus feeding, high osmolality, infection, lactose intolerance, antibiotic therapy, high fat content
- Constipation
- Metabolic: dehydration, hyperglycaemia, electrolyte imbalance

Parenteral nutrition

Feed composition

Carbohydrate is normally provided in the form of concentrated glucose. While it is possible to provide the body's energy requirements with glucose alone, it is advantageous to provide 30–40% of total calories as lipid (e.g. soya bean emulsion). The nitrogen source is synthetic, crystalline L-amino acids. The nitrogen source should contain appropriate quantities of all essential and most of the non-essential amino acids. There should be a high branched-chain amino acid content and a high concentration of glycine should be avoided. Carbohydrate, lipid and nitrogen sources are usually mixed into a large bag in a sterile pharmacy unit. Vitamins, trace elements and appropriate electrolyte concentrations can be achieved in a single infusion, thus avoiding multiple connections.

Choice of parenteral feeding route

Central venous
A dedicated central venous catheter (or lumen of a multi-lumen catheter) is placed under sterile conditions. A subcutaneous tunnel is often used to separate the skin and vein entry sites. This probably reduces the risk of infection and certainly identifies the special purpose of the catheter. It is important that blood samples are not taken and other injections or infusions are not given through the feeding lumen. The main advantage of the central venous route is that it allows infusion of hyperosmolar solutions, providing adequate energy intake in reduced volume.

Peripheral venous
Parenteral nutrition via the peripheral route requires a solution with osmolality < 800mOsm/kg. Either the volume must be increased or the energy content (particularly from carbohydrate) reduced. Peripheral cannulae sites must be changed frequently.

Complications

- Catheter related   misplacement
                             infection
                             thromboembolism
- Fluid excess
- Hyperosmolar hyperglycaemic state
- Electrolyte imbalance
- Hypophosphataemia
- Metabolic acidosis   hyperchloraemia
                             metabolism of cationic amino acids
- Rebound hypoglycaemia   high endogenous insulin levels
- Vitamin deficiency   folate: pancytopenia
                             thiamine: encephalopathy
                             vitamin K: hypoprothrombinaemia
- Vitamin excess   vitamin A: dermatitis
                             vitamin D: hypercalcaemia
- Fatty liver

Infection Control

Infection control

Infection acquired within the ICU is a major cause of mortality, morbidity and increased duration of stay. Steps should be taken to minimise the risk and prevent the spread of bacteria between patients, staff and relatives.

ICU design

- Ample wash hand basins with elbow operated mixer taps, soap and antiseptic dispensers.
- Separate clean-treatment and sluice areas.
- Some isolation cubicles with positive / exhaust air flow facility.
- Ample space around bed areas.

Staff measures

- Remove watches and jewellery, remove long-sleeve white coats and jackets, roll shirt sleeves up to elbow.
- Hand and forearm washing before and after touching patient.
- Wear disposable aprons & gloves if in contact with patient known or suspected to be infected with communicable organism, e.g. TB, MRSA, multi-resistant pseudomonas, vancomycin-resistant enterococcus.
- Wear gloves and aprons when handling any body fluid and eye protection when any danger of fluid or droplet splash.
- Strict aseptic technique for invasive procedures (e.g. central venous catheter insertion) and clean technique during basic procedures such as endotracheal suction, changing ventilator circuits or drug infusions.
- Previous immunisation against hepatitis B, tuberculosis.
- Stethoscopes should be cleaned between patients.
- Clear sign posting of precautions to be taken on cubicle doors.

Visitors

- Non-ICU medical and paramedical staff, relatives and friends should adhere to the guidelines in force regarding the patient being visited, e.g. hand washing, gowns and gloves as directed.
- Traffic through the ICU should be minimised.

Cross-infection

- Inform the Infection Control nurse should cross-infection arise with more than one patient infected by indistinguishable strains of bacteria.
- For MRSA, nasal swabs should be taken from staff to detect carriers. If identified, they should not return to work until adequate treatment has cleared the bacterium as confirmed by three negative cultures.
- Affected patients should be source isolated, treated with antibiotics and topical antiseptics if necessary, and barrier-nursed.
- If cross-infection persists or spreads, other sources should be sought, e.g. taps and sinks, reusable equipment (rebreathing bags, ventilators).

Protective isolation

- Some patients carry potentially contagious or infective organisms and require source isolation, e.g. HIV, hepatitis B.
- Immunosuppressed patients, e.g. neutropenic following chemotherapy, are at risk of acquiring infection and thus require protective isolation.

Microbiological surveillance

Policies vary; some ICUs routinely screen sputum, bronchoalveolar lavage, blood, urine and drain fluid every 2–4 days while others screen only when indicated, e.g. deteriorating cardiorespiratory status, pyrexia, neutrophilia. Take samples promptly to the laboratory for analysis and culture.

Care of intravascular catheters

- Sites should be covered with transparent semi-permeable dressings to allow observation and prevent secretions from accumulating.
- No consensus exists on routine changes of intravascular catheters. Some ICUs routinely change all catheters (some using the same site over a guidewire, others a fresh insertion site) at 5–7 day intervals, others adopt a 'wait-and-see' approach.
- Catheters can be changed over a guidewire if signs of moderate infection are present, e.g. pyrexia or unexplained neutrophilia but without major cardiorespiratory disturbance.
- Catheters should be changed to fresh site if:
  - old site appears infected
  - patient shows signs of severe infection
  - a positive growth is obtained from a blood culture drawn through the catheter.

Routine changes of disposables

	frequency
ventilator circuit (if using bacterial filters)	weekly or between patients
ventilator circuit (if using water bath humidifier)	daily
ET tube catheter mount and bacterial filter	daily
disposable oxygen masks	daily
CPAP circuits	weekly or between patients
rebreathing bags and masks	weekly or between patients
intravenous infusion giving sets	48h
intermittent infusion giving sets	daily
parenteral nutrition giving sets	daily
enteral feeding giving sets	daily
arterial/venous pressure transducer sets	48h
wound dressings	depends on type of dressing
tracheostomy site	as necessary
urinary catheter bags	weekly

79

See also:
Bacteriology, 148; Virology, serology & assays, 150; Antimicrobials, 248; Acute chest infection 1, 276; Acute chest infection 2, 278; Sepsis / infection, 490; ICU layout, 522

Special Support Surfaces

Special support surfaces

Pressure sores

Pressure sores occur due to compression of tissue between bone and the support surface and due to shearing forces, friction and maceration of tissues against the support surface. The use of special beds attempts to reduce the pressure at the contacting skin surface to a level lower than the capillary occlusion pressure. In the majority of cases it is sufficient to minimise the time that the support surface contacts any one area of skin by position changes.

Factors suggesting the need for a special bed

- Patients with severely restricted mobility due to traction or haemodynamic instability cannot be turned frequently, if at all.
- Patients with decreased skin integrity, e.g. burns, pressure sores already present, chronic steroid use, diabetes mellitus.
- Patients on vasoactive drug infusions.

Types of special support surface

Air mattress
An air mattress either replaces or is placed on top of a standard hospital bed mattress. These provide significant reduction in contact pressure. An air mattress should be considered as minimum support for any patient with the above factors.

Low air loss bed
The low air loss bed is a purpose built pressure relieving bed. It allows easier patient mobility than other support surfaces. Contact pressure may still be higher than capillary occlusion pressure so positioning is still required. Patients who are haemodynamically unstable should usually be managed on a low air loss bed, particularly if receiving vasoconstrictor drugs. The presence of pressure sores with intact skin is an indication for a low air loss bed. Rotating low air loss beds are also available allowing limited, automated lateral rotation. These may be useful where manual positioning is not practical.

Air fluidised bed
The air fluidised bed is the only support surface that consistently lowers contact pressure to below capillary occlusion pressure. Consequently, patients with severe haemodynamic instability, who cannot be turned, and patients with pressure sores with broken skin benefit most. In addition, the ability to control the temperature of the immediate environment is an advantage in patients with large surface area burns and hypothermic patients. Any exudate from the skin is adsorbed into the silicone beads on which the patient floats. This drying effect is particularly useful in major burns (although it must be taken into account for fluid replacement therapy). The air fluidised bed also has a role in pain relief.

Respiratory Monitoring

Pulse oximetry

Continuous non-invasive monitoring of arterial oxygen saturation by placement of a probe emitting red and near-infra red light over pulse on digit, earlobe, cheek or bridge of nose. It is unaffected by skin pigmentation, hyperbilirubinaemia or anaemia (unless profound).

Physics

The colour of blood varies with oxygen saturation due to the optical properties of the haem moiety. As the Hb molecule gives up O_2 it becomes less permeable to red light and takes on a blue tint. Saturation is determined spectrophotometrically by measuring the 'blueness', utilising the ability of compounds to absorb light at a specific wavelength. The use of two wavelengths (650 & 940 nm) permits the relative quantities of reduced and oxyhaemoglobin to be calculated, thereby determining saturation. The arterial pulse is used to provide time points to allow subtraction of the constant absorption of light by tissue and venous blood.

The accuracy of pulse oximetry is within 2% above 70% SaO_2.

Indications

- Continuous monitoring of arterial oxygen saturation.

Complications

Nil though ensure that probe is designed for long-term use as some 'perioperative' probes have a heating element which can result in superficial burns.

Cautions

- As only two wavelengths are used, pulse oximetry measures functional rather than fractional oxyhaemoglobin saturation. Erroneously high readings are given with carboxyhaemoglobin and methaemoglobin.
- With poor peripheral perfusion or intense vasoconstriction the reading may be inaccurate ('fail soft') or, in newer models, absent ('fail hard').
- Motion artefact and high levels of ambient lighting may affect readings.
- Erroneous signals may be produced by significant venous pulsation from tricuspid regurgitation or venous congestion. Venous pulsatility accounts for differences between ear and finger SpO_2 in the same subject.
- Ensure a good LED signal indicator or a pulse waveform (if available) is seen on the monitor.
- Vital dyes (e.g. methylene blue, indocyanine green) may affect SpO_2 readings.

Capnography

Methods

For capnography respiratory gases must be sampled continuously and measured by a rapid response device. Since CO_2 has an absorption band in the infra-red spectrum, measurement is facilitated in gas mixtures. Other gases do interfere with the infra-red absorption by CO_2, the effect depending on the concentration of CO_2. This may be overcome by calibrating the instrument with known concentrations of CO_2 in the required measurement range, diluted with a gas mixture similar to exhaled gas. Alternatively, mass spectrometry may be used but the technique is relatively expensive and subject to condensation in the sampling device.

The capnogram

The CO_2 concentration of exhaled gas displayed continuously consists of 4 phases (figure). The presence of significant concentrations of CO_2 in phase 1 implies rebreathing of exhaled gas. Failure of an expiratory valve to open is the most likely cause of rebreathing during manual ventilation, although an inadequate flow of fresh gas into a rebreathing bag is a common cause. The slope of phase 3 is dependent on the rate of alveolar gas exchange. A steep slope may indicate ventilation perfusion mismatch since alveoli that are poorly ventilated but well perfused discharge late in the respiratory cycle. A steep slope is seen in patients with significant auto-PEEP.

End-tidal PCO_2

End-tidal PCO_2 approximates arterial PCO_2 in patients with normal lung function. A large difference between end-tidal and arterial PCO_2 may represent an increased dead space to tidal volume ratio, poor pulmonary perfusion or intra-pulmonary shunting. A progressive rise in end-tidal PCO_2 may represent hypoventilation, airway obstruction or increased CO_2 production due to increased metabolic rate. Pulmonary function is rarely normal in ICU patients, therefore the end-tidal PCO_2 is a poor approximation of arterial PCO_2.

Dead space to tidal volume ratio

The difference between arterial and end-tidal PCO_2 may be used to calculate the physiological dead space to tidal volume ratio via the Bohr equation:

$$\frac{V_D}{V_T} = \frac{PaCO_2}{PetCO_2}$$

In health a value between 30 and 45% should be expected.

The components of the normal capnogram

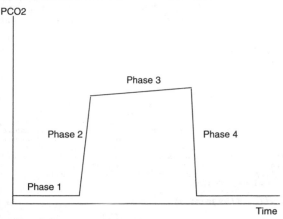

PCO2

Phase 3

Phase 2

Phase 4

Phase 1

Time

Phase 1
During the early part of the exhaled breath anatomical dead space and sampling device dead space gas are sampled. There is negligible CO_2 in phase 1.

Phase 2
As alveolar gas begins to be sampled there is a rapid rise in CO_2 concentration.

Phase 3
Phase 3 is known as the alveolar plateau and represents the CO_2 concentration in mixed expired alveolar gas. There is normally a slight increase in PCO_2 during phase 3 as alveolar gas exchange continues during expiration. End-tidal PCO_2 will be less than the PCO_2 of ideal alveolar gas since the sampled exhaled gas is mixed with alveolar dead space gas.

Phase 4
As inspiration begins there is a rapid fall in sample PCO_2.

See also:
Ventilatory support—indications, 4; IPPV—description of ventilators, 6; IPPV—modes of ventilation, 8; Blood gas analysis, 94

Pulmonary function tests

Few of the numerous pulmonary function tests available currently impact upon clinical management of the critically ill, particularly if the patient has to be moved to a laboratory. A number of other tests require highly specialised equipment and fulfil a predominant research role.

Clinically relevant tests

Measurement	Test	Common clinical use
PaO_2, SaO_2, $PaCO_2$	arterial blood gases	
SpO_2	pulse oximetry	
end-tidal PCO_2	capnography	
vital capacity, tidal volume	spirometry, electronic flowmetry	serial measurement of borderline function (VC < 10–15ml/kg) e.g. Guillain–Barré syndrome (spontaneous ventilation) asthma
peak expiratory flow rate	Wright peak flow meter	(spontaneous ventilation) asthma
FEV_1, FVC	spirometry, electronic flowmetry	(spontaneous ventilation) asthma, obstructive/restrictive disease
lung/chest wall compliance (see equations opposite)	pressure-volume curve	ventilator adjustments, monitoring disease progression
flow-volume loop, pressure-volume loop	pneumotachograph, manometry	ventilator adjustments

Research tests (examples)

Measurement	Test	Research use
diaphragmatic strength (transdiaphragmatic pressure)	gastric and oesophageal manometry	respiratory muscle function, weaning
pleural (intrathoracic) pressure	oesophageal manometry	ventilator trauma, work of breathing, weaning
functional residual capacity	closed circuit helium dilution, (bag-in-a-box) open circuit N_2 washout	lung volumes, compliance
ventilation–perfusion relationship	multiple inert gas elimination technique, isotope techniques	regional lung ventilation–perfusion, pulmonary gas exchange
pulmonary diffusing capacity	carbon monoxide uptake	pulmonary gas exchange

Equations

- Compliance equals the change in pressure during a linear increase of 1Litre in volume above FRC.
- The alveolar-arterial oxygen difference is < 2kPa in youth and < 3.3kPa in old age.
- The Bohr equation calculates physiological deadspace, V_D. The normal value is below 30%.
- The shunt equation estimates the proportion of blood shunted past poorly ventilated alveoli (Q_S) compared to total lung blood flow (Q_T).

These equations allow estimation of ventilation/perfusion mismatch:
- V/Q = 1—ventilation and perfusion are well-matched.
- V/Q > 1—increased deadspace (where alveoli are poorly perfused but well ventilated).
- V/Q < 1—increased venous admixture or shunt (where alveolus is perfused but poorly ventilated).

The normal range is < 15%.

Lung volumes and capacities

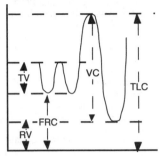

TLC = total lung capacity
VC = vital capacity
FRC = functional residual capacity
TV = tidal volume
RV = residual volume

Equations

Compliance:
Lung compliance (l/cmH_2O) = $\Delta V_L/\Delta P_L$ where L, the litre above FRC, is the slope of the linear portion of the curve.

Total respiratory system compliance is derived from the equation:
(1/total compliance) = (1/Lung compliance) + (1/chest wall compliance)

Total compliance can be calculated in well sedated, ventilated patients as tidal volume/(end-inspiratory pause pressure minus PEEP).

Alveolar gas equation
P_AO_2 = FIO_2-($PaCO_2$/respiratory quotient) [RQ often approximated to 0.8]

Alveolar-arterial oxygen difference
(A-a) difference = $FIO_2 \times 94.8 - PaCO_2 - PaO_2$

Bohr equation:
V_D/V_T = ($PaCO_2$ − expired PCO_2)/$PaCO_2$

Shunt equation
$Q_S/Q_T = (CcO_2 - CaO_2)/(CcO_2 - CvO_2)$
where CcO_2 = end-capillary O_2 content, a = arterial, v = mixed venous

See also:
Ventilatory support—indications, 4; IPPV—description of ventilators, 6; IPPV—modes of ventilation, 8; Pulse oximetry, 86; Capnography, 88; Blood gas analysis, 94; Acute weakness, 356; Guillain- Barré syndrome, 370; Myasthenia gravis, 372; Rheumatic disorders, 506; Vasculitides, 508

Blood gas machine

A small amount of heparinised blood is either injected from a syringe or aspirated from a capillary tube into the machine. The blood comes into contact with three electrodes which measure pH, PO_2 and PCO_2.

- pH—measured by the potential across a pH-sensitive glass membrane separating a sample of known pH and the test sample.
- PO_2—the partial oxygen pressure, is measured by applying a polarizing voltage between a platinum cathode and a silver anode. Oxygen is reduced, generating a current proportional to the oxygen tension.
- PCO_2—the partial pressure of carbon dioxide, utilises a pH electrode with a Teflon membrane which allows through uncharged molecules (CO_2) but not charged ions (H^+). CO_2 alone thus changes the pH of a bicarbonate electrolyte solution, the change being linearly related to the PCO_2.
- Hb—estimated photometrically—this is not as accurate as co-oximetry (see below).
- Bicarbonate—calculated by the Henderson–Hasselbach equation

$$pH = 6.1 + \log_{10} \frac{\text{arterial } [HCO_3^-]}{PaCO_2 \times 0.03}$$

Actual HCO_3^- includes bicarbonate, carbonate and carbamate.
- Actual base excess (deficit)—the difference in concentration of strong base (acid) in whole blood and that titrated to pH 7.4, at PCO_2 5.33kPa and 37°C.
- Standard base excess (deficit)—a calculated *in vivo* base excess (deficit).
- Standard bicarbonate—the plasma concentration of hydrogen carbonate equilibrated at PCO_2 5.33 kPa, PO_2 13.33 kPa and temperature 37°C.

Blood gas values can be given either as 'pHstat' or 'alphastat', the former correcting for body temperature by shifting the calculated Bohr oxyhaemoglobin dissociation curve (hyperthermia to the right, hypothermia to the left). Alphastat measures true blood gas levels in the sample.

Co-oximeter

This differs from a blood gas machine in that the blood is haemolysed to calculate (i) total Hb and fetal Hb and (ii) oxyHb, carboxyhaemoglobin (COHb), methaemoglobin and sulphaemoglobin by utilising absorbance at six wavelengths (535, 560, 577, 622, 636, 670 nm).

Taking a good blood gas sample

Use a 1ml syringe containing preferably a dry heparin salt (if not, liquid sodium heparin 1000IU/ml solution just filling the hub). Take sample, expel air, mix sample thoroughly and insert without delay.

Cautions

- Too much heparin causes dilution errors and is acidic.
- Nitrous oxide or halothane anaesthesia may give unreliable PO_2 values.
- Intravenous lipid administration may affect pH values.
- Abnormal (high/low) plasma protein concentrations affect the base deficit.

Blood gas analysis

A heparinised (arterial, venous, capillary) blood sample can be inserted into a blood gas machine and/or Co-oximeter for measurement of gas tensions and saturations, and acid–base status.

Measurements

- Identification of arterial hypoxaemia and hyperoxia, hypercapnia and hypocapnia—enabling monitoring of disease progression and efficacy of treatment. Ventilator and FIO_2 adjustments can be made precisely.
- pH, $PaCO_2$ and base deficit (or bicarbonate) values can be reviewed in parallel for diagnosis of acidosis and alkalosis, whether it is respiratory or metabolic in origin, and whether any compensation has occurred. (See Figure opposite).
- Using a Co-Oximeter, accurate measurement can be made of haemoglobin oxygen saturation and the total Hb level. The more sophisticated Co-oximeters permit measurement of the fraction of metHb, COHb, deoxyHb and fetal Hb.
- Measurement of mixed venous oxygen saturation—for calculation of oxygen consumption and monitoring of oxygen supply:demand balance.

Causes of acid-base disturbances

Respiratory acidosis—excess CO_2 production and/or inadequate excretion e.g. hypoventilation, excess narcotic

Respiratory alkalosis—reduction in PCO_2 due to hyperventilation

Metabolic acidosis—usually lactic, keto, renal or tubular
Consider tissue hypoperfusion, ingestion of acids (e.g. aspirin),
loss of alkali (e.g. diarrhoea, renal tubular acidosis),
diabetic ketoacidosis

Metabolic alkalosis—excess alkali (e.g. bicarbonate or buffer
infusion), loss of acid (e.g. large gastric aspirate, renal),
hypokalaemia, drugs (e.g. diuretics)

Normal values

pH	7.35–7.45
PCO_2	4.6–6 kPa
PO_2	10–13.3 kPa
HCO_3^-	22–26mmol/L
ABE	−2.4 to +2.2
Arterial O_2 saturation	95–98%
Mixed venous oxygen saturation	70–75%

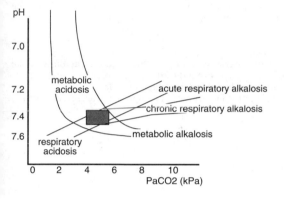

Invasive blood gas monitoring

Continuous blood gas monitoring can be achieved via an intra-arterial heparin-bonded catheter with on-line display of directly measured and computed blood gas variables. Results are updated every 20–30sec. Recalibration is generally recommended at 12–hourly intervals.

Technology

Systems utilise either electrode, tonometric or optode technology. Electrode technology is similar to that described for blood gas machine measurement. Optical sensors utilise either absorbance or fluorescence spectrophotometry to measure the signal from the chemical interaction between the analyte (O_2, CO_2 and H^+) and an indicator phase.

Problems

Damping of the arterial pressure waveform can occur through the presence of the catheter within the arterial cannula. A dedicated, non-tapering 20G cannula reduces this damping effect.

An increasing drift in accuracy is recognised after several days.

Extravascular lung water measurement

Standard methods of assessing pulmonary oedema are indirect. The chest X-ray allows qualitative assessment only and is slow to change in response to clinical treatment. Assessment of cardiac filling pressures does not take into account the degree of capillary permeability or lymphatic adaptation. Consequently, a relatively low CVP or PAWP may be associated with pulmonary oedema formation. and high filling pressures in chronic heart failure may be associated with no oedema and be entirely appropriate. Extravascular lung water (EVLW) measurement provides a technique for quantifying pulmonary oedema and monitoring the response to treatment.

Measurement technique

The normal value of 4–7ml/kg for extravascular lung water has been derived by gravimetric techniques performed post-mortem. During life a double indicator technique may be used. Two indicators are injected via a central vein; one distributes within the vascular space and the other throughout the intra- and extra-vascular space. The volume of distribution of the indicators are derived from the dilution curves detected at the femoral artery. Cooled 5% glucose is used as a thermal indicator for intra- and extravascular volume and indocyanine green bound to albumin as a colorimetric indicator for intravascular volume. Detection at the femoral artery is by a fibreoptic catheter with a thermistor tip. The cardiac output is measured by thermodilution at the femoral artery. The rate of exponential decay of the thermodilution curve allows the derivation of the volume of distribution between the injection and detection sites (the heart and lungs).

Pulmonary thermal volume = thermodilution CO × rate of exponential decay of thermodilution curve (intra- and extravascular volume)

Similar principles may be applied to the dye dilution curve produced on injection of the indocyanine green which is assumed to distribute within the vascular space only.

Pulmonary blood volume = dye dilution CO × rate of exponential decay of dye dilution curve (intravascular volume)

EVLW may be calculated by subtracting pulmonary blood volume from pulmonary thermal volume.

Limitations of EVLW measurement

Since it is known that albumin can exchange across capillary membranes, pulmonary blood volume is over-estimated by this technique and extravascular lung water is therefore underestimated. However, the corresponding error is small and not particularly significant clinically. A more serious drawback is in the limitation of treatment options. Treatment of pulmonary oedema by diuresis and ultrafiltration have been shown to be less effective at reducing EVLW in capillary leak, compared to congestive heart failure. Similarly, the strategy of preventing oedema formation by diuresis while maintaining the circulation with catecholamine infusions appears to be futile; vasoconstriction so produced increases EVLW.

See also:

Cardiovascular Monitoring

ECG monitoring

Continuous ECG monitoring is routine in every intensive care unit. The standard technique is to display a three lead ECG (commonly lead II). Other limb leads may be used although the electrodes are placed at the shoulders and left side of the abdomen. Other lead configurations can be used for specific purposes:

Chest—Shoulder—V5   Early detection of left ventricular strain
Chest—Manubrium—V5 Early detection of left ventricular strain
Chest—Back—V5   P wave monitoring

Modern, continuous monitors include alarm functions for bradycardia and tachycardia monitoring, and software routines for arrhythmia detection or ST segment analysis.

Causes of changes in heart rate or rhythm

Changes in heart rate or rhythm may be an indication of:

Sympathetic activity   circulatory insufficiency
                        pain
                        anxiety
                        hypoxaemia
                        hypercapnia
Adverse drug effects   antiarrhythmics
                        sedatives

Electrolyte imbalance
Fever

Blood pressure monitoring

Non-invasive techniques

Non-invasive techniques are intermittent but automated. They include oscillotonometry (detection of cuff pulsation as the systolic pressure), detection of arterial turbulence under the cuff, ultrasonic detection of arterial wall motion under the cuff and detection of blood flow distal to the cuff. Any cuff system should use a cuff large enough to cover 2/3 of the surface of the upper arm.

Invasive (direct) arterial monitoring

Blood pressure is most usefully monitored from larger limb arteries, e.g. femoral or brachial. However, the potential for damage to these arteries is considerable and most consider it safer to use the radial or dorsalis pedis arteries, the pressure in which is higher. The arterial cannula is connected to an appropriate transducer system via a short length of non-compliant manometer tubing. The transducer should be matched to the monitor, i.e. as recommended by the manufacturer of the monitor. The transducer must be zeroed to atmospheric pressure. The transducer should be positioned at the level of the 4th intercostal space in the mid-axillary line. The transducer, manometer tubing and cannula should be continuously flushed with 3ml/h heparinised saline (1000IU/L).

Damping errors
It is important that the monitoring system is correctly damped. An under-damped system will over-estimate systolic and under-estimate diastolic blood pressure. The converse is true for an over-damped system. Moreover, it is not possible to interpret correctly the waveform shape if damping is not correct. A correctly damped system will return immediately to the pressure waveform after flushing. Return is slow in an over-damped system and there is often resonance around the baseline before return to the pressure waveform in an under-damped system.

Interpretation of waveform
The shape of the arterial pressure waveform gives useful qualitative information about the state of the heart and circulation:

Short systolic time	hypovolaemia
	high peripheral resistance
Marked respiratory swing	hypovolaemia
	pericardial effusion
	airways obstruction
	high intra-thoracic pressure
Slow systolic upstroke	poor myocardial contractility
	high peripheral resistance

Limitations of blood pressure monitoring
It is important not to rely on arterial blood pressure monitoring alone in the critically ill. A normal blood pressure does not guarantee adequate blood flow to all organs. Conversely, a low blood pressure may be acceptable if perfusion pressure is adequate for all organs and blood flow is high. Measurement of cardiac output, in addition to blood pressure, is necessary where there is doubt about the adequacy of the circulation.

Examples of arterial waveform shape

Normal arterial waveform

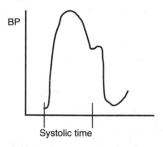

Short systolic time

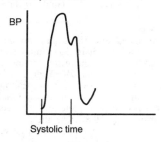

Slow systolic upstroke

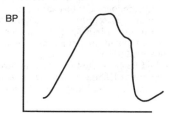

See also:
Arterial cannulation, 106; Hypotension, 300; Hypertension, 302

Arterial cannulation

Indications

Performed correctly, arterial cannulation is a safe technique allowing continuous monitoring of blood pressure and frequent sampling of blood. It is indicated in any patient with unstable or potentially unstable haemodynamic or respiratory status.

Radial artery cannulation

The radial artery is most frequently chosen because it is accessible and has good collateral blood flow. Allen's test may be used to confirm the ulnar blood supply to the hand before the radial artery is punctured. However, it is not highly reliable.

Allen's test

Both the radial and ulnar arteries are compressed at the wrist. The patient is instructed to form a fist so blanching the skin of the hand. The hand is then relaxed and the ulnar artery is released. The hand should become pink within 5–10seconds. The radial artery should not be cannulated if there is a delay > 15seconds to the hand becoming pink.

Technique of cannulation

The wrist is hyperextended and the thumb abducted. After skin cleansing local anaesthetic (1% plain lignocaine) is injected into the skin and subcutaneous tissue over the most prominent pulsation. The course of the artery is noted and a 20G Teflon cannula is inserted along the line of the vessel. The usual technique is to enter the vessel in the same way as an intravenous cannula would be inserted. There is usually some resistance to skin puncture. To avoid accidentally puncturing the posterior wall of the artery, the skin and artery should be punctured as two distinct manoeuvres. Alternatively a small skin nick may be made to facilitate skin entry.

In the case of elderly patients with mobile, atheromatous vessels a technique that involves deliberate transfixation of the artery may be employed. The cannula is passed through the anterior and posterior walls of the vessel, thus immobilising it. The needle is removed and the cannula withdrawn slowly into the lumen of the vessel, before being advanced into the lumen.

The cannula should be connected to a continuous flushing device after successful puncture. Flushing with a syringe should be avoided since the high pressures generated may lead to a retrograde cerebral embolus.

Complications

- Digital ischaemia due to arterial spasm, thrombosis, or embolus
- Bleeding in cases with altered coagulation status
- Infection is a risk in prolonged cannulation

Alternative sites for cannulation

Brachial artery
End artery supplying a large volume of tissue. Thus thrombosis has potentially severe consequences.

Ulnar artery
Should be avoided if the radial artery is occluded.

Femoral artery
May be difficult to keep clean. Also supplies a large volume of tissue. A longer catheter should be used to avoid displacement.

Dorsalis pedis artery
Blood pressure will be at least 10–20mmHg higher than in the central circulation.

107

Central venous catheter—use

Types of catheter
- Single, double or triple lumen.
- Sheaths for insertion of pulmonary artery catheter or pacing wire
- Tunnelled catheter for long term use.
- Triple lumen catheters allow multiple infusions given separately ± continuous pressure monitoring. Minimises risk of accidental bolus.
- 12Fr double lumen catheters used for venovenous dialysis/filtration.
- Common routes are internal jugular, subclavian and femoral.
- 'Long' catheters can be inserted via medial brachial or axillary veins though are generally not recommended due to the risk of thrombosis.

Uses
- Invasive haemodynamic monitoring.
- Infusion of drugs liable to cause peripheral phlebitis or tissue necrosis if tissue extravasation occurs (e.g. TPN, dopamine, amiodarone).
- Rapid volume infusion, n.b. the rate of flow is inversely proportional to the length of the cannula.
- Access, e.g. for pacing wire insertion.
- Emergency access when peripheral circulation is 'shut down'.
- Renal replacement therapy, plasmapheresis, exchange transfusion.

Contraindications / cautions
- Coagulopathy.
- Undrained pneumothorax on contralateral side.
- Agitated, restless patient.

Complications
- Arterial puncture.
- Haemorrhage.
- Arrhythmias.
- Infection (usually skin, occasionally sepsis or endocarditis).
- Pneumothorax.
- Air embolism, venous thrombosis, haemothorax, chylothorax (all rare).

Central venous pressure measurement

Use of an electronic pressure transducer is preferable to manometry which incorporates a three-way tap, a fluid reservoir bag and a fluid-filled vertical column, the height of which corresponds to CVP. The pressure transducer should be placed and 'zeroed' at the level of the left atrium (approximately mid-axillary line) rather than the sternum which is more affected by patient position (supine/semi-erect/prone). Venous pulsation and some respiratory swing should be seen in the trace but not a RV pressure waveform (i.e. catheter inserted too far).

Troubleshooting

Excessive bleeding at the insertion site is usually controlled by direct compression. If not controlled, correct any coagulopathy, If post-thrombolysis, consider tranexamic acid.

The incidence of local infection (usually *Staph. epidermidis* or *Staph. aureus*) rises > 5 days. Routine change of catheter at 5 days is not necessary though change over a wire may be sufficient if patient develops an unexplained pyrexia or neutrophilia. However, removal ± change of site is needed if site is cellulitic or blood cultures taken through the catheter are positive.

109

See also:
Parenteral nutrition, 74; Temporary internal pacing, 46; Central venous catheter—insertion, 110; Pulmonary artery catheter—insertion, 114; Fluid challenge, 262; Pneumothorax, 288; Haemothorax, 290; Acute renal failure—management, 322

Central venous catheter—insertion

Landmarks

Various landmarks have been described. For example:
- Internal jugular: Halfway between mastoid process and sternal notch, lateral to carotid pulsation and medial to medial border of sternocleidomastoid. Aim toward ipsilateral nipple, advancing under body of sternocleidomastoid until vein entered.
- Subclavian: 3cm below junction of lateral third and medial two thirds of clavicle. Turn head to contralateral side. Aim for point between jaw and contralateral shoulder tip. Advance needle subcutaneously to hit clavicle. Scrape needle around clavicle and advance further until vein entered.
- Femoral: Locate femoral artery in groin. Insert needle 3cm medially and angled rostrally. Advance until vein entered.

Insertion technique

The Seldinger technique (described below) is safer than the "catheter-over-needle" technique and should generally be used in ICU patients.

1. Use aseptic technique throughout. Clean area with antiseptic and surround with sterile drapes. Anaesthetise local area with 1% lignocaine. Flush lumen(s) of catheter with saline.
2. Use metal needle to locate central vein.
3. Pass wire (with 'J' or floppy end leading) through needle into vein. Only minimal resistance at most should be felt. If not, remove wire and confirm needle tip is still located within vein lumen. Monitor for arrhythmias. If these occur, wire is probably at tricuspid valve. Usually responds to pulling wire back a few cm.
4. Remove needle leaving wire extruding from skin puncture site.
5. Depending on size/type of catheter to be inserted, a rigid dilator ($\pm$ preceded by a scalpel incision to enlarge puncture site) may be passed over the wire to form a track through the subcutaneous tissues to the vein. Remove dilator.
6. Thread catheter over wire. Ensure end of wire extrudes from catheter to prevent accidental loss of wire in vein. Insert catheter into vein to depth of 15–20cm. Remove wire.
7. Check for flashback of blood down each lumen and respiratory swing, then flush with saline.
8. Suture catheter to skin. Clean & dry area. Cover with sterile transparent semi-permeable dressing.
9. A chest X-ray is usually performed to verify correct position of tip (junction of superior vena cava & right atrium) and to exclude a pneumothorax. Unless in an emergency situation, a satisfactory position should generally be confirmed before use of the catheter.

Pulmonary artery catheter—use

Uses

- Pressure monitoring—RA, RV, PA, PAWP
- Flow monitoring—(right ventricular) cardiac output
- Oxygen saturation—'mixed venous' (i.e. in RV outflow tract/PA), determination of left to right shunts (ASD, VSD)
- Derived variables—SVR, PVR, LVSW, RVSW, DO_2, VO_2, O_2ER
- Temporary pacing
- Right ventricular ejection fraction and end-diastolic volume

Specialised catheters

- Continuous mixed venous oxygen saturation measurement
- Continuous cardiac output measurement
- RV end-diastolic volume, RV ejection fraction calculation
- Ventricular ($\pm$ atrial) pacing

Management

Monitor PA pressure continuously to recognise forward catheter migration and pulmonary arterial occlusion. If so, correct immediately by partial catheter withdrawal to prevent infarction.

The incidence of local infection (usually *Staph. aureus* or *Staph. epidermidis*) rises after 5 days. Recent studies suggest change of catheter over a wire may be sufficient if patient develops unexplained pyrexia or neutrophilia. However, removal $\pm$ change of insertion site is needed if site is cellulitic or cultures of blood taken through line are positive.

Samples of pulmonary artery blood should be withdrawn slowly from the distal lumen to prevent 'arterialization', i.e. pulmonary venous sampling.

Wedge pressure measurements

Inflate balloon slowly, monitoring the waveform to avoid overwedging and potential arterial rupture (especially elderly and pulmonary hypertension). The trace should not 'wedge' until $\geqslant 1.3$ml of air has been injected into the balloon.

Take readings at end-expiration when intrathoracic pressure approximates closest to atmospheric pressure. For ventilated patients end expiration $\equiv$ lowest wedge reading; during spontaneous breathing end expiration $\equiv$ highest reading. Measurement is difficult in the dyspnoeic patient; the authors suggest using a 'mean' wedge reading in this instance.

The PAWP cannot be higher than the PA diastolic pressure.

CVP, PAWP and CO should not be measured during rapid volume infusion but after a period of equilibration (5–10min).

The PAWP does not equal the LVEDP in mitral stenosis.

In mitral regurgitation the PAWP is measured at the end of the 'a' wave.

West's Zones

The catheter tip should lie in a zone III region (where pulmonary arterial pressure > pulmonary venous pressure > alveolar pressure and which will be below left atrial level on a lateral CXR).

A non-zone III position should be suspected if (i) following an increment in PEEP, the PAWP rises by greater than half that increment, (ii) no detectable cardiac pulsation and/or excessive respiratory variation is seen in the wedge trace.

A non-zone III position is more likely with PEEP and/or hypovolaemia.

Normal values

Stroke volume	70–100ml
Cardiac output	4–6L/min
Right atrial pressure	0–5mmHg
Right ventricular pressure	20–25/0–5mmHg
Pulmonary artery pressure	20–25/10–15mmHg
Pulmonary artery wedge pressure	6–12mmHg
Mixed venous oxygen saturation	70–75%

113

Derived variables

Variable	Calculation	Normal range
cardiac index	$\dfrac{CO}{\text{Body surface area}}$	$2.5\text{–}3.5\text{L/min/m}^2$
stroke index	$\dfrac{SV}{\text{Body surface area}}$	$40\text{–}60\text{ml/m}^2$
systemic vascular resistance	$\dfrac{MAP-RAP \times 79.9}{CO}$	$960\text{–}1400\text{dyn.sec/cm}^5$
pulmonary vascular resistance	$\dfrac{MPAP-PAWP \times 79.9}{CO}$	$25\text{–}125\text{dyn.sec/cm}^5$
left ventricular stroke work	$(MAP-PAWP) \times SV \times 0.0136$	$44\text{–}68\text{g-m.m}^2$
right ventricular stroke work	$(MPAP-RAP) \times SV \times 0.0136$	$4\text{–}8\text{g-m.m}^2$
oxygen delivery	$0.134 \times CO \times Hb_a \times SaO_2$	$950\text{–}1300\text{ml/min}$
oxygen consumption	$0.134 \times CO \times (Hb_a \times SaO_2 - Hb_v \times SvO_2)$	$180\text{–}320\text{ml/min}$
oxygen extraction ratio	$1 - \dfrac{SaO_2 - SvO_2}{SaO_2}$	$0.25\text{–}0.30$

See also:
Positive end expiratory pressure, 20; Blood gas analysis, 94; Extravascular lung water measurement, 98; Central venous catheter—use, 108; Pulmonary artery catheter—insertion, 114; Cardiac output—thermodilution, 116; Cardiac output—other invasive, 118; Fluid challenge, 262; Heart failure—assessment, 312; Heart failure—management, 314; Systemic inflammatory response, 488

Pulmonary artery catheter—insertion

Insertion

1 Insert 8Fr central venous introducer sheath under strict aseptic technique. Pulmonary artery catheterisation is easier via the internal jugular and subclavian veins than the femoral vein.

2 Prepare catheter pre-insertion—3-way taps on all lumens, flush lumens with crystalloid, inflate balloon with 1.6ml air and check for concentric inflation and leaks, place transparent sleeve over catheter to maintain future sterility, pressure transduce distal lumen and zero to a reference point (usually mid-axillary line). Depending on catheter used, other pre-insertion calibration steps may be required, e.g. oxygen saturation.

3 Insert catheter 15cm (i.e. beyond the length of the introducer sheath) before inflating balloon. Advance catheter smoothly through the right heart chambers using the bend on the catheter tip to aid passage. Pause to record pressures and note waveform shape in RA, RV and PA. When a characteristic PAWP waveform is obtained, stop advancing catheter, deflate balloon and ensure that PA waveform reappears. If not, withdraw catheter by a few cm.

4 Slowly re-inflate balloon, observing waveform trace. The wedge recording should not be obtained until at least 1.3ml of air has been injected into the balloon. If not, withdraw catheter 1–2cm and repeat. If 'overwedged' (pressure continues to climb on inflation), catheter is inserted too far and balloon has inflated forward over distal lumen. Immediately deflate, withdraw catheter 1–2cm and repeat.

5 After insertion, a chest X-ray is usually performed to verify catheter position and to exclude pneumothorax.

Contraindications / cautions

- Coagulopathy
- Tricuspid valve prosthesis or disease

Complications

- Problems of central venous catheterisation
- Arrhythmias (especially when traversing tricuspid valve)
- Infection (including endocarditis)
- Pulmonary artery rupture
- Pulmonary infarction
- Knotting of catheter
- Valve damage (do not withdraw catheter unless balloon deflated)

Troubleshooting

Excessive catheter length in a heart chamber causes coiling and a risk of knotting. No more than 15–20cm should be passed before the waveform changes. If not, deflate balloon, withdraw catheter, repeat. A knot can be managed by (i) 'unknotting' with an intraluminal wire, (ii) pulling taut and removing catheter + introducer sheath together, or (iii) surgical or angiographic intervention.

If catheter fails to advance to next chamber, consider (i) 'stiffening' catheter by injecting iced crystalloid through distal lumen (ii) rolling patient to left lateral (iii) advancing catheter slowly with balloon deflated.

The catheter should never be withdrawn with the balloon inflated.

Arrhythmias on insertion usually occur when the catheter tip is at the tricuspid valve. These usually resolve on withdrawing the catheter or, occasionally, following a slow bolus of 1.5mg/kg lignocaine.

Waveforms

mmHg

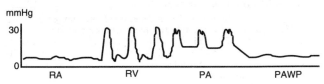

Cardiac output—thermodilution

Thermodilution is the technique utilised by the pulmonary artery catheter to measure right ventricular cardiac output. The principle is a modification of the Fick principle whereby a bolus of cooled 5% glucose is injected through the proximal lumen into the central circulation (right atrium) and the temperature change is detected by a thermistor at the catheter tip, some 30cm distal. A modification of the Hamilton–Stewart equation, utilising the volume, temperature and specific heat of the injectate, enables cardiac output to be calculated by an on-line computer from a curve measuring temperature change in the pulmonary artery.

A recent development has been 'continuous' thermodilution measurement using a modified catheter that emits heat pulses from a thermal filament lying within the right ventricle and right atrium, 14–25cm from the tip. 7.5 watts of heat are added to the blood intermittently every 30–60sec and these temperature changes are measured by a thermistor 4cm from the tip. Although updated frequently, the cardiac output displayed is usually an average of the previous 3–6min.

Thermodilution injection technique

The computer constant must be set for the volume and temperature of the 5% glucose used. Ten ml of ice-cold glucose provides the most accurate measure. Five ml of room temperature injectate is sufficiently precise for normal and high output states however its accuracy does worsen at low output values.

1 Press 'Start' button on computer.
2 Inject fluid smoothly over 2–3seconds.
3 Repeat at least twice more at random points in the respiratory cycle.
4 Average 3measurements falling within 10% of each other. Reject outputs obtained from curves which are irregular/non-smooth.

Erroneous readings

- Valve lesions—tricuspid regurgitation will allow some of the injectate to reflux back into the right atrium. With aortic regurgitation a proportion will regurgitate back into the left ventricle.
- Septal defects.
- Loss of injectate. Check that all connections are tight and not leaking.

Advantages

Most commonly used and familiar ICU technique, computer warnings of poor curves

Disadvantages

- Non-continuous (by injection technique)
- 5–10% inter- and intra-observer variability
- Erroneous readings with tricuspid regurgitation, intra-cardiac shunts
- Frequently repeated measurements may result in considerable volumes of 5% glucose being injected.

See also:
Pulmonary artery catheter—use, 112; Cardiac output—other invasive, 118;
Cardiac output—non-invasive, 120; Fluid challenge, 262; Hypotension, 300;
Heart failure—assessment, 312; Heart failure—management, 314; Metabolic
acidosis, 420; Systemic inflammatory response, 488

Cardiac output—other invasive

Dye dilution

The mixing of a given volume of indicator to an unknown volume of fluid allows calculation of this volume from the degree of dilution of the indicator. The time elapsed for the indicator to pass some distance in the cardiovascular system yields a cardiac output value. The cardiac output is calculated as

$$\frac{60 \times I}{C_m \times t}$$

where I is the amount of indicator injected, C_m is the mean concentration of the indicator and t is the total duration of the curve. The standard dye dilution technique is to inject indocyanine green into a central vein followed by repeated sampling of arterial blood to enable construction of a time–concentration curve with a rapid upstroke and an exponential decay. Plotting the dye decay curve semi-logarithmically and extrapolating values to the origin produces the cardiac output. A recent advance using the COLD-Pulsion device measures the concentration decay directly from an indwelling arterial probe and automatically computes cardiac output.

Advantages
Reasonably accurate

Disadvantages
Invasive, re-circulation of dye prevents multiple repeated measurements, lengthy, requires initial calibration with known dye dilutions, underestimates low output values

Direct Fick

Based on the principle that the amount of a substance passing into a flowing system is equal to the difference in concentration of the substance on each side of the system multiplied by the flow within the system. Cardiac output is thus usually calculated by dividing total body oxygen consumption by the difference in oxygen content between arterial and mixed venous blood. Alternatively, CO_2 production can be used instead of VO_2 as the indicator. Arterial CO_2 can be derived non-invasively from end-tidal CO_2 while mixed venous CO_2 can be determined by rapid rebreathing into a bag until CO_2 levels have equilibrated.

Advantages
'Gold standard' for cardiac output estimation

Disadvantages
For VO_2: Invasive (requires measurement of mixed venous blood), requires leak-free open circuit or an unwieldy closed circuit technique, oxygen consumption measurements via metabolic cart are unreliable if FIO_2 is high, lung oxygen consumption is not measured by the pulmonary artery catheter technique (may be high in ARDS, pneumonia...)

For CO_2: Non-invasive but requires normal lung function and is thus not generally applicable in ICU patients.

Cardiac output—non-invasive

Doppler ultrasound

An ultrasound beam of known frequency will be reflected by moving red blood corpuscles with a shift in frequency proportional to the velocity of blood flow. The actual velocity can be calculated from the Doppler equation which requires the cosine of the vector between the direction of the ultrasound beam and that of blood flow. This has been applied to blood flow in the ascending aorta and aortic arch (via a suprasternal approach), descending thoracic aorta (oesophageal approach) and intracardiac flow (e.g. transmitral from an apical approach). Spectral analysis of the Doppler frequency shifts produces velocity-time waveforms, the area of which represents the 'stroke distance', i.e. the distance travelled by a column of blood with each left ventricular systole. (See figure opposite.). The product of stroke distance and aortic (or mitral valve) cross-sectional area is stroke volume. Cross-sectional area can be measured echocardiographically however, as both operator expertise and equipment is required, this additional measurement can be either ignored or assumed from nomograms to provide a reasonable *estimate* of stroke volume.

Advantages
Quick, safe, minimally invasive, reasonably accurate, continuous (via oesophageal approach), other information on contractility, preload and afterload from waveform shape (see figure opposite).

Disadvantages
Non-continuous (unless via oesophagus), learning curve, operator-dependent

Thoracic bioimpedance

Impedance changes originate in the thoracic aorta when blood is ejected from the left ventricle. This effect is used to determine stroke volume from formulae utilising the electrical field size of the thorax, base thoracic impedance and fluctuation related to systole, and ventricular ejection time. A correction factor for sex, height and weight is also introduced. The technique simply utilises four pairs of electrodes placed in proscribed positions on the neck and thorax; these are connected to a dedicated monitor which measure thoracic impedance to a low amplitude, high frequency 70KHz 2.5mA current applied across the electrodes.

Advantages
Quick, safe, totally non-invasive, reasonably accurate in normal, spontaneously breathing subjects

Disadvantages
Discrepancies in critically ill patients, (especially those with arrhythmias, tachycardias, intrathoracic fluid shifts, anatomical deformities, aortic regurgitation, metal within the thorax), inability to verify signal

Doppler blood flow velocity waveform variables

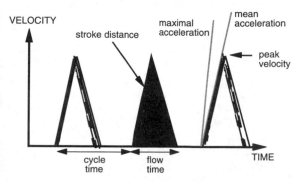

Changes in Doppler flow velocity waveform shape

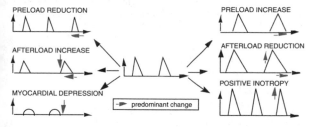

See also:
Cardiac output—thermodilution, 116; Cardiac output—other invasive, 118; Fluid challenge, 262; Acute chest infection 1, 276; Acute chest infection 2, 278; Adult respiratory distress syndrome 1, 280; Adult respiratory distress syndrome 2, 282; Hypotension, 300; Heart failure—assessment, 312; Heart failure—management, 314; Metabolic acidosis, 420; Systemic inflammatory response, 488

Gut tonometry

A gas permeable silicone balloon attached to a gas-impermeable sampling tube is passed into the lumen of the gut. Devices exist for tonometry in the stomach or sigmoid colon. The tonometer allows indirect measurement of the PCO_2 of the gut mucosa and calculation of the pH of the mucosa.

Indications

Gut mucosal hypoperfusion is an early consequence of hypovolaemia. Covert circulatory inadequacy due to hypovolaemia may be detected as gut mucosal acidosis and has been related to post-operative complications after major surgery. In critically ill patients there is some evidence that the prevention of gut mucosal acidosis improves outcome. The sigmoid colon tonometer is useful to detect ischaemic colitis early (e.g. after abdominal vascular surgery).

Technique

Saline tonometry
The tonometer balloon is prepared by degassing and filling with 2.5ml 0.9% saline. The saline is withdrawn into a syringe connected to the sampling tube prior to insertion. After insertion the saline is passed back into the balloon. The PCO_2 of the saline in the balloon equilibrates with the PCO_2 of the gut lumen over a period of 30–90minutes. At steady state it is assumed that the PCO_2 gut lumen and gut mucosa are in equilibrium. Time correction factors have been derived for partial equilibration between the balloon saline and the gut lumen. The measurement is completed by sampling the saline from the balloon and an arterial blood sample for measurement of arterial $[HCO_3^-]$. The pH of the gut mucosa (pHi) is calculated in a modified Henderson–Hasselbach equation:

$$pH = 6.1 + \log_{10} \frac{\text{arterial } [HCO_3^-]}{PCO_2 \text{(tonometer)} \times K}$$

where K is the time-dependent equilibration constant. Although the technique is quite simple it is labour intensive and requires attention to detail when filling the balloon. The need for an arterial blood sample is also a disadvantage for a technique which has its main importance in preventing critical illness.

Gas tonometry
Using air in the tonometry balloon allows more rapid equilibration between the tonometer and the luminal PCO_2. A recent development is to use a modified capnometer to automatically fill the balloon with air and sample the PCO_2 after 5minutes equilibration. For covert circulatory inadequacy the arterial $[HCO_3^-]$ will not be abnormal for most patients. Thus it is the tonometric PCO_2 which provides the greater part of variation in the measurement. This may be compared with end-tidal PCO_2 (measured with the same capnometer) as an estimate of arterial PCO_2. With a normal capnogram, a balloon PCO_2 significantly higher than end-tidal PCO_2 implies gut mucosal hypoperfusion.

Neurological Monitoring

Intracranial pressure monitoring

Indications

To confirm the diagnosis of raised intracranial pressure (ICP) and monitor treatment. May be used in cases of head injury particularly if ventilated, Glasgow Coma Score < 7, or with an abnormal CT scan. Also used in encephalopathy, post-neurosurgery and in selected cases of intracranial haemorrhage. Although a raised ICP can be related to poor prognosis after head injury the converse is not true. Sustained reduction of raised ICP in head injury may improve outcome although controlled trials are lacking.

Methods of monitoring intracranial pressure

Ventricular monitoring
A catheter is inserted into the lateral ventricle via a burr hole. The catheter may be connected to a pressure transducer or may contain a fibreoptic pressure monitoring device. Fibreoptic catheters require regular calibration according to the manufacturer's instructions. Both systems should be tested for patency and damping by temporarily raising intracranial pressure (e.g. with a cough or by occluding a jugular vein). CSF may be drained through the ventricular catheter to reduce intracranial pressure.

Subdural monitoring
The dura is opened via a burr hole and a hollow bolt inserted into the skull. The bolt may be connected to a pressure transducer or admit a fibreoptic or hi-fidelity pressure monitoring device. A subdural bolt is easier to insert than ventricular monitors. The main disadvantages of subdural monitoring are a tendency to underestimate ICP and damping effects. Again, calibration and patency testing should be frequent.

Complications

Infection   —particularly after 5 days
Haemorrhage —particularly with coagulopathy or difficult insertion

Using ICP monitoring

- Normal ICP is < 10mmHg.
- A raised ICP is usually treated when > 25mmHg in head injury.
- As ICP increases there are often sustained rises in ICP to 50–100mmHg lasting for 5–20min, increasing with frequency as the baseline ICP rises. This is associated with 60% mortality.
- Cerebral perfusion pressure (CPP) is the difference between mean BP and mean ICP. Treatment aimed at reducing ICP may also reduce mean BP. It is important to maintain CPP at > 50mmHg.

See also:
Intracranial haemorrhage, 364; Subarachnoid haemorrhage, 366; Raised intracranial pressure, 368; Head injury 1, 462; Head injury 2, 464

Jugular venous bulb saturation

Retrograde passage of a fibre-optic catheter from the internal jugular vein into the jugular bulb enables continuous monitoring of jugular venous bulb saturation (SjO_2). This can be used in conjunction with other monitors of cerebral haemodynamics such as middle cerebral blood flow, cerebral arterio-venous lactate difference and intracranial pressure to direct management.

Principles of SjO_2 management

Normal values are approximately 65–70%. In the absence of anaemia and with maintenance of normal SaO_2 values, values of $SjO_2 > 75\%$ suggest luxury perfusion or global infarction with oxygen not being utilised; values $< 54\%$ correspond to cerebral hypoperfusion while values $< 40\%$ suggest global ischaemia and are usually associated with increased cerebral lactate production. Knowledge of SjO_2 allows optimisation of brain blood flow to avoid (i) either excessive or inadequate perfusion and (ii) iatrogenically-induced hypoperfusion through treating raised intracranial pressure aggressively with diuretics and hyperventilation. Studies in trauma patients have found (i) a higher mortality with episodes of jugular venous desaturation and (ii) a significant relationship between cerebral perfusion pressure (CPP) and SjO_2 when the CPP was $< 70mmHg$. A falling SjO_2 may be an indication to increase CPP though no prospective randomised trial has yet been performed to study outcome effect.

Approximately 85% of cerebral venous drainage passes down one of the internal jugular veins (usually right). SjO_2 usually represents drainage from both hemispheres and is equal on both sides however, after focal injury, this pattern of drainage may alter.

Insertion technique

1 Insert introducer sheath rostrally in internal jugular vein.
2 Calibrate fibre-optic catheter pre-insertion.
3 Insert catheter via introducer sheath; advance to jugular bulb.
4 Withdraw introducer sheath.
5 Confirm (i) free aspiration of blood via catheter, (ii) satisfactory light intensity reading, (iii) satisfactory positioning of catheter tip by lateral cervical X-ray (high in jugular bulb, above level of 2nd cervical vertebra).
6 Perform *in vivo* calibration, repeat calibration 12-hourly.

Troubleshooting

If the catheter is sited too low in the jugular bulb, erroneous SjO_2 values may result from mixing of intracerebral and extracerebral venous blood. This could be particularly pertinent when cerebral blood flow is low.

Ensure light intensity reading is satisfactory; if too high the catheter may be abutting against a wall and if low the catheter may not be patent or have a small clot over the tip. Before treating the patient always confirm the veracity of low readings against a blood sample drawn from the catheter and measured in a co-oximeter.

Formulae

$$SjO_2(\%) = SaO_2(\%) \frac{CMRO_2 \times 104}{CBF \times Hb \times 1.34}$$

where
SjO_2 = jugular bulb oxygen saturation
$SaO_2(\%)$ = arterial oxygen saturation
$CMRO_2$ = cerebral metabolism of oxygen
CBF = cerebral blood flow

$$\text{cerebral oxygen extraction ratio} = \frac{SaO_2 - SjO_2}{SaO_2}$$

cerebral perfusion pressure = systemic BP − intracranial pressure

129

See also:
Intracranial pressure monitoring, 126; Other neurological monitoring, 132;
Intracranial haemorrhage, 364; Subarachnoid haemorrhage, 366; Raised
intracranial pressure, 368; Head injury 1, 462; Head injury 2, 464

EEG / CFM monitoring

EEG monitoring

The EEG reflects changes in cortical electrical function. This, in turn, is dependent on cerebral perfusion and oxygenation. EEG monitoring can be useful to assess epileptiform activity as well as cerebral well-being in patients who are sedated and paralysed. The latter aim is to detect depression of cortical activity and subsequent recovery. The conventional EEG can be used intermittently but is expensive and impractical for continuous use. Large amounts of paper, difficult interpretation and susceptibility to electrical interference are the main drawbacks. Data reduction and artefact suppression are necessary to allow successful use of EEG recordings in the ICU.

Cerebral function monitor (CFM)

The CFM is a single channel, filtered trace from 2 recording electrodes placed over the parietal regions of the scalp. A third electrode may be used in the midline to help with interference detection. The parietal recording electrodes are usually placed close to watershed areas of the brain in order to allow maximum sensitivity for ischaemia detection. Voltage is displayed against time on a paper chart running at 6–30cm/h.

Use of CFM

The CFM may be used to detect cerebral ischaemia; depressed cerebral activity is associated with reduced cortical electrical activity. Burst suppression (periods of electrical silence which become increasingly prolonged) provide an early warning.

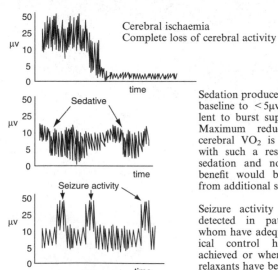

Sedation produces a fall in baseline to < 5µv, equivalent to burst suppression. Maximum reduction in cerebral VO_2 is achieved with such a response to sedation and no further benefit would be gained from additional sedation.

Seizure activity may be detected in patients in whom have adequate clinical control has been achieved or where muscle relaxants have been used.

Patients with 'locked in' syndrome, who appear completely unconscious, may be detected by the presence of normal cerebral electrical activity.

Typical CFM patterns

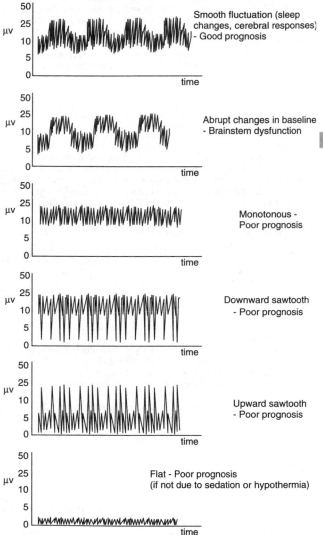

Other neurological monitoring

Cerebral blood flow (CBF)

CBF can be measured by radioisotopic techniques utilising tracers such as [133]Xenon given intravenously or by inhalation. This remains a research tool in view of the radioactivity exposure and the usual need to move the patient to a gamma-camera. However, portable monitors are now available. Middle cerebral artery (MCA) blood flow can be determined non-invasively by transcranial Doppler ultrasonography. The pulsatility index(PI) relates to cerebrovascular resistance with a rise in PI indicating a rise in resistance and cerebral vasospasm.

$$PI = \frac{\text{systolic flow velocity} - \text{diastolic flow velocity}}{\text{mean flow velocity}}.$$

Vasospasm can also be designated when the MCA blood flow velocity exceeds 120cm/sec and severe vasospasm when velocities > 200cm/sec. Low values of common carotid end-diastolic blood flow and velocity have been shown to be highly discriminating predictors of brain death. Impaired reactivity of CBF to changes in PCO_2 (in normals 3–5% per mmHg PCO_2 change) is another marker of poor outcome.

Near-infra-red spectroscopy (NIRS)

- near-infra-red (700–1000nm) light propagated across the head is absorbed by haemoglobin (oxy- and de-oxy), myoglobin and oxidised cytochrome aa_3 (the terminal part of the respiratory chain involved in oxidative phosphorylation).
- the sum of (oxy + deoxy) haemoglobin is considered an index of cerebral blood volume (CBV) change, and the difference as an index of change in haemoglobin saturation assuming no variation occurs in CBV. CBV and flow can be quantified by changing the FIO_2 and measuring the response.
- cerebral blood flow is measured by a modification of the Fick principle. Oxy-haemoglobin is the intravascular non-diffusible tracer, its accumulation being proportional to the arterial inflow of tracer. Good correlations have been found with the [133]Xenon technique.
- cytochrome aa_3 cannot be quantified by NIRS but its redox status may be followed to provide some indication of mitochondrial function.
- movement artefact must be avoided and some devices require reduction of ambient lighting.

Lactate

The brain normally utilises lactate as a fuel however in states of severely impaired cerebral perfusion the brain may become a net lactate producer with the venous lactate rising above the arterial value. A lactate oxygen index can be derived by dividing the venous-arterial lactate difference by the arterio-jugular venous oxygen difference. Values > 0.08 are consistently seen with cerebral ischaemia.

See also:
  Lactate, 160; Intracranial haemorrhage, 364; Subarachnoid haemorrhage, 366;
Raised intracranial pressure, 368; Head injury 1, 462; Head injury 2, 464; Brain
stem death, 516

Laboratory Monitoring

34

Urea & creatinine

Measured in blood, urine and, occasionally, in other fluids such as abdominal drain fluid (e.g. ureteric disruption, fistulae)

Urea

A product of the urea cycle resulting from ammonia breakdown, it depends upon adequate liver function for its synthesis and adequate renal function for its excretion. Low levels are thus seen in cirrhosis and high levels in renal failure. Uraemia is a clinical syndrome including lethargy, drowsiness, confusion, pruritus and pericarditis resulting from high plasma levels of urea (or, more correctly, nitrogenous waste products—azotaemia).

The ratio of urine:plasma urea may be useful in distinguishing oliguria of renal or pre-renal origins. Higher ratios (> 10:1) are seen in pre-renal conditions e.g. hypovolaemia whereas low levels (< 4:1) occur with direct renal causes.

24–hour measurement of urinary urea (or nitrogen) excretion has been previously used as a guide to nutritional protein replacement but is currently not considered a useful routine tool.

Creatinine

A product of creatine breakdown, it is predominantly derived from skeletal muscle and is also renally excreted. Low levels are found with malnutrition and high levels with muscle breakdown (rhabdomyolysis) and impaired excretion (renal failure).

The usual ratio for plasma urea:creatinine is approximately 1:10. A much lower ratio in a critically ill patient is suggestive of rhabdomyolysis whereas higher ratios are seen in cirrhosis, malnutrition, hypovolaemia and hepatic failure.

The ratio of urine:plasma creatinine may help distinguish between oliguria of renal or pre-renal origins. Higher ratios (> 40) are seen in pre-renal conditions and low levels (< 20) with direct renal causes.

Creatinine clearance is a measure of glomerular filtration. Once filtered, only small amounts of creatinine are re-absorbed. Normally > 100ml/min.

$$\text{Creatinine clearance} = \frac{(\text{Urine creatinine} \times \text{flow rate})}{\text{Plasma creatinine}}$$

Normal plasma ranges

Urea   2.5–6.5mmol/L
Creatinine 70–120μmol/L (depends on lean body mass)

137

Electrolytes (Na^+, K^+, Cl^-, HCO_3^-)

Measured accurately by direct-reading ion-specific electrodes from plasma or urine, though are sensitive to interference by excess liquid heparin.

Sodium, potassium

Plasma levels may be elevated but poorly reflect intracellular (approximately 3–5mmol/L for Na^+, 140–150mmol/L for K^+) or total body levels. Plasma potassium levels are affected by plasma H^+ levels; a metabolic acidosis reduces urinary potassium excretion while an alkalosis will increase excretion.

Older measuring devices such as flame photometry or indirect-reading ion-specific electrodes gave spuriously low plasma Na^+ levels with concurrent hyperproteinaemia or hypertriglyceridaemia.

Urinary excretion depends on intake, total body balance, acid-base balance, hormones (including anti-diuretic hormone, aldosterone, corticosteroids, atrial natriuretic peptide), drugs (particularly diuretics, non-steroidal anti-inflammatories and ACE inhibitors), and renal function.

In oliguria, a urinary Na^+ level < 10mmol/L suggests a pre-renal cause whereas > 20mmol/L is seen with direct renal damage. This does not apply if diuretics have been given previously.

Chloride, bicarbonate

Bicarbonate levels vary with acid-base balance.

In the kidney, Cl^- reabsorption is increased when HCO_3^- reabsorption is decreased, and vice versa. Plasma $[Cl^-]$ thus tends to vary inversely with plasma $[HCO_3^-]$, keeping the total anion concentration normal.

Anion gap

The anion gap is the difference between unestimated anions (e.g. phosphate, ketones, lactate) and cations.

In metabolic acidosis an increased anion gap occurs with renal failure, ingestion of acid, ketoacidosis and hyperlactataemia whereas a normal anion gap (usually associated with hyperchloraemia) is found with decreased acid excretion (e.g. Addison's disease, renal tubular acidosis) and loss of base (e.g. diarrhoea, pancreatic/biliary fistula, acetazolamide, ureterosigmoidostomy). Hyperchloraemia is found with experimental salt water drowning but rarely seen in actual cases.

Normal plasma ranges

Sodium	135–145mmol/L
Potassium	3.5–5.3mmol/L
Chloride	95–105mmol/L
Bicarbonate	23–28mmol/L

Anion gap = plasma $[Na^+] + [K^+] - [HCO_3^-] - [Cl^-]$.
Normal range 8–16mmol/L

Calcium, magnesium & phosphate

Calcium

Plasma calcium levels have been traditionally corrected to plasma albumin levels; this is now considered irrelevant, particularly at the low albumin levels seen in critically ill patients. Measurement of the ionised fraction is probably more pertinent.

High calcium levels occur with hyperparathyroidism, certain malignancies, sarcoidosis while low levels are seen in renal failure, severe pancreatitis and hypoparathyroidism.

Magnesium

Plasma levels poorly reflect intracellular or whole body stores, 65% of which is in bone and 35% in cells. The ionised fraction is approximately 50% of the total level.

High magnesium levels are seen with renal failure and excessive administration; this rarely requires treatment unless serious cardiac conduction problems or neurological complications (respiratory paralysis, coma) intervene.

Low levels occur following severe diarrhoea, diuretic therapy, alcohol abuse, and accompany hypocalcaemia.

Magnesium is used therapeutically for a number of conditions including ventricular and supraventricular arrhythmias, eclampsia, seizures, asthma, and after post-myocardial infarction. Supranormal plasma levels of 1.5–2.0mmol/L are often sought.

Phosphate

High levels are seen with renal failure and in the presence of an ischaemic bowel. Low levels (sometimes < 0.1mmol/L) occur with critical illness, chronic alcoholism and diuretic usage and may result in muscle weakness, failure to wean and myocardial dysfunction.

Normal plasma ranges

Calcium	2.2–2.6mmol/L
Ionised calcium	0.95–1.2mmol/L.
Magnesium	0.7–1.0mmol/L
Phosphate	0.7–1.4mmol/L

141

Liver function tests

Hepatic metabolism proceeds via Phase I enzymes (oxidation and phosphorylation) and then subsequently to Phase II enzymes (glucuronidation, sulphation, acetylation). Phase I enzyme reactions involve cytochrome P450.

Markers of hepatic damage

- Alanine aminotransferase (ALT)
- Aspartate aminotransferase (AST)
- Llactate dehydrogenase (LDH)

Patterns and ratios of various enzymes are variable and unreliable diagnostic indicators. Measurement of ALT alone is usually sufficient. It is more liver-specific but less sensitive than AST and has a longer half-life.

AST is not liver-specific but is a sensitive indicator of hepatic damage. The plasma level is proportional to the degree of hepatocellular damage. Low levels occur in extrahepatic obstruction and inactive cirrhosis.

LDH is insensitive and non-specific. Isoenzyme electrophoresis is needed to distinguish cardiac, erythrocyte, skeletal muscle and liver injury.

Acute phase reactants such as C-reactive protein (CRP) are also produced by the liver. Levels increase during critical illness and following hepatocellular injury.

Markers of cholestasis

- Bilirubin
- Alkaline phosphatase
- Gamma-glutamyl transferase (γ-GT)

Bilirubin is derived from Hb released from erythrocyte breakdown and conjugated with glucuronide by the hepatocytes. The conjugated fraction is water-soluble whereas the unconjugated fraction is lipid-soluble. Levels are increased with intra- and extra-hepatic biliary obstruction (predominantly conjugated), hepatocellular damage and haemolysis (usually mixed picture). Jaundice is detected when levels $>45\mu mol/L$.

Alkaline phosphatase is released from bone, liver, intestine and placenta. In the absence of bone disease (check Ca^{2+} and PO_4^{3-}) and pregnancy, raised levels usually indicate biliary tract dysfunction.

A raised γ-GT is a highly sensitive marker of hepatobiliary disease. Increased synthesis is induced by obstructive cholestasis, alcohol, various drugs and toxins, acute and chronic hepatic inflammation.

Markers of reduced synthetic function

- Albumin
- Clotting factors
- Cholinesterase

Albumin levels fall during critical illness due to protein catabolism, capillary leak, decreased synthesis, dilution with artificial colloids. Coagulation factors II, VII, IX and X are liver-synthesised. Over 33% of functional hepatic mass must be lost before any abnormality is seen.

Indicators of function

- Lignocaine metabolites (MegX)

Indicators of hepatic blood flow

- Indocyanine green clearance
- Bromosulphthalein clearance

Normal plasma ranges

Albumin	35–53g/L
Bilirubin	3–17μmol/L
Conjugated bilirubin	0–6μmol/L
Alanine aminotransferase	5–50 U/L
Alkaline phosphatase	100–280 U/L
Aspartate aminotransferase	11–55 U/L
Cholinesterase	2.3–9.0 KU/L
γ-Glutamyl-transferase	5–37 U/L
Lactate dehydrogenase	230–460 U/L

See also:
Parenteral nutrition, 74; Jaundice, 346; Acute liver failure, 348; Chronic liver failure, 352; Paracetamol poisoning, 442; HELLP syndrome, 480

Full blood count

Haemoglobin

A raised haemoglobin occurs in polycythaemia (primary and secondary to chronic hypoxaemia) and in haemoconcentration. Anaemia may be due to reduced red cell mass (decreased red cell production or survival) or haemodilution. The latter is common in critically ill patients. In severe anaemia there may be a hyperdynamic circulation which, if severe, may decompensate to cardiac failure. In this case blood transfusion must be performed with extreme care to avoid fluid overload, or in association with plasmapheresis. Differential diagnosis of anaemia includes:

Reduced MCV	iron deficiency (anisocytosis and poikilocytosis)
Raised MCV	vitamin B_{12} or folate deficiency
	alcohol excess
	liver disease
	hypothyroidism.
Normal MCV	anaemia of chronic disease
	bone marrow failure (including acute folate deficiency)
	hypothyroidism
	haemolysis (increased reticulocytes and bilirubin)

White blood cells

A raised white cell count is extremely common in critical illness. Causes of changes in the differential count include:

Neutrophilia	Lymphocytosis	Eosinophilia
bacterial infection	brucellosis	asthma
trauma and surgery	typhoid	allergic conditions
burns	myasthenia gravis	parasitaemia
haemorrhage	hyperthyroidism	
inflammation	leukaemia	
steroid therapy		
leukaemia		

Neutropenia	Lymphopenia
viral infections	steroid therapy
brucellosis	SLE
typhoid	Legionnaire's disease
tuberculosis	AIDS
sulphonamide treatment	
severe sepsis	
hypersplenism	
bone marrow failure	

Barrier nursing is required for neutropenia $< 1.0 \times 10^9/L$.

Platelets

Correct interpretation of platelet counts requires blood to be taken from a venepuncture (not capillary blood). Arterial blood is commonly taken from an indwelling cannula but is not ideal. Thrombocytopenia is due to decreased platelet production (bone marrow failure, vitamin B_{12} or folate deficiency), decreased platelet survival (ITP, TTP, infection, hypersplenism, heparin therapy), increased platelet consumption (haemorrhage, DIC) or in vivo aggregation giving an apparent thrombocytopenia; this should be checked on a blood film. Spontaneous bleeding is associated with platelet counts $< 20 \times 10^9/L$ and platelet cover is required for procedures or traumatic bleeds at counts $< 50 \times 10^9/L$.

Normal ranges

Haemoglobin	13–17g/dL (men), 12–16g/dL (women)
MCV	76–96fL
White cell count	$4–11 \times 10^9/L$
Neutrophils	$2–7.5 \times 10^9/L$
Lymphocytes	$1.3–3.5 \times 10^9/L$
Eosinophils	$0.04–0.44 \times 10^9/L$
Basophils	$0–0.1 \times 10^9/L$
Monocytes	$0.2–0.8 \times 10^9/L$
Platelets	$150–400 \times 10^9/L$

145

See also:
Blood transfusion, 172; Blood products, 240; Anaemia, 386; Sickle cell disease, 388; Haemolysis, 390; Neutropenia, 394; Platelet disorders, 392; Leukaemia, 396; Vasculitides, 508

Coagulation monitoring

Basic coagulation screen

The basic screen consists of a platelet count, prothrombin time, activated partial thromboplastin time and thrombin time. Close attention to blood sampling technique is very important for correct interpretation of coagulation tests. Drawing blood from indwelling catheters should, ideally, be avoided since samples may be diluted or contaminated with heparin. The correct volume of blood must be placed in the sample tube to avoid dilution errors. Laboratory coagulation tests are usually performed on citrated plasma samples taken into glass tubes.

Specific coagulation tests

Activated clotting time (ACT)
Sample tube contains celite, a diatomaceous earth, which activates the contact system; thus the ACT predominantly tests the intrinsic pathway. The ACT is prolonged by heparin therapy, thrombocytopenia, hypothermia, haemodilution, fibrinolysis and high dose aprotinin. Normal is 100–140sec.

Thrombin time (TT)
Sample tube contains lyophilised thrombin and calcium. Thrombin bypasses the intrinsic and extrinsic pathways such that the coagulation time tests the common pathway with conversion of fibrinogen to fibrin. The TT is prolonged by fibrinogen depletion, e.g. fibrinolysis or thrombolysis and heparin via antithrombin III dependent interaction with thrombin. A high dose TT is more sensitive to heparin anticoagulation than fibrinogen levels. Normal is 12–16sec.

Prothrombin time (PT)
Sample tube contains tissue factor and calcium. Tissue factor activates the extrinsic pathway. The PT is prolonged with coumarin anticoagulants, liver disease and vitamin K deficiency. Normal is 12–16sec.

Activated partial thromboplastin time (APTT)
Sample tube contains kaolin and cephalin as a platelet substitute to activate the intrinsic pathway. The APTT is prolonged by heparin therapy, DIC, severe fibrinolysis, von Willebrand factor, factor VIII, factor X1 or factor XIII deficiencies. Normal is 30–40sec.

D-dimers and Fibrin degradation products (FDPs)
Fibrin fragments are released by plasmin lysis. FDPs can be assayed by an immunological method; they are often measured in the critically ill to confirm disseminated intravascular coagulation. A level of 20–40µg/ml is common post-operatively, in sepsis, trauma, renal failure and DVT. Raised levels do not distinguish fibrinogenolysis and fibrinolysis. Assay of the d-dimer fragment is more specific for fibrinolysis, e.g. in DIC since it is only released after fibrin is formed.

Coagulation factor assays
Assays are available for all coagulation factors and may be used for diagnosis of specific defects. Heparins inhibit factor Xa activity. Factor Xa assay is therefore the most specific method of controlling low molecular weight heparin therapy. Since this assay is not dependent on contact system activation it also avoids the effects of aprotinin when monitoring heparin therapy.

The coagulation cascade

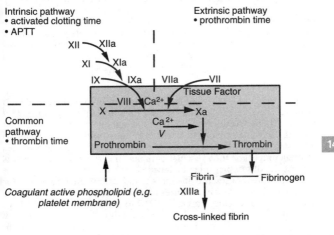

Intrinsic pathway
• activated clotting time
• APTT

Extrinsic pathway
• prothrombin time

XII — XIIa
XI — XIa
IX — IXa   VIIa — VII
VIII   Ca²⁺   Tissue Factor
X → Xa
Common pathway
• thrombin time
Ca²⁺
V
Prothrombin → Thrombin

Coagulant active phospholipid (e.g. platelet membrane)

Fibrin ← Fibrinogen
XIIIa
Cross-linked fibrin

147

Bacteriology

Microbiology samples should, if possible, be taken prior to commencement of antimicrobial therapy. In severe infections broad spectrum antimicrobials should be started without awaiting results. Sampling sites include those suspected clinically of harbouring infection or, if a specific site cannot be identified clinically, blood, urine and sputum samples. In severe infection indwelling, intravascular catheters should be replaced and the catheter tips sent for culture. Samples should be sent to the laboratory promptly to allow early incubation and to prevent potentially misleading growth. Swabs must be sent in the appropriate transport media.

Blood cultures

In order to avoid skin contamination the skin should be cleaned with alcohol. The skin preparation should be allowed to dry thoroughly before venepuncture. A 5–20ml blood sample is withdrawn and divided into anaerobic and aerobic culture bottles. It is usual to take samples from several venepunctures, in addition to cultures through indwelling intravascular catheters if catheter related sepsis is suspected. All samples must be labelled with the site they were taken from. Culture bottles are incubated and examined frequently for bacterial growth. Positive cultures must be interpreted in light of the clinical picture; an early pure growth from multiple bottles is likely to be significant, although cultures from critically ill patients may appear later or not at all due to antibiotic therapy. Any Gram negative isolates or *Staph aureus* are taken as significant.

Urine

A catheter specimen is usual from critically ill patients. The sampling site should be prepared aseptically prior to sampling. The specimen should be sent to the laboratory immediately and examined microscopically for organisms, casts and crystals. Urine is plated onto culture medium with a calibrated loop and incubated for 18–24h prior to examination. Bacteria $> 10^8/L$ (or a pure growth of $10^5/L$) represents a significant growth. All catheter specimens show bacterial growth if the catheter has been in place for > 2 days. Isolation of the same organism from blood confirms a significant culture.

Sputum

Sputum samples are easily contaminated during collection, particularly specimens from non-intubated patients. Suction specimens from intubated patients can be taken via a sterile suction catheter, protected catheter brush or from specific lung segments via a bronchoscope. Gram negative bacteria are frequently isolated from tracheal aspirates of intubated patients; only deep suction specimens are significant. Blood cultures should accompany sputum specimens in the diagnosis of pneumonia. Samples must be sent to the laboratory immediately.

Pus samples and wound swabs

Aspirated pus must be sent to the laboratory immediately or a swab sample may be taken and sent in transport medium. Pus is preferable for bacterial isolation.

Typical nosocomial infections

Pneumonia due to *Ps. aeruginosa*, *Staph aureus*, *Klebsiella* spp., *Enterobacter* spp., *E. coli*, *Proteus* spp.
Urinary infection with *E. coli*, *Ps. aeruginosa*, *Klebsiella* spp., *Proteus* spp.
Catheter related sepsis—*Staph aureus*, *Staph epidermidis*

149

See also:
   Pleural aspiration, 36; Bronchoscopy, 38; Chest physiotherapy, 40; Atelectasis and pulmonary collapse, 272; Acute chest infection 1, 276; Acute chest infection 2, 278; Abdominal sepsis, 340; Meningitis, 362; Tetanus, 376; Botulism, 378; Burns—fluid management, 468; Burns—general management, 470; Neutropenia, 394; Sepsis / infection, 490; Pyrexia, 500; HIV related disease, 512; Malaria, 514

Virology, serology & assays

Antibiotic assays

Antibiotic assays are usually performed when the drug in question has a narrow therapeutic range. The most commonly requested antibiotic assays are for aminoglycosides and vancomycin. It is not usual to request an assay on day 1 of treatment. Thereafter, samples are taken daily prior to giving a dose and at 1hour after an intravenous injection or infusion.

Serology

A clotted blood specimen allows antibodies to viral and atypical antigens to be assayed. It is usual to send acute and convalescent (14 days) serum to determine rising antibody titres. Single sample titres may be used to determine previous exposure and carrier status.

Hepatitis B

Serology includes hepatitis B surface antigen as a screening test and hepatitis B e core antigen to determine infectivity. There is a 10% carrier rate in South East Asians. Serology should be sent in all patients at high risk, e.g. jaundice, intravenous drug abuse, homosexuals, prostitutes, those with tattoos or unexplained hepatic enzyme abnormalities. In addition, it is important to ensure that hepatitis B status is known in staff and patients who suffer accidental exposure to body fluids, e.g. through needlestick injury. Those who are not immune may be treated with immunoglobulin.

HIV

Since an HIV positive status has grave consequences for lifestyle it should rarely be assessed without prior counselling and consent. The CD4 count may be used to assess the likelihood of symtomatology being AIDS related; again, consent is required before this is done. Patients should be considered for testing with the following risk factors: homosexual or bisexual males, intravenous drug abusers, haemophiliacs, Central African or West Indian origin, sexual partners of those at high risk and patients presenting with an AIDS related illness. In critically ill patients such consent can rarely be obtained and unconsented testing may be used where a significant change in management may arise with knowledge of the HIV status or where organ donation is being considered. Most AIDS related infections can be adequately treated without knowledge of the HIV status. However, patients or staff who are recipients of a needlestick injury can be treated with zidovudine if the donor is known to be HIV positive; unconsented testing is therefore reasonable.

Viral culture

Most commonly used for CMV. Samples of blood, urine or bronchial aspirate may be sent for DEAFF (detection of early antigen fluorescent foci). Herpes virus infections may be detected by electron microscopy of samples (including pustule fluid).

Fungi

Candida and Aspergillus can be assessed by culture ± antigen tests. Cryptococcus can be detected by Indian ink stain in biopsy samples.

Common serology for critically ill patients

Hepatitis A
Hepatitis B
Hepatitis C
HIV
CMV
Mycoplasma pneumoniae
Legionella pneumophila

Antibiotic therapeutic levels

	Trough (mg/L)	Peak (mg/L)
Amikacin	< 8	30
Gentamicin	< 2	4–10*
Tobramycin	< 2	4–10
Vancomycin	< 8	20–30

*Seek microbiological advice if once daily gentamicin is used

See also:
Acute chest infection 1, 276; Acute chest infection 2, 278; Jaundice, 346;
Acute liver failure, 348; HIV related disease, 512

Toxicology

Purpose

Samples taken from blood, urine, vomitus or gastric lavage (depending on drug or poison ingested) for:

- Monitoring of therapeutic drug levels (usually plasma) and avoidance of toxicity, e.g. digoxin, aminoglycosides, lithium, phenytoin
- Identification of unknown toxic substances (e.g. cyanide, amphetamines, opiates) causing symptomatology and/or pathology. Always take a urine sample for analysis.
- Confirmation of toxic plasma levels and monitoring of treatment effect, e.g. paracetamol, aspirin
- Medicolegal, e.g. alcohol, recreational drugs following road trauma

Samples

Confirm with chemistry laboratory ± local poisons unit as to which, how, and when body fluid samples should be taken for analysis e.g. peak/trough levels for aminoglycosides, urine samples for out-of-hospital poisoning, repeat paracetamol levels to monitor efficacy of treatment

See also:
Virology, serology & assays, 150; Poisoning—general principles, 438

Miscellaneous Monitoring

Urinalysis

Techniques

- Biochemical/metabolic:
  (i) colorimetric 'dipsticks' read manually from reference chart or by automated machine within 15sec—2min of dipping in urine (see manufacturers' instructions). Usually performed at the bedside.
  (ii) sodium and potassium levels can be measured in most analysers used for plasma electrolyte measurement. Re-calibration of the machine or special dilution techniques may be required.
  (iii) laboratory analysis.
- Haematological—either by dipstick or laboratory testing
- Microbiological—microscopy, culture, sensitivity; antigen tests
- Renal disease—usually by microscopy + laboratory testing

Associated tests

Some of the above investigations are performed in conjunction with a blood test, e.g. urine:plasma ratios of urea, creatinine and osmolality to distinguish renal from pre-renal causes of oliguria, 24h urine collection plus plasma creatinine for creatinine clearance estimation.

Cautions

- White blood cells, proteinuria and mixed bacterial growths are routine findings in catheterised patients and do not necessarily indicate infection.
- A 'positive' dipstick test for blood does not differentiate between haematuria, haemoglobinuria or myoglobinuria.
- Only conjugated bilirubin is excreted into the urine.
- Urinary sodium and potassium levels are increased by diuretic usage.

Urinalysis tests

Biochemical/metabolic:

pH	dipstick
glucose	dipstick
ketones	dipstick
protein	dipstick, laboratory
bilirubin	dipstick
sodium, potassium	electrolyte analyser, laboratory
urea, creatinine, nitrogen	laboratory
osmolality	laboratory
specific gravity	bedside gravimeter, laboratory
myoglobin	laboratory, positive dipstick to blood
drugs, poisons	sent to Poisons Reference Laboratory

Haematological:

red blood cells	microscopy, positive dipstick to blood
haemoglobin	laboratory, positive dipstick to blood
neutrophils	dipstick, laboratory

Microbiological:

bacteriuria	microscopy, culture
TB	microscopy, culture (early morning specimens)
Legionnaire's disease	laboratory

Nephro-urological:

haematuria	microscopy
granular casts	microscopy
protein	laboratory
sodium, potassium	electrolyte analyser, laboratory
malignant cells	cytology

Indirect calorimetry

Calorimetry refers to the measurement of energy production. Direct calorimetry is the measurement of heat production in a sealed chamber but is impractical for critically ill patients. Indirect calorimetry measures the rate of oxidation of metabolic fuels by detecting the volume of O_2 consumed and CO_2 produced. The ratio of CO_2 production to O_2 utilisation (respiratory quotient or RQ) defines which fuels are being utilised (see table). Knowledge of the oxygen utilisation by the various fuels allows calculation of the energy production. Carbohydrate and fat are oxidised to CO_2 and water producing 15–17 and 38–39kJ/g respectively. Protein is oxidised to CO_2, water and nitrogen (subsequently excreted as urea) producing 15–17kJ/g.

Technique of indirect calorimetry

Inspiratory and mixed expiratory gases must be sampled. O_2 concentration may be measured by a fuel cell sensor or a fast response, paramagnetic sensor. CO_2 is usually measured by infrared absorption. Sensors may be calibrated with reference to known concentrations of standard gas or by burning a pure fuel with a predictable O_2 consumption. Measurements are usually made at ambient temperature, pressure and humidity prior to conversion to standard temperature, pressure and humidity. In order to calculate metabolic rate (energy expenditure) inspired and expired minute volumes are required. It is common for one minute volume to be measured and the other to be derived from a Haldane transformation:

$$V_I = V_E \times \frac{N_E}{N_I}$$

The nitrogen concentrations are assumed to be the concentration of gas which is not O_2 or CO_2. Calculation of energy expenditure utilises a modification of the de Weir formula:

$$\text{Energy expenditure} = (3.94 VO_2 + 1.11 VCO_2) \times 1.44$$

Although it is possible to calculate the rate of protein metabolism by reference to the urinary urea concentration, and therefore to separate non-protein from protein energy expenditure, the resulting modification of the above formula is not usually clinically significant.

Errors associated with indirect calorimetry

Underestimate of VCO_2	H^+ ion loss, haemodialysis, haemofiltration
Overestimate VCO_2	hyperventilation, HCO_3^- infusion
Underestimate VO_2	free radical production, unmeasured O_2 supply
$FIO_2 > 0.6$	small difference between inspired and expired O_2
Loss of volume	circuit leaks, bronchopleural fistula

Use of indirect calorimetry

Helps to match nutritional intake to energy expenditure. It is important to feed critically ill patients appropriately, avoiding both underfeeding and overfeeding (see table). Indirect calorimetry may also be used to assess work of breathing by assessing the change in VO_2 during weaning from mechanical ventilation. VO_2 change may also be used to assess appropriate levels of sedation and analgesia.

Respiratory quotients for various metabolic fuels

Ketones	0.63
Fat	0.71
Protein	0.80
Carbohydrate	1.00

The whole body RQ depends on the fuel or combination of fuels being utilised. Normally a combination of fat and carbohydrate are utilised with a RQ of 0.8.

Lipogenesis associated with overfeeding may give a RQ of 1.1–1.3

159

See also:
IPPV—description of ventilators, 6; Nutrition—use and indications, 70; Enteral nutrition, 72; Parenteral nutrition, 74; Capnography, 88; Opioid analgesics, 222; Non-opioid analgesics, 224; Sedatives, 226; Pain, 496; Pyrexia, 500

Lactate

Measurement of blood lactate

Analysers are available to allow rapid measurement of blood or plasma lactate on small samples, using enzyme based methods. The enzymatic conversion of lactate to pyruvate is an oxygen utilising reaction. The extraction of oxygen from the sample can be detected by a sensitive oxygen fuel cell sensor and is directly proportional to the sample lactate concentration. A whole blood sample (venous or arterial since there is no practical difference) is collected into a heparin fluoride tube to prevent coagulation and glycolysis (lactate producing). Nitrite may be used in the sample tube to convert haemoglobin to the met-form, thus avoiding uptake of oxygen during the enzyme reaction. The enzymatic method is specific for the L-isomer and will not, therefore, detect d-lactate (e.g. in short bowel syndrome). Normal arterial whole blood lactate concentration is < 1.5mmol/L. Lactate may also be measured from regional sites as an aid to the assessment of regional perfusion (e.g. arterial—jugular bulb difference)

Biochemistry of lactate production

The cytoplasmic glycolytic pathway produces pyruvate which would normally be metabolised to CO_2 and water in the mitochondria. In conditions of cellular hypoxia mitochondrial metabolism is impaired and pyruvate is converted to lactate by lactate dehydrogenase in the cytoplasm.

$$\text{pyruvate} + NADH + H^+ \xleftrightarrow{\text{LDH}} \text{lactate} + NAD^+$$

Lactate is a base not an acid so a high blood lactate is not, therefore, synonymous with lactic acidosis; there needs to be a concurrent metabolic acidosis for diagnosis. In continuous haemofiltration the replacement fluid is usually buffered with lactate at 35–45mmol/L; thus blood lactate levels will rise without acidosis.

Causes of lactic acidosis

Lactic acidosis occurs when production of lactic acid is in excess of removal. The major sources are skeletal muscle, brain and red blood cells. Removal is mainly by metabolism to glucose in the liver and kidney. Hepatic removal is impaired by poor perfusion and acidosis. Lactic acidosis is traditionally classified as type A or type B. Type A refers to excess production when tissue oxygenation is inadequate. Type B occurs where there is no systemic tissue hypoxia. Treatment of metabolic acidosis with sodium bicarbonate solution increases lactate production. A severe and persistent lactic acidosis is associated with a poor outcome.

Identifying type A lactic acidosis

Evidence of poor tissue perfusion may be obvious clinically. Calculation of arterial DO_2 may confirm inadequate tissue oxygen delivery but a normal DO_2 does not guarantee adequacy of supply.

See also:
   Haemo(dia)filtration 1, 54; Haemo(dia)filtration 2, 56; Blood gas analysis, 94;
Arterial Cannulation, 106; Other neurological monitoring, 132; Metabolic acidosis,
420; Systemic inflammatory response, 488

Colloid osmotic pressure

Colloid osmotic pressure (COP) is the pressure required to prevent net fluid movement between two solutions separated by a selectively permeable membrane when one contains a greater colloid concentration than the other. The selectively permeable membrane should impede the passage of colloid molecules but not small ions and water. COP is determined by number of molecules rather than type. However, most solutions exhibit non-ideal behaviour due to intermolecular interactions and electrostatic effects. Hence COP cannot be inferred from plasma protein concentrations; it must be measured.

Measurement of COP

In a membrane oncometer the plasma sample is separated from a reference 0.9% saline solution by a membrane with a molecular weight exclusion between 10 000 and 30 000 dalton. The reference solution is in a closed chamber containing a pressure transducer. Saline will pass to the sample chamber by colloid osmosis creating a negative pressure in the reference chamber. When the negative pressure prevents any further flow across the membrane, it is equal to the COP of the sample. Normal plasma COP is 25–30mmHg.

Clinical use of COP measurement

Assessing significance of reduced plasma proteins
Plasma albumin levels are almost invariably reduced in critically ill patients. Causes include interstitial leakage, failed synthesis and increased metabolism. However, the same group of patients often have raised levels of acute phase proteins which contribute to COP. Since there is no evidence that correction of plasma albumin levels is beneficial, many clinicians correct plasma volume deficit with artificial colloid. These will contribute to COP while also reducing hepatic albumin synthesis. If COP is maintained > 20mmHg it is likely that reduced plasma albumin levels are of no significance.

Avoiding pulmonary oedema
It has been suggested that a difference between COP and pulmonary artery wedge pressure > 6mmHg minimises the risk of pulmonary oedema. However, in the face of severe capillary leak it is unlikely that pulmonary oedema can be avoided if plasma volumes are to be maintained compatible with circulatory adequacy. Conversely, a normal COP would not necessarily prevent pulmonary oedema in severe capillary leak; the contribution of COP to fluid dynamics in this situation is much reduced.

Selection of appropriate fluid therapy
It is difficult not to support the use of colloid fluids in hypo-oncotic patients. In patients with renal failure the repeated use of colloid fluid may lead to a hyper-oncotic state. This is associated with tissue dehydration and failure of glomerular filtration (thus prolonging the renal failure). Measurement of a high COP in patients who have been treated with artificial colloids should direct the use of crystalloid fluids. It is important to note that excessive diuresis may also lead to a hyper-oncotic state for which crystalloid replacement may be necessary.

See also:
Liver function tests, 142; Fluid challenge, 262

Fluids

Crystalloids

Types

- Saline: e.g. 0.9% saline, Hartmann's solution, 0.18% saline in 4% glucose
- Glucose: e.g. 5% glucose, 10% glucose, 20% glucose
- Potassium chloride
- Sodium bicarbonate: e.g. 1.26%, 8.4%

Uses

- Crystalloid fluids are used to provide the daily requirements of water and electrolytes. They should be given to critically ill patients as a continuous background infusion to supplement fluids given during feeding or to carry drugs.
- Higher concentration glucose infusions are used to prevent hypoglycaemia.
- Potassium chloride is used to supplement crystalloid fluids.
- Correction of metabolic acidosis (sodium bicarbonate)

Routes

- IV

Notes

Plasma volume should be maintained or replaced with colloid solutions since crystalloids are rapidly lost from the plasma. It should be noted that plasma substitutes are carried in 0.9% saline. so that the majority of critically ill patients only require 0.9% saline infusions for excess loss.

Sodium content of 0.9% saline is equivalent to that of extracellular fluid. A daily requirement of 70–80mmol sodium is normal although there may be excess loss in sweat and from the gastrointestinal tract.

Hartmann's solution has no practical advantage over 0.9% saline for fluid maintenance. It may, however, be useful if large volumes of crystalloid are exchanged (e.g. during continuous haemofiltration) to maintain acid–base balance.

5% glucose is used to supply intravenous water requirements, the 50g/L glucose being present to ensure an isotonic solution. Normal requirement is 1.5–2.0L/day. Water loss in excess of electrolytes is uncommon but occurs in excess sweating, fever, hyperthyroidism, diabetes insipidus and hypercalcaemia.

Potassium chloride must be given slowly since rapid injection may cause fatal arrhythmias. No more than 40mmol/h may be given although 20mmol/h is more usual. Frequency of infusions are predicted by plasma potassium measurements.

Ion content of crystalloids (mmol/L)

	Na^+	K^+	HCO_3^-	Cl^-	Ca^{2+}
0.9% saline	150			150	
Hartmann's	131	5	29	111	2
0.18% saline in 4% glucose	30			30	

Ion content of gastrointestinal fluids (mmol/L)

	H^+	Na^+	K^+	HCO_3^-	Cl^-
Gastric	40–60	20–80	5–20		150	100–150
Biliary		120–140	5–15	30–50	80–120
Pancreatic		120–140	5–15	70–110	40–80
Small bowel		120–140	5–15	20–40	90–130
Large bowel		100–120	5–15	20–40	90–130

167

See also:
  Nutrition—use and indications, 70; Urea & creatinie, 136; Electrolytes (Na^+, K^+, Cl^-, HCO_3^-), 138; Colloids, 170; Hypernatraemia, 402; Hyponatraemia, 404; Hyperkalaemia, 406; Diabetic ketoacidosis, 428; Hyperosmolar diabetic emergencies, 430

Sodium bicarbonate

Types

- Isotonic sodium bicarbonate 1.26%,
- Hypertonic sodium bicarbonate (1mmol/ml) 8.4%

Uses

- Correction of metabolic acidosis
- Alkalinisation of urine

Routes

- IV

Notes

Sodium bicarbonate may be given as an isotonic (1.26%) solution to correct acidosis associated with renal failure or to induce a forced alkaline diuresis. The hypertonic (8.4%) solution is rarely required in intensive care practice to raise the pH to >7.0 in severe metabolic acidosis. Bicarbonate therapy is inappropriate when tissue hypoperfusion or necrosis is present.

Administration may be indicated as either specific therapy (e.g. alkaline diuresis for salicylate overdose), or if the patient is symptomatic (usually dyspnoeic) in the absence of tissue hypoperfusion (e.g. renal failure).

The $PaCO_2$ may rise if minute volume is not increased. Bicarbonate cannot cross the cell membrane without dissociation so the increase in $PaCO_2$ may result in intracellular acidosis and depression of myocardial cell function.

The decrease in plasma ionised calcium may also cause a decrease in myocardial contractility. Significantly worse haemodynamic effects have been reported with bicarbonate compared to equimolar saline in patients with severe heart failure.

Convincing human evidence that bicarbonate improves myocardial contractility or increases responsiveness to circulating catecholamines in severe acidosis is lacking though anecdotal success has been reported. Acidosis relating to myocardial depression is related to intracellular changes which are not accurately reflected by arterial blood chemistry.

Excessive administration may cause hyperosmolality, hypernatraemia, hypokalaemia and sodium overload.

Bicarbonate may decrease tissue oxygen availability by a left shift of the oxyhaemoglobin dissociation curve.

Sodium bicarbonate does have a place in the management of acid retention or alkali loss, e.g. chronic renal failure, renal tubular acidosis, fistulae, diarrhoea. Fluid and potassium deficit should be corrected first.

Ion content of sodium bicarbonate (mmol/L)

	Na^+	K^+	HCO_3^-	Cl^-	Ca^{2+}
1.26% sodium bicarbonate	150		150		
8.4% sodium bicarbonate	1000		1000		

See also:
  Blood gas analysis, 94; Electrolytes (Na^+, K^+, Cl^-, HCO_3^-), 138; Crystalloids, 166; Metabolic acidosis, 420; Salicylate poisoning, 440

Colloids

Types

- Albumin: e.g. 4.5–5%, 20–25% human albumin solution
- Dextran: e.g. 6% Dextran 70
- Gelatin: e.g. 3.5% polygeline (Haemaccel), 4% succinylated gelatin (Gelofusin)
- Hydroxyethyl starch: e.g. 6% hetastarch (Elo-HAES, Hespan), 6 &10% pentastarch (Pentaspan, HAES-steril)

Uses

Used for maintenance of plasma volume and acute replacement of plasma volume deficit.

- Short term volume expansion (gelatin, dextran)
- Medium term volume expansion (albumin, pentastarch)
- Long term volume expansion (hetastarch)

Routes

- IV

Side effects

- Dilution coagulopathy
- Anaphylaxis
- Interference with blood cross matching (Dextran 70)

Notes

Smaller volumes of colloid are required for resuscitation with less contribution to oedema. Maintenance of plasma colloid osmotic pressure (COP) is a useful effect not seen with crystalloids but they contain no clotting factors or other plasma enzyme systems.

Albumin is the main provider of COP in the plasma and has a number of other functions. However, there is no evidence that maintenance of plasma albumin levels, as opposed to maintenance of plasma COP with artificial plasma substitutes, is advantageous.

Albumin 20–25% and Pentaspan 10% are hyperoncotic and used to provide colloid where salt restriction is necessary. This use is rarely necessary in intensive care where it has been shown that plasma volume expansion is related to the weight of colloid infused rather than the concentration. Artificial colloids used with ultrafiltration or diuresis are just as effective in oedema states.

Polygeline is a 3.5% solution and contains calcium (6.25mmol/L). The calcium content prevents the use of the same administration set for blood transfusions. Succinylated gelatin is a 4.5% solution with a larger molecular weight range than polygeline giving a slightly longer effect. This and the lack of calcium in solution make this a more useful solution than polygeline for short term plasma volume expansion.

In patients with capillary leak there is considerable leak of albumin and smaller molecular weight colloids to the interstitium. In these cases it is probably better to use larger molecular weight colloids such as hydroxyethyl starch.

Hetastarch is usually a 6% solution with a high degree of protection from metabolism. The molecular weight ranges vary but molecular sizes are large enough to ensure a prolonged effect. These are the most useful colloids in capillary leak.

Pentastarch has a lower degree of protection from metabolism and therefore a shorter effect.

Unique features of albumin

Transport of various molecules
Free radical scavenging
Binding of toxins
Inhibition of platelet aggregation

Relative persistence of colloid effect

Albumin	+ + +
Dextran 70	+ +
Gelofusin	+
Haemaccel	+
Hespan	+ + + +
Pentaspan	+ +
Elo-HAES	+ + + +
HAES-steril	+ +

- Persistence is dependent on molecular size and protection from metabolism

171

- All artificial colloids are polydisperse (i.e. there is a range of molecular sizes).

See also:
Crystalloids, 166; Blood transfusion, 172; Fluid challenge, 262; Anaphylactoid reactions, 492

Blood transfusion

Blood storage

Blood cells are eventually destroyed due to oxidant damage during storage of whole blood. Since white cells and plasma enzyme systems are of importance in this cellular destruction, effects are correspondingly less severe for packed red cells. Microaggregate formation is associated with platelets, white cells and fibrin and range in size from 20–170μm; the risk of microaggregate damage is also reduced with packed red cells. In addition to spherocytosis and haemolysis, prolonged storage depletes ATP and 2,3–DPG levels thus increasing the oxygen affinity of the red cells. If whole blood is to be used in critically ill patients it should be as fresh as possible.

Compatibility

In an emergency, with massive blood loss that threatens life, it is permissible to transfuse O negative packed cells but a sample must be taken for grouping prior to transfusion. With modern laboratory procedures it is possible to obtain ABO compatibility for group specific transfusion within 5–10min and a full cross match in 30min.

Hazards of blood transfusion.

- Citrate toxicity—hypocalcaemia is rarely a problem and the prophylactic use of calcium supplementation is not recommended
- Potassium load—potassium returns to cells rapidly but hyperkalaemia may be a problem if blood is stored at room temperature
- Sodium load—from citrate if the transfusion is massive
- Hypothermia—can be avoided by warming blood as it is transfused
- Jaundice—haemolysis of incompatible or old blood
- Pyrexia—immunological transfusion reactions to incompatible red or white cells
- DIC—partial activation of clotting factors and destruction of stored cells, either in old blood or when transfusion is incompatible
- Anaphylactoid reaction—urticaria is common and probably due to a reaction to transfused plasma proteins; if severe it may be treated by slowing the transfusion and giving chlorpheniramine 10mg IV/IM. In severe anaphylaxis, in addition to standard treatment, the transfusion should be stopped and saved for later analysis and a sample taken for further cross-matching.

Respiratory Drugs

Bronchodilators

Types

- β_2 agonists: e.g. salbutamol, adrenaline, terbutaline
- Anticholinergics: e.g. ipratropium
- Theophyllines: e.g. aminophylline
- Steroids: e.g. hydrocortisone, prednisolone
- Others: e.g. ketamine, isoflurane, halothane

Uses

Relief of bronchospasm

Routes

- Inhaled (salbutamol, adrenaline, terbutaline, ipratropium, isoflurane, halothane)
- Nebulised (salbutamol, adrenaline, terbutaline, ipratropium)
- IV (salbutamol, adrenaline, terbutaline, ipratropium, aminophylline, hydrocortisone, ketamine)
- PO (aminophylline, prednisolone)

Side effects

- CNS stimulation (salbutamol, adrenaline, terbutaline, aminophylline)
- Tachycardia (salbutamol, adrenaline, terbutaline, aminophylline, ketamine)
- Hypotension (salbutamol, terbutaline, aminophylline, isoflurane, halothane)
- Hyperglycaemia (salbutamol, adrenaline, terbutaline, hydrocortisone, prednisolone)
- Hypokalaemia (salbutamol, adrenaline, terbutaline, hydrocortisone, prednisolone)
- Lactic acidosis (salbutamol)

Notes

Selective β_2 agonists are usually used by inhalation via a pressurised aerosol or a nebulizer. Inhalation usually gives rapid relief of bronchospasm, although the aerosol is not of benefit in severe asthma due to incomplete exhalation.

Nebulized drugs require a minimum volume of 4ml and a driving gas flow of 6–8L/min.

In extremis, adrenaline may be used IV, SC or injected down the endotracheal tube. Adrenaline is not selective and therefore arrhythmias are more likely. However, the α agonist effect may reduce mucosal swelling by vasoconstriction.

Ipratropium bromide has no systemic effects, does not depress mucocilliary clearance and is synergistic with β_2 agonists but with a slower onset of action.

Aminophylline is synergistic with β_2 agonists. Dosages must be adjusted according to plasma levels (range 10–20mg/L) since toxic effects may be severe. Dose requirements are reduced by heart failure, liver disease, chronic airflow limitation, fever, cimetidine, erythromycin. Dose requirements are increased in smokers and those with a moderate to high alcohol intake.

Drug dosages

	Aerosol[*]	Nebulizer[*]	IV bolus	IV infusion
Salbutamol	100–200µg	2.5–5mg		3–20µg/min
Terbutaline	250–500µg	5–10mg	1.5–5µg/min	
Adrenaline		0.5mg		
Ipratropium		250µg		
Aminophylline			5mg/kg over 20min	0.5mg/kg/h
Hydrocortisone			200mg qds	

[*] Aerosols and nebulizers are usually given four times daily but may be given more frequently if necessary.

In extremis adrenaline may be given as 0.1–0.5mg subcutaneously, injected down the endotracheal tube or by IV infusion.

177

See also:
Steroids, 250; Asthma—general management, 284; Asthma—ventilatory management, 286

Respiratory stimulants

Types
- Drug antagonists: e.g. naloxone, flumazenil
- CNS stimulants: e.g. doxapram
- Almitrine

Uses
- Acute respiratory failure due to failure of ventilatory drive
- Drug induced ventilatory failure, e.g. as a result of excessive sedation or post-operatively.

Routes
- IV

Modes of action
- Naloxone—short acting opiate antagonist.
- Flumazenil—short acting benzodiazepine antagonist.
- Doxapram—generalised central nervous system stimulant with predominant respiratory stimulation at lower doses. Stimulation of carotid chemoreceptors at very low doses with increased tidal volumes.
- Almitrine—increases the sensitivity of carotid chemoreceptors to hypoxaemia and hypercapnia.

Side effects
- Seizures (flumazenil, doxapram)
- Tachyarrhythmias (naloxone, flumazenil)
- Hallucinations (doxapram)

Notes
The use of respiratory stimulants in hypercapnic respiratory failure in chronic airflow limitation is questionable.

Naloxone may be used in respiratory depression due to opiate drugs. Since it reverses all opiate effects it may be better to reverse respiratory depression with non-specific respiratory stimulants leaving pain relief intact. May need to be repeated where long acting opiates are involved.

Most benzodiazepines are long acting compared to flumazenil so repeated doses may be necessary.

Effects of doxapram are short lived so infusion is necessary. After about 12h infusion the effects on ventilatory drive become markedly reduced.

Almitrine does not produce central respiratory stimulation but there is an improvement in ventilation perfusion matching by augmentation of hypoxic pulmonary vasoconstriction. Effects continue for several hours after injection.

Drug dosages

	IV bolus	IV infusion
Naloxone	0.1–0.4mg	
Flumazenil	0.2mg over 15min (0.1mg/min to max 2mg)	
Doxapram	1–1.5mg/kg over 30sec	2–3mg/min
Almitrine	0.25–0.5mg/kg over 30min	

179

See also:
   Opioid analgesics, 222; Sedatives, 226; Respiratory failure, 270; Generalised
seizures, 360; Sedative poisoning, 444; Post-operative intensive care, 510

Nitric oxide (NO)

NO is now recognised as a fundamental mediator in many physiological processes. One of the most important effects is smooth muscle relaxation; nitric oxide is the major local controller of vascular tone via effects on cyclic GMP.

Inhaled nitric oxide

NO is provided for inhalation from cylinders (1000ppm NO in nitrogen). It is diluted with inspiratory gases either at the gas supply to the ventilator or in the inspiratory limb of the ventilator circuit, to provide an inhaled concentration of 1–40ppm although most patients require less than 20ppm. Inhalation produces vasodilatation at the site of gas exchange improving ventilation perfusion matching and reducing pulmonary artery pressure.

Side effects

NO is immediately bound to haemoglobin ensuring local effects only. There is no tolerance but patients can become dependent on continued inhalation with rebound pulmonary hypertension and hypoxaemia on withdrawal. For this reason withdrawal must be slow. Ideally, a reserve NO source should be used when patients are disconnected from the ventilator, e.g. for manual inflation during physiotherapy, unless FIO_2 can be increased to compensate. Excessive humidification of inspired gases may form nitric acid with NO; the use of heat-moisture exchangers rather than water baths is recommended.

Monitoring

NO and nitrogen dioxide concentrations may be monitored conveniently with portable fuel cell analysers. Alternatively, chemiluminescence analysers may be used. It is important to monitor concentrations of both gases in the inspiratory limb of the ventilator circuit. Monitoring of nitrogen dioxide is important to ensure that toxic doses are not formed with the oxygen in the inspired gas and subsequently inhaled by the patient. Although it is extremely rare to see toxic nitrogen dioxide concentrations (> 5ppm) it is possible to remove nitrogen dioxide from the inspired gas by using a soda lime adsorber. Methaemoglobin is formed when NO binds to haemoglobin. Prolonged inhalation at higher doses may rarely produce significant methaemoglobinaemia ($> 5\%$) and this should therefore be monitored daily.

Achieving the correct dose

Approximately 50% of patients with severe respiratory failure respond to NO. However, the most effective dose varies. It is usual to start at 1ppm for 10min and monitor the change in PaO_2/FIO_2 ratio. An increase should be followed by an increase in nitric oxide concentration to 5ppm for a further 10min. Thereafter, the dose is adjusted according to response at 10min intervals until the most effective dose is found. Since the underlying pathophysiology may change, it is important to assess the dose response at daily intervals, aiming to keep the dose at the lowest effective level.

Scavenging

Since the concentrations used are so small dilution of exhaled gases into the atmosphere are unlikely to produce important environmental concentrations. In the air-conditioned intensive care environment air changes are so frequent as to make scavenging unnecessary.

See also:
Vasodilators, 186; Adult respiratory distress syndrome 1, 280; Adult respiratory distress syndrome 2, 282

Cardiovascular Drugs

Inotropes

Types

- Catecholamines: e.g. adrenaline, noradrenaline, dobutamine, dopamine
- Phosphodiesterase (PDE) inhibitors: e.g. milrinone, enoximone
- Dopexamine
- Cardiac glycosides: e.g. digoxin (weak)

Modes of action

- Increase force of myocardial contraction, either by stimulating cardiac β_1 adrenoreceptors (catecholamines), decreasing cAMP breakdown (PDE inhibitors), directly increasing contractility (digoxin), or inhibiting neuronal re-uptake of noradrenaline (dopexamine). All agents with the exception of digoxin have, to greater or lesser degrees, associated dilator or constrictor properties via α_1 & β_1 adrenoreceptors or dopaminergic receptors.
- Digoxin may cause splanchnic vasoconstriction and, for an inotropic effect, requires plasma levels at the top of the therapeutic range.
- The increase in cardiac work is usually reduced in those drugs possessing associated dilator effects.
- Other than adrenaline (when used for its vasoconstrictor effect in cardiopulmonary resuscitation) or digoxin (for long-term use in chronic heart failure), inotropes are usually given by continuous IV infusion titrated for effect.

Uses

- Myocardial failure, e.g. post-myocardial infarction, cardiomyopathy
- Myocardial depression, e.g. sepsis
- Augmentation of oxygen delivery in high-risk surgical patients

Side-effects

- Arrhythmias (usually associated with concurrent hypovolaemia)
- Tachycardia (usually associated with concurrent hypovolaemia)
- Hypotension (related to dilator properties ± concurrent hypovolaemia)
- Hypertension (related to constrictor properties)
- Anginal chest pain, or ST-segment and T-wave changes on ECG

Notes

Adrenaline, noradrenaline, dobutamine and dopamine should be given via a central vein as tissue necrosis may occur secondary to peripheral extravasation.

Drug dosages

Adrenaline	infusion starting from 0.05µg/kg/min
Noradrenaline	infusion starting from 0.05µg/kg/min
Dobutamine	infusion from 2.5–25µg/kg/min
Dopamine	infusion from 2.5–50µg/kg/min
Dopexamine	infusion from 0.5–6µg/kg/min
Milrinone	loading dose of 50µg/kg over 10min followed by infusion from 0.375–0.75µg/kg/min
Enoximone	loading dose of 0.5–1mg/kg over 10min followed by infusion from 5–20µg/kg/min
Digoxin	0.5mg given PO or IV over 10–20min. Repeat at 4–8h intervals until loading achieved (assessed by clinical response). Maintenance dose thereafter is 0.0625–0.25mg/day depending on plasma levels and clinical response.

185

See also:
  Intra-aortic balloon counterpulsation, 50; Cardiac output—thermodilution, 116; Cardiac output—other invasive, 118; Cardiac output—non-invasive, 120; Basic resuscitation, 258; Fluid challenge, 262; Hypotension, 300; Heart failure—assessment, 312; Heart failure—management, 314; Systemic inflammatory response, 488

Vasodilators

Types

- Nitrates: e.g. glyceryl trinitrate, isosorbide dinitrate,
- Angiotensin converting enzyme (ACE) inhibitors: e.g. captopril
- Smooth muscle relaxants: e.g. sodium nitroprusside, hydralazine
- α-adrenergic antagonists: e.g. phentolamine
- β_2-adrenergic agonists: e.g. salbutamol
- Calcium antagonists: e.g. nifedipine, diltiazem
- Dopaminergic agonists: e.g. 'low dose' ($\leqslant 3\mu g/kg/min$) dopamine, dopexamine
- Phosphodiesterase inhibitors: e.g. enoximone, milrinone
- Prostaglandins: e.g. epoprostenol (PGI_2), alprostadil (PGE_1)

Modes of action

- Increase cyclic GMP concentration (by nitric oxide donation or by inhibiting cGMP breakdown), or acts directly on dopaminergic receptors leading to vasodilatation
- Reduce (to varying degrees) ventricular preload and/or afterload.
- Reduce cardiac work.

Uses

- Myocardial failure, e.g. post-myocardial infarction, cardiomyopathy
- Angina/ischaemic heart disease
- Systemic hypertension (including phaeochromocytoma)
- Vasoconstriction
- Peripheral vascular disease/hypoperfusion
- Splanchnic perfusion (dopexamine, dopamine)
- For myocardial/gut ischaemia during vasopressin treatment
- Pulmonary hypertension—(inhaled NO or prostaglandins)

Side-effects / complications

- Hypotension (often associated with concurrent hypovolaemia)
- Tachycardia (often associated with concurrent hypovolaemia)
- Symptoms include headache, flushing, postural hypotension
- Renal failure (ACE inhibitors)—especially with renal artery stenosis, hypovolaemia, non-steroidals

Notes

Glyceryl trinitrate and isosorbide dinitrate reduce both preload and afterload. At higher dose the afterload effect is more prominent.

Tolerance to nitrates usually commences within 24–36h. unless intermittent oral dosing is used. Progressive increases in dose are required to achieve same effect.

Prolonged (> 24–36h) dose-related administration of sodium nitroprusside can produce a metabolic acidosis related to cyanide accumulation.

ACE inhibitor tablets can be crushed and given either SL or via a nasogastric tube.

Dopaminergic drugs improve splanchnic blood flow though clinical benefits are unproved. Dopamine also has a diuretic action.

Hydrallazine has an unpredictable effect on blood pressure and, if given IV, should be used with caution.

Drug dosages

Nitrates	glyceryl trinitrate 2–40mg/h
isosorbide dinitrate	2–40mg/h
Sodium nitroprusside	20–400µg/min
Hydralazine	5–10mg by slow IV bolus, repeat after 20–30min.
	Alternatively, by infusion starting at 200–300µg/min and reducing to 50–150µg/min.
ACE inhibitors	captopril: 6.25mg test dose increasing to 25mg tds
	enalapril: 2.5mg test dose increasing to 40mg od
	lisinopril: 2.5mg test dose increasing to 40mg od
Nifedipine:	5–20mg PO. Capsule fluid can be injected down nasogastric tube or given sublingually.
Phentolamine	2–5mg IV slow bolus. Repeat as necessary.
Dopexamine	infusion from 0.5–6µg/kg/min.
Milrinone	loading dose of 50µg/kg over 10min followed by infusion from 0.375–0.75µg/kg/min.
Enoximone	loading dose of 0.5–1mg/kg over 10min followed by infusion from 5–20µg/kg/min.
Epoprostenol, alprostadil	infusion from 2–30 ng/kg/min
Nitric oxide	by inhalation: 2–40 ppm

187

Vasopressors

Types
- α-adrenergic: e.g. noradrenaline, adrenaline, dopamine, ephedrine, phenylephrine, methoxamine,
- Drugs reducing production of cyclic GMP (in septic shock): e.g. methylene blue, nitric oxide synthase inhibitors (e.g. L-NMMA)
- Angiotensin II

Modes of action
- Acting on peripheral α-adrenergic receptors
- Blocking cGMP production directly (methylene blue) or indirectly (NO synthase inhibition).
- Increase afterload, mainly by arteriolar vasoconstriction
- Venoconstriction

Uses
- To increase organ perfusion pressures, particularly in high output, low peripheral resistance states, e.g. sepsis, anaphylaxis
- To raise coronary perfusion pressures in cardiopulmonary resuscitation

Side-effects / complications
- Increase cardiac work
- Decreased cardiac output, especially with agents where pressor effects predominate
- Myocardial ischaemia
- Increased myocardial irritability, especially with concurrent hypovolaemia, leading to arrhythmias and tachycardia
- Decreased peripheral perfusion possibly leading to distal ischaemia
- With NO blockade, potential removal of beneficial effects of NO
- Cytotoxicity

Notes
Methoxamine, phenylephrine and angiotensin are the 'purest' pressor agents; the other α-adrenergic agents have inotropic properties to greater or lesser degrees. Ephedrine is similar to adrenaline but its effects are more prolonged as it is not metabolised by monoamine oxidase.

Effects of pressor agents on splanchnic, renal and cerebral circulations are variable and unpredictable.

Pulmonary vascular resistance is also raised by these agents.

Methylene blue, L-NMMA and angiotensin are currently unlicensed as pressor agents in patients.

Drug dosages

Noradrenaline	infusion starting from 0.05μg/kg/min
Adrenaline	infusion starting from 0.05μg/kg/min
Dopamine	infusion from 5–50μg/kg/min
Methoxamine	3–10mg by slow IV bolus (rate of 1mg/min)
Ephedrine	3–30mg by slow IV bolus
Methylene blue	1–2mg/kg over 15–30min
Angiotensin II	infusion starting from 0.05μg/kg/min

189

Hypotensive agents

Types

- Vasodilators
- β-blockers

In routine ICU practice β-blockers are used infrequently because most have a long half-life and the negative inotropic effects are generally undesirable. Exceptions are esmolol and labetalol, both of which have short half-lives and vasodilating properties.

Modes of action

- Vasodilators reduce preload and afterload to variable degrees depending on type and dose
- β-blockers reduce the force of myocardial contractility

Uses

- Hypertension—systemic and pulmonary
- Heart failure—to reduce afterload ± preload (caution with β-blockers)
- Control of blood pressure, e.g. dissecting aortic aneurysm

Side-effects / complications

- Excessive hypotension
- Heart failure (with β-blockers)
- Peripheral hypoperfusion (with β-blockers)
- Bronchospasm (with β-blockers)
- Decreased sympathetic response to hypoglycaemia (with β-blockers)

Notes

In critically ill patients it is generally advisable to use short-acting β-blockers by infusion.

Drug dosages

Nitrates	glyceryl trinitrate 2–40mg/h
	isosorbide dinitrate 2–40mg/h
Sodium nitroprusside	20–400µg/min.
ACE inhibitors	captopril: 6.25mg test dose increasing to 25mg tds
	enalapril: 2.5mg test dose increasing to 40mg o.d. lisinopril: 2.5mg test dose increasing to 40mg o.d.
Nifedipine:	5–20mg PO. Capsule fluid can be injected down nasogastric tube or given sublingually.
Phentolamine	2–5mg IV slow bolus. Repeat as necessary.
Esmolol	A titrated loading dose regimen is commenced followed by an infusion rate of 50–200µg/kg/min.
Propranolol	Initially given as slow IV 1mg boluses repeated at 2min intervals until effect is seen (to maximum 5mg)
Labetalol	0.25–2mg/min

Antiarrhythmics

Only the antiarrhythmics likely to be used in the ICU are described.
For supraventricular tachyarrhythmias:

adenosine, verapamil, amiodarone, digoxin, β-blockers, Mg^{2+}

For ventricular tachyarrhythmias:

amiodarone, lignocaine, flecainide, bretylium, β-blockers, Mg^{2+}

Uses

- Correction of supraventricular and ventricular tachyarrhythmias which either compromise the circulation or could potentially do so.
- Differentiation between supraventricular and ventricular arrhythmias using adenosine

Notes

All antiarrhythmic agents have side-effects; other than digoxin they are negatively inotropic to greater or lesser degrees and may induce profound hypotension (e.g. verapamil, β-blockers) or bradycardia (e.g. β-blockers, amiodarone, digoxin, lignocaine). β-blockers in particular should be used with caution because of these effects.

All A-V blockers are contraindicated in re-entry tachycardia (e.g. Wolff–Parkinson–White syndrome).

- Adenosine: very short-acting; may revert paroxysmal SVT to sinus rhythm. Ineffective for atrial flutter and fibrillation, ventricular tachycardia. Contraindicated in 2° and 3° heart block, sick sinus syndrome, asthma. May cause flushing, bronchospasm and occasional severe bradycardia.

- Amiodarone: effective against all types of tachyarrhythmia. Usually given by IV infusion for rapid effect but requires initial loading dose. When converting from IV to oral dosing, initial high oral dosing (200mg tds) is still required. Contraindicated in patients with thyroid dysfunction. Has low acute toxicity though may cause severe bradycardia. Avoid with other Class III agents (e.g. sotalol). Must be given via central vein as causes peripheral phlebitis.
- β-blockers: for SVT, esmolol is preferred due to its short half-life though may cause marked vasodilatation. Requires initial, increasing loading doses; an infusion may be needed thereafter. Propranolol can be given by slow IV boluses of 1mg repeated at 2min intervals until effect is seen (maximum 5mg).
- Bretylium: may take 15–20min to take effect; now used predominantly for resistant VF/VT. CPR should be continued for at least 20min.
- Digoxin: slow-acting, requires loading (1–1.5g) to achieve therapeutic plasma levels which can be monitored. Loading ideally given over 12–24h but can be done over 4–6h. Contraindicated in 2° and 3° heart block. May cause severe bradycardia. Low K^+ and Mg^{2+} and markedly raised Ca^{2+} increase myocardial sensitivity to digoxin. Amiodarone raises digoxin levels.
- Lignocaine: 10ml of 1% solution contains 100mg. It has no effect on supraventricular arrhythmias. Loading achieved by 1mg/kg slow IV bolus followed by infusion. Contraindicated in 2° and 3° heart block. May cause bradycardia and CNS side-effects, e.g. drowsiness, seizures.
- Verapamil: should not be given with β-blockers as profound hypotension and bradyarrhythmias may result. Pre-treatment with 3–5ml 10% calcium gluconate by slow IV bolus prevents hypotension without affecting its antiarrhythmic properties.

Modes of action (Vaughan-Williams classification)

Class	Action	Examples
I	Reduces rate of rise of action potential:	
	• Ia: increases action potential duration	• Ia: disopyramide
	• Ib: shortens duration	• Ib: lignocaine
	• Ic: little effect	• Ic: flecainide
II	Reduces rate of pacemaker discharge	β-blockers
III	Prolongs duration of action potential and hence length of refractory period	Amiodarone Sotalol
IV	Antagonises transport of calcium across cell membrane	Verapamil Diltiazem

Drug dosages

Adenosine	3mg rapid IV bolus. If no response after 1min give 6mg. If no response after 1min give 12mg.
Amiodarone	5mg/kg over 20min (or 150–300mg over 3min in emergency) then IV infusion of 15mg/kg/24h in 5% glucose via central vein. Reduce thereafter to 10mg/kg/24h (approx. 600mg/day) for 3–7 days then maintain at 5mg/kg/24h (300–400mg/day)
β-blockers	Esmolol: A titrated loading dose regimen is commenced followed by an infusion rate of 50–200µg/kg/min.
	Propranolol: Initially given as slow IV boluses of 1mg repeated at 2min intervals until effect is seen to a maximum of 5mg.
	Labetalol: 0.25–2mg/min
Bretylium	In emergency 5mg/kg by rapid IV bolus. If no response after 5min, repeat or increase to 10mg/kg.
Digoxin	0.5mg given IV over 10–20min. Repeat at 4–8h intervals until loading achieved (assessed by clinical response). Maintenance dose thereafter is 0.0625–0.25mg/day depending on plasma levels and clinical response.
Lignocaine	1mg/kg slow IV bolus for loading then 2–4mg/min infusion. Should be weaned slowly over 24h.
MgSO$_4$	10–20mmol over 1–2h. Can be given over 5min in emergency.
Verapamil	2.5mg slow IV. If no response repeat to a maximum of 20mg. An IV infusion of 1–10mg/h may be tried. 10% calcium gluconate solution should be readily available.

193

See also:
Defibrillation, 44; ECG monitoring, 102; Basic resuscitation, 258; Cardiac arrest, 260; Tachyarrhythmias, 304

Chronotropes

Types
- Anticholinergic: e.g. atropine, glycopyrrolate
- β_2-agonist: e.g. isoprenaline

Modes of action
- The anticholinergic drugs act by competitive antagonism of acetylcholine at peripheral muscarinic receptors and decreases atrioventricular conduction time.
- Isoprenaline enhances atrioventricular nodal conduction as well as having inotropic and vasodilating properties.

Uses
- All types of bradycardia including 3° heart block
- High dose atropine is used in cardiopulmonary resuscitation protocols for treatment of asystole.

Side-effects / complications
- Anticholinergic drugs produce dry mouth, reduction and thickening of bronchial secretions, and inhibition of sweating. Urinary retention may occur but parenteral administration does not lead to glaucoma.
- Isoprenaline may induce hypotension, palpitations, dysrhythmias and sweating.

Notes
The anticholinergic agents are usually given by IV bolus, repeated as necessary, whereas isoprenaline is given by continuous infusion.

They are frequently used as a bridge to temporary pacing but should not be considered a substitute. External or internal pacing should be readily accessible.

Atropine nebulizers have been used successfully in patients developing symptomatic bradycardia during endotracheal suction.

Neurological effects are seen with atropine but not glycopyrrolate.

Drug dosages

Atropine	0.3–0.6mg IV bolus. 3mg is needed for complete vagal blockade.
Glycopyrrolate	0.2–0.4mg IV bolus.
Isoprenaline	infusion from 1–10µg/min

See also:
  Temporary internal pacing, 46; External pacing, 48; ECG monitoring, 102; Basic resuscitation, 258; Cardiac arrest, 260; Bradyarrhythmias, 306

Anti-anginal agents

Types
- Vasodilators: e.g. nitrates, calcium antagonists
- β-blockers
- Potassium channel openers: e.g. nicorandil
- Heparin

Modes of action
- Calcium channel blockers cause competitive blockade of cell membrane slow calcium channels leading to decreased influx of calcium ions into cells. This leads to inhibition of contraction and relaxation of cardiac and smooth muscle fibres resulting in coronary and systemic vasodilatation
- Nitrates may cause efflux of calcium ions from smooth muscle and cardiac cells and also increases cGMP synthesis resulting in coronary and systemic vasodilatation.
- β-blockers inhibit β-adrenoreceptor stimulation, reducing myocardial work and oxygen consumption. This effect is somewhat offset by compensatory peripheral vasoconstriction.
- Potassium channel openers cause vasodilatation by relaxation of vascular smooth muscle. The potassium channel opening action works on the arterial circulation while a nitrate action provides additional venodilatation.
- Though heparin has no direct anti-anginal effect, patients with unstable angina benefit from heparinisation which reduces platelet aggregation by fibrin.

Uses
- Angina pectoris

Side-effects / complications
- See Dilators, Hypotensive agents.
- Nicorandil is contraindicated in hypotension and cardiogenic shock. It should be avoided in hypovolaemia. Headache and flushing are the major reported side-effects.

Notes
Combination therapy involving intravenous nitrates, calcium antagonists, β-blockade and heparinisation has been shown to be beneficial in unstable angina; thrombolytic therapy confers no added advantage.

Potassium channel openers belong to a new class of drug yet to be extensively evaluated in critically ill patients and should be thus used with caution, especially when hyperkalaemia is a concern.

Angina may occasionally be worsened by a 'coronary steal' phenomenon where blood flow is diverted away from stenosed coronary vessels. This does not however occur with nicorandil.

Drug dosages

Glyceryl trinitrate	0.3mg sublingually, 0.4–0.8mg by buccal spray, 2–40mg/h by IV infusion
Isosorbide dinitrate	10–20mg tds orally, 2–40mg/h by IV infusion
Nifedipine:	5–20mg PO. The capsule fluid can be aspirated then injected down nasogastric tube or given sublingually.
Propranolol:	Given either orally at doses of 10–100mg tds or IV as slow boluses of 1mg repeated at 2min intervals to a maximum of 5mg until effect is seen. This can be repeated every 2–4h as necessary.
Nicorandil	10–20mg bd

197

See also:
Angina, 310

Renal Drugs

Diuretics

Types

- Osmotic diuretics: e.g. mannitol
- Thiazides: e.g. metolazone
- Loop diuretics: e.g. frusemide, bumetanide
- Potassium sparing diuretics: e.g. amiloride, spironolactone, potassium canrenoate

Uses

- To increase urine volume
- Control of chronic oedema (thiazides)
- Control of hypertension (thiazides)
- To promote renal excretion (e.g. forced diuresis, hypercalcaemia)

Routes

- IV (mannitol, frusemide, bumetanide, potassium canrenoate)
- PO (metolazone, frusemide, bumetanide, amiloride, spironolactone)

Modes of action

- Osmotic diuretics—reduce distal tubular water reabsorption
- Thiazides—inhibit distal tubular Na^+ loss and carbonic anhydrase and increase Na^+ and K^+ exchange. This reduces the supply of H^+ ions for exchange with Na^+ ions producing and alkaline natriuresis with potassium loss
- Loop diuretics—inhibit Na^+ and Cl^- reabsorption in the ascending loop of Henle
- Potassium sparing diuretics—inhibit distal tubular Na^+ and K^+ exchange

Side effects

- Hyponatraemia or hypernatraemia
- Hypokalaemia
- Oedema formation (mannitol)
- Reduced catecholamine effect (thiazides)
- Hyperglycaemia (thiazides)
- Metabolic alkalosis (loop diuretics)
- Hypomagnesaemia (loop diuretics)
- Pancreatitis (frusemide)

Notes

It is important to correct pre-renal causes of oliguria before resorting to diuretic use.

Diuretics do not prevent renal failure but may convert oliguric to polyuric renal failure.

If there is inadequate glomerular filtration mannitol is retained and passes to the extracellular fluid to promote oedema formation.

Bumetanide may be used in porphyria where thiazides and other loop diuretics are contraindicated.

Potassium sparing diuretics should be avoided with ACE inhibitors.

Drug Dosages

	Oral	IV	Infusion
Mannitol		100g over 20min 6hrly	
Metolazone	5–10mg od		
Frusemide	20–40mg 6–24hrly	5–80mg 6–24hrly	1–10mg/h
Bumetanide	0.5–1mg 6–24hrly	0.5–2mg 6–24hrly	1–5mg/h
Amiloride	5–10mg 12–24hrly		
Spironolactone	100–400mg od		
K^+ Canrenoate		200–400mg od	

See also:

Dopamine

The effects of dopamine are dependent on the dose infused. Dopamine is used widely at low doses in an attempt to secure preferential DA1 stimulation and increase renal perfusion. Higher doses increase cardiac contractility via β_1 stimulation and produce vasoconstriction via α stimulation. Where vasoconstriction is inappropriate this will reduce renal perfusion. Despite the widespread use of low dose dopamine ($< 3\mu g/kg/min$) there is no definite evidence of increased renal perfusion in man. There is, however, evidence of natriuresis and diuresis by enhanced Na^+ transport in the ascending loop of Henlé. This effect is similar to that of a loop diuretic. In addition to the renal effects of DA1 stimulation there may be preferential perfusion of the splanchnic bed which may help maintain the integrity of the gut mucosa and prevent inflammatory activation associated with gut mucosal hypoperfusion.

See also:
Heart failure—assessment, 312; Heart failure—management, 314; Oliguria, 318;
Acute renal failure—management, 322

Gastrointestinal Drugs

H₂ blockers & proton pump inhibitors

Types
- H₂-antagonists: e.g. ranitidine, cimetidine
- Proton pump inhibitors: e.g. omeprazole

Modes of action
These agents inhibit secretion of gastric acid, reducing both volume and acid content, either by antagonism of the histamine H_2 receptor or by inhibiting H^+K^+-APase which fuels the parietal cell proton pump on which acid secretion depends.

Uses
- Peptic ulceration, gastritis, duodenitis
- Reflux oesophagitis
- Prophylaxis against stress ulceration
- Upper gastrointestinal haemorrhage of peptic/stress ulcer origin
- With non-steroidal anti-inflammatory agents in patients with dyspepsia
- Gastric tonometry measurement

Side-effects / complications
- The major concern voiced against these agents is the increased risk of nosocomial pneumonia by removal of the acid barrier. However, this remains an area of controversy.
- H₂-antagonists: rare but include arrhythmias, altered liver function tests, confusion (in the elderly)
- Proton pump inhibitors: altered liver function tests

Notes
Although licensed and frequently used for stress ulcer prophylaxis, overwhelming supportive evidence is scanty. Enteral nutrition has been shown to be as effective.

Some studies have shown efficacy in upper gastrointestinal haemorrhage secondary to stress ulceration or peptic ulceration.

Dosages should be modified in renal failure.

Cimetidine can affect metabolism of other drugs, in particular, warfarin, phenytoin, theophylline and lignocaine (related to hepatic cytochrome P450–linked enzyme systems). This does not occur with ranitidine.

Omeprazole can delay elimination of diazepam, phenytoin and warfarin.

Intravenous omeprazole is currently unlicensed.

Drug dosages

Ranitidine	50mg tds by slow IV bolus, 150mg bd PO
Cimetidine	200–400mg qds by slow IV bolus, 400mg bd PO
Omeprazole	40mg od (over 20–30min), 20–40mg PO

Sucralfate

Modes of action

- Sucralfate is a basic aluminium salt of sucrose octasulphate and is probably not absorbed from the gastrointestinal tract.
- Exerts a cytoprotective effect by preventing mucosal injury. A protective barrier is formed both over normal mucosa and any ulcer lesion providing protection against penetration of gastric acid, bile and pepsin as well as irritants such as aspirin and alcohol.
- Directly inhibits pepsin activity and absorbs bile salts
- Weak antacid activity

Uses

- Peptic ulceration, gastritis, duodenitis
- Reflux oesophagitis
- Prophylaxis against stress ulceration

Side-effects / complications

- Constipation
- Reduced bioavailability of some drugs given orally e.g. digoxin, phenytoin. Can be overcome by giving agents at least 2h apart.
- Use with caution in renal failure due to risk of increased aluminium absorption.

Notes

Although licensed and frequently used for stress ulcer prophylaxis, overwhelming supportive evidence is scanty. Enteral nutrition and gastric acid blockers have been shown to be as effective.

Evidence for a reduced incidence of nosocomial pneumonia compared to H_2 blocker therapy is also conflicting. Significant reduction in nosocomial pneumonia has been shown compared to a combination of H_2 blocker plus antacid but not against H_2 blocker alone.

Antacids should not be given for 30min before and after sucralfate.

Drug dosages

Sucralfate   1g six times a day PO or via NG tube.

209

Antacids

Types
- Sodium bicarbonate
- Magnesium-based antacids: e.g. magnesium trisilicate
- Aluminium-based antacids: e.g. aluminium hydroxide (Aludrox)
- Proprietary combinations: e.g. Gaviscon

Modes of action
- Neutralises gastric acid
- Provides protective coating on upper gastrointestinal mucosa

Uses
- Symptomatic relief of gastritis, duodenitis, oesophagitis
- Stress ulcer prophylaxis (contentious)

Side-effects / complications
- Possible increased risk of nosocomial pneumonia
- Aluminium toxicity (if aluminium-containing antacids are used long-term in patients with renal dysfunction).
- Diarrhoea (magnesium-based antacids)
- Constipation (aluminium-based antacids).
- Metabolic alkalosis if large amounts are administered.
- Milk–alkali syndrome resulting in hypercalcaemia, metabolic alkalosis and renal failure is very rare.

Notes

As their main use is for symptomatic relief, antacids are rarely needed in mechanically ventilated patients.

Continual nasogastric infusion of a weak sodium bicarbonate solution has been used successfully in treating stress ulcer-related haemorrhage.

Drug dosages

Magnesium trisilicate	10–30ml qds
Aluminium hydroxide	10–30ml qds
Gaviscon	10–30ml qds

211

See also:
  Upper gastrointestinal endoscopy, 66; H$_2$ blockers & proton pump inhibitors, 206; Sucralfate, 208; Upper gastrointestinal haemorrhage, 332; Bleeding varices, 334; Bowel perforation and obstruction, 336

Anti-emetics

Types
- Phenothiazines: e.g. prochlorperazine, chlorpromazine
- Benzamides: e.g. metoclopramide, domperidone
- Anti-histamines: e.g. cyclizine
- Ondansetron

Modes of action
- Phenothiazines increase the threshold for vomiting at the chemoreceptor trigger zone via central DA_2-dopaminergic blockade; at higher doses there may also be some effect on the vomiting centre
- Metoclopramide acts centrally and by increasing gastric motility
- The exact mechanism of cyclizine action is unknown. It increases lower oesophageal sphincter tone and may inhibit the midbrain emetic centre.
- Domperidone is a butyrophenone derivative acting both centrally and on gastrointestinal motility by blocking peripheral DA_2-dopaminergic receptors
- Ondansetron is a highly selective $5HT_3$ receptor antagonist; its precise mode of action is unknown but may act both centrally and peripherally

Uses
- Nausea
- Vomiting

Side-effects / complications
- Dystonic or dyskinetic reactions, oculogyric crises (prochlorperazine, metoclopramide, domperidone)
- Arrhythmias (metoclopramide, prochlorperazine)
- Headaches, flushing (ondansetron)
- Urticaria, drowsiness, dry mouth, blurred vision, urinary retention (cyclizine)
- Postural hypotension (prochlorperazine, cyclizine)
- Rarely neuroleptic malignant syndrome (prochlorperazine, metoclopramide)

Notes
The initial choice should fall between prochlorperazine, metoclopramide or cyclizine. Prochlorperazine and cyclizine are preferable when vomiting is related to drugs and metabolic disturbances acting at the chemoreceptor trigger zone while metoclopramide should be tried first if a gastrointestinal cause is implicated.

Metoclopramide and prochlorperazine dosage should be reduced in renal and hepatic failure.

Ondansetron dosage should be reduced in hepatic failure.

Drug dosages

Prochlorperazine	5–10mg tds PO, 12.5mg qds IM or by slow IV bolus (note: not licensed for IV use)
Metoclopramide	10mg tds by slow IV bolus, IM or PO
Cyclizine	50mg tds slow IV bolus, IM or PO
Domperidone	10–20mg tds PO
Ondansetron	4–8mg tds by slow IV bolus, IM or PO

213

See also:
Enteral nutrition, 72; Vomiting / gastric stasis, 326

Gut motility agents

Types
- Metoclopramide
- Cisapride
- Erythromycin

Modes of action
- Metoclopramide probably acts by blocking peripheral DA_2-dopaminergic receptors
- Cisapride stimulates whole bowel motility probably by enhancing acetylcholine release at the gut wall myenteric plexus; effects are largely abolished by atropine.
- Erythromycin is a motilin agonist acting on antral enteric neurones

Uses
- Ileus, large nasogastric aspirates
- Vomiting

Side-effects / complications
- Dystonic or dyskinetic reactions, oculogyric crises (metoclopramide)
- Arrhythmias (cisapride, metoclopramide)
- Diarrhoea, abdominal cramps (cisapride)

Notes
Metoclopramide and cisapride dosage should be reduced in renal failure and hepatic failure and erythromycin in hepatic failure.

Cisapride should not be co-administered with azole antifungals (e.g. ketoconazole) and may prolong prothrombin times in patients taking warfarin.

Drug dosages

Metoclopramide	10mg tds by slow IV bolus, IM or PO
Cisapride	10mg qds
Erythromycin	250mg qds PO or IV

215

See also:
 Enteral nutrition, 72; Vomiting / gastric stasis, 326; Bowel perforation and obstruction, 336

Antidiarrhoeals

Types
- Loperamide
- Codeine phosphate

Modes of action
Loperamide and codeine phosphate bind to gut wall opiate receptors, reducing propulsive peristalsis and increasing anal sphincter tone

Side-effects / complications
- Abdominal cramps, bloating
- Constipation (if excessive amounts given)

Notes
Should not be used when abdominal distension develops, particularly with ulcerative colitis or pseudomembranous colitis, or as sole therapy in infective diarrhoea.

Caution with liver failure for loperamide and renal failure for codeine.

Drug dosages

Loperamide	2 capsules (20ml) initially, then 1 capsule (10ml) after every loose stool for up to 5 days
Codeine phosphate	30–60mg 4–6hrly PO, IM or by slow IV bolus

217

See also:
Enteral nutrition, 72; Diarrhoea, 328; Sepsis / infection, 490

Anti-constipation agents

Types
- Laxatives: e.g. lactulose, propantheline, mebeverine, castor oil
- Bulking agents: e.g. dietary fibre (bran), hemicelluloses (methylcellulose, ispaghula husk)
- Suppositories: e.g. glycerine
- Enemata: e.g. warmed normal saline, olive oil or arachis oil retention enemata,

Modes of action
- Laxatives include
  (i) antispasmodic agents such as anticholinergics (e.g. propantheline) and mebeverine (a phenylethylamine derivative of reserpine)
  (ii) non-absorbable disaccharides (e.g. lactulose) which soften the stool by an osmotic effect and by lactic acid production from a bacterial fermenting effect
  (iii) irritants, such as castor oil, which is hydrolysed in the small intestine releasing ricinoleic acid
- Bulking agents are hydrophilic and thus increase water content of the stool.

Side-effects / complications
- Bloating and abdominal distension
- Diarrhoea if excessive amounts given

Notes
Surgical causes presenting as constipation such as bowel obstruction must be excluded. Other measures should be taken if possible to improve bowel function e.g. reducing concurrent opiate dosage, starting enteral nutrition.

The agent of choice is lactulose.

Larger doses of lactulose are used in hepatic failure as the pH of the colonic contents is reduced; this markedly lowers formation and absorption of ammonium ions and other nitrogenous products into the portal circulation.

Anthraquinone glycosides (e.g. senna) and liquid paraffin are no longer recommended for use.

Drug dosages

Lactulose   15–50ml tds PO

See also:
Enteral nutrition, 72; Failure to open bowels, 330

Neurological Drugs

Opioid analgesics

Types

- Natural opiates: e.g. morphine, codeine
- Semi-synthetic: e.g. diamorphine, dihydrocodeine, papaveretum
- Synthetic: e.g. pethidine, fentanyl, alfentanil

Uses

- Analgesia. Strong analgesics are extracts from opium or synthetic substances with similar properties. They are useful for continuous pain rather than sharp, intermittent pain.
- Sedation
- Mild vasodilatation in heart failure (diamorphine, morphine)
- Anti-diarrhoeal (codeine)

Routes

- IV (morphine, diamorphine, papaveretum, pethidine, fentanyl, alfentanil)
- IM/SC (morphine, codeine, diamorphine, dihydrocodeine, papaveretum, pethidine)
- PO (morphine, codeine, diamorphine, dihydrocodeine, pethidine)
- Epidural (morphine, diamorphine, fentanyl, alfentanil)

Side effects

- Respiratory depression
- Central nervous system depression
- Addiction (rare in the critically ill)
- Withdrawal syndrome (withdraw slowly)
- Stimulation of the vomiting centre
- Appetite loss
- Dry mouth
- Decreased gastric emptying and gut motility
- Histamine release and itching
- Increased muscular tone

Notes

Morphine is poorly absorbed from the gastrointestinal tract and is, therefore, usually administered parenterally. It is metabolised to morphine-6–glucuronide in the liver which is 6 times more potent than morphine and accumulates in renal failure.

Codeine is a weak analgesic but is favoured by some in head injury since it is less sedative than morphine.

Papaveretum is a natural mixture of opiates which has been reformulated as a semi-synthetic product without noscopine.

Pethidine has local anaesthetic properties associated with cardiac depression and vasodilatation. It is metabolised to norpethidine which may lead to seizures on accumulation. Respiratory depression occurs despite maintenance of respiratory rate.

Fentanyl and alfentanil are good, short acting analgesics with poor sedative quality. They cause severe respiratory depression and muscular rigidity.

Drug dosages

Intravenous

	Bolus	Infusion
Morphine	0.1–0.2mg/kg	0.05–0.07mg/kg/h
Diamorphine	0.05–0.1mg/kg	0.03–0.06mg/kg/h
Pethidine	0.5mg/kg	0.1–0.3mg/kg/h
Fentanyl	5–7.5µg/kg	5–20µg/kg/h
Alfentanil	15–30µg/kg	20–120µg/kg/h

Other routes

Morphine	10mg IM/SC 4hrly	5–20mg PO 4hrly
Codeine	30–60mg IM 4hrly	30–60mg PO 4hrly
Diamorphine	5mg IM/SC 4hrly	5–10mg PO 4hrly
Dihydrocodeine	50mg IM/SC 4–6hrly	30mg PO 4–6hrly
Pethidine	25–100mg IM/SC 4hrly	50–150mg PO 4hrly

Note that the above doses are a guide only and may need to be altered widely according to individual circumstances. The correct dose of an opiate analgesic is generally enough to ablate pain.

223

See also:
IPPV—modes of ventilation, 8; IPPV—failure to tolerate ventilation, 10; Non-opioid analgesics, 224; Sedatives, 226; Pain, 496; Post-operative intensive care, 510

Non-opioid analgesics

Types
- Non-steroidal anti-inflammatory drugs: e.g. aspirin, indomethacin, diclofenac
- Paracetamol
- Ketamine
- Nitrous oxide
- Local anaesthetics: e.g. lignocaine, bupivacaine

Uses
- Pain associated with inflammatory conditions (aspirin, indomethacin, diclofenac)
- Post-operative pain and musculoskeletal pain (aspirin, indomethacin, diclofenac, paracetamol, ketamine, nitrous oxide, lignocaine, bupivacaine)
- Opiate sparing effect (aspirin, indomethacin, diclofenac used with strong analgesics)
- Antipyretic (aspirin, paracetamol)

Routes
- IV (ketamine)
- IM (diclofenac)
- PO (aspirin, indomethacin, diclofenac, paracetamol)
- PR (aspirin, diclofenac, paracetamol)
- Local /regional (lignocaine, bupivacaine)
- Inhaled (nitrous oxide)

Side effects
- Gastrointestinal bleeding (aspirin, indomethacin, diclofenac)
- Renal dysfunction (indomethacin, diclofenac if any hypovolaemia)
- Reduced platelet aggregation (aspirin, indomethacin, diclofenac)
- Reduced prothrombin formation (aspirin, indomethacin, diclofenac)
- Myocardial depression (lignocaine, bupivacaine)
- Hypertension and tachycardia (ketamine)
- Seizures (lignocaine, bupivacaine)
- Hallucinations and psychotic tendencies (ketamine—prevented by concurrent use of benzodiazepines or droperidol)

Notes
Paracetamol overdose can cause severe hepatic failure due to the effects of alkylating metabolites. These are normally removed by conjugation with glutathione but stores are rapidly depleted in overdose.

Ketamine is a derivative of phencyclidine used as an intravenous anaesthetic agent. In sub-anaesthetic doses it is a powerful analgesic. Ketamine has several advantages over opiates in that it is associated with good airway maintenance, allows spontaneous respiration and provides cardiovascular stimulation. It is also a bronchodilator.

Nitrous oxide is a powerful, short acting analgesic which is useful to cover short, painful procedures. It is particularly useful when delivered via an intermittent positive pressure breathing system as an adjunct to chest physiotherapy. Nitrous oxide should not be used in cases of undrained pneumothorax since it may diffuse into the pneumothorax resulting in tension.

Drug dosages

Aspirin	600mg PO/PR 4hrly
Indomethacin	50–100mg PO/PR 12hrly
Diclofenac	25–50mg PO 8hrly, 100mg PR 12–24hrly, 75mg IM 12hrly
Paracetamol	0.5–1g PO/PR 4–6hrly
Ketamine	5–25µg/kg/min IV
Lignocaine	Maximum 200mg or 500mg if given with adrenaline*
Bupivacaine	Maximum 150mg*

* Local anaesthetic doses vary according to area to be anaesthetised.
Maximum doses are given to avoid toxic effects.

225

Sedatives

Types
- Benzodiazepines: e.g. diazepam, midazolam
- Chlormethiazole
- Major tranquillisers: e.g. chlorpromazine, haloperidol
- Anaesthetic agents: e.g. propofol, isoflurane

Uses
- Sedation anxiolysis

Routes
- IV (diazepam, midazolam, chlormethiazole, chlorpromazine, haloperidol, propofol)
- IM (diazepam, chlorpromazine, haloperidol)
- PO (diazepam, chlorpromazine, haloperidol)
- Inhaled (isoflurane)

Side effects
- Hypotension (diazepam, midazolam, chlormethiazole, chlorpromazine, haloperidol, propofol)
- Respiratory depression (diazepam, midazolam, chlormethiazole, chlorpromazine, haloperidol, propofol)
- Arrhythmias (chlorpromazine, haloperidol)
- Hypersalivation (chlormethiazole)
- Extrapyramidal disorder (chlorpromazine, haloperidol)
- Fluoride toxicity (isoflurane)

Notes

226

Sedation is necessary for most ICU patients. While the appropriate use of sedative drugs can provide comfort for patients, most of the drugs available have severe cardiovascular and respiratory side effects. Objective assessment of depth of sedation is necessary to ensure that comfort does not give way to excessive levels of sedation. All drugs used are cumulative and infusion doses must be kept to a minimum.

Benzodiazepines have the advantage that they are amnesic. Diazepam is most often administered as an emulsion in intralipid; organic solvents are extremely irritant to veins. Effects of diazepam can be particularly prolonged in hepatic or renal failure and are potentiated by cimetidine. Midazolam is usually shorter acting than diazepam. Some patients suffer severe respiratory depression with hypotension; this effect is unpredictable.

Propofol is an intravenous anaesthetic agent that has gained popularity in intensive care when used in sub-anaesthetic doses. It is short acting although, in common with other sedatives, effects are cumulative when infusions are prolonged or when there is hepatic or renal failure. As propofol is administered as an emulsion in 10% intralipid, infusion volumes may contribute to the calorie load administered.

Chlorpromazine antagonises adrenaline and noradrenaline causing vasodilatation and hypotension. It also has a local anaesthetic effect with may cause cardiac depression.

Isoflurane is largely exhaled unchanged and is therefore short acting. However, cumulative effects have been recorded with prolonged use. Exhaled isoflurane must be adequately scavenged.

Drug dosages

	Bolus	Infusion
Diazepam	0.05–0.15mg/kg	Excessive half-life
Midazolam	50µg/kg	10–50µg/kg/h
Propofol	0.5–2mg/kg	1–3mg/kg/h
Chlormethiazole	0.1–0.2ml/kg/min*	0.5–1.0ml/min
Chlorpromazine	12.5–100mg	Excessive half-life

Note that the above doses are a guide only and may need to be altered widely according to individual circumstances.
*Chlormethiazole is given as a rapid infusion rather than a bolus

Monitoring sedation

Frequent, objective reassessment of sedation depth with corresponding adjustment of infusion doses is necessary to avoid severe cardiovascular and respiratory depression. Simple sedation scores are available to aid assessment.

UCL Hospitals Sedation Score

Agitated and restless	+3
Awake and uncomfortable	+2
Aware but calm	+1
Roused by voice, remains calm	0
Roused by movement	−1
Roused by painful or noxious stimuli	−2
Unrousable	−3
Natural sleep	A

227

Sedation doses are adjusted to achieve a score as close as possible to 0. Positive scores require increased sedation doses and negative scores require reduced sedation doses.

See also:
Ventilatory support—indications, 4; IPPV—modes of ventilation, 8; IPPV—failure to tolerate ventilation, 10; Indirect calorimetry, 158; Opioid analgesics, 222; Hypotension, 300; Agitation / confusion, 358; Sedative poisoning, 444; Post-operative intensive care, 510

Muscle relaxants

Types
- Depolarising: e.g. suxamethonium
- Non-depolarising: e.g. pancuronium, atracurium, vecuronium

Mode of action
- Suxamethonium is structurally related to acetylcholine and causes initial stimulation of muscular contraction seen clinically as fasciculation. During this process, the continued stimulation leads to desensitisation of the post-synaptic membrane of the neuro-muscular junction with efflux of potassium ions. Subsequent flaccid paralysis is short acting (2–3min) and cannot be reversed (is actually potentiated) by anticholinesterase drugs. Prolonged effects are seen where there is congenital or acquired pseudocholinesterase deficiency.
- Non-depolarising muscle relaxants prevent acetylcholine from depolarising the post-synaptic membrane of the neuro-muscular junction by competitive blockade. The effects can be reversed by anticholinesterase drugs (e.g. neostigmine). They have a slower onset and longer duration of action than depolarising muscle relaxants.

Uses
- To facilitate endotracheal intubation
- To facilitate mechanical ventilation where optimal sedation does not prevent patient interference with the function of the ventilator.

Routes
- IV

Side effects
- Hypertension (suxamethonium, pancuronium)
- Bradycardia (suxamethonium)
- Tachycardia (pancuronium)
- Hyperkalaemia (suxamethonium)

Notes
Modern intensive care practice and developments in ventilator technology have rendered the use of muscle relaxants less common. Furthermore, it is rarely necessary to paralyse muscles fully to facilitate mechanical ventilation.

Requirement for muscle relaxants should be reassessed frequently. Ideally, relaxants should be stopped intermittently to allow depth of sedation to be assessed. If mechanical ventilation proceeds smoothly when relaxants have been stopped they probably should not be restarted.

Suxamethonium is contraindicated in spinal neurological disease, hepatic disease and for 5–50 days after burns.

Atracurium is non-cumulative and popular for infusion. Non-enzymatic (Hoffman) degradation allows clearance independent of renal or hepatic function, although effects are prolonged in hypothermia.

Drug dosages

	Bolus	Infusion
Suxamethonium	50–100mg	2–5mg/min
Pancuronium	4mg	1–4mg/h
Atracurium	25–50mg	25–50mg/h
Vecuronium	5–7mg	Excessive half life

Anticonvulsants

Types
- Benzodiazepines: e.g. diazepam, clonazepam
- Phenytoin
- Carbamazapine
- Sodium valproate
- Chlormethiazole
- Magnesium sulphate
- Thiopentone

Uses
- Control of status epilepticus
- Intermittent seizure control
- Myoclonic seizures (clonazepam, sodium valproate)

Routes
- IV (diazepam, clonazepam, phenytoin, sodium valproate, chlormethiazole, magnesium sulphate, thiopentone)
- PO (diazepam, clonazepam, phenytoin, carbamazapine, sodium valproate)
- PR (diazepam)

Side effects
- Sedation (diazepam, clonazepam, chlormethiazole, thiopentone)
- Respiratory depression (diazepam, clonazepam, chlormethiazole, thiopentone)
- Nausea and vomiting (phenytoin, sodium valproate)
- Ataxia (phenytoin, carbamazapine)
- Visual disturbance (phenytoin, carbamazapine)
- Hypotension (diazepam, thiopentone)
- Arrhythmias (phenytoin, carbamazapine)
- Pancreatitis (thiopentone)
- Hepatic failure (sodium valproate)

Notes

Common insults causing seizures include cerebral ischaemic damage, space occupying lesions, metabolic encephalopathy and neurosurgery. Anticonvulsants provide control of seizures but do not replace removal of the cause where this is possible.

Onset of seizure control may be delayed by up to 24h with phenytoin but a loading dose is usually given during the acute phase of seizures.

Magnesium sulphate is especially useful in seizures due to pre-eclampsia and eclampsia.

Phenytoin has a narrow therapeutic range and a non-linear relationship between dose and plasma levels. It is therefore essential to monitor plasma levels frequently. Enteral feeding should be stopped temporarily while oral phenytoin is administered. Intravenous use should only occur if the ECG is monitored continuously.

Carbamazapine has a wider therapeutic range than phenytoin and there is a linear relationship between dose and plasma levels. It is not, therefore, critical to monitor plasma levels frequently.

Plasma concentrations of sodium valproate are not related to effects so monitoring of plasma levels is not useful.

Intravenous drug dosages

	Bolus	Infusion
Diazepam	2.5mg repeated to 20mg	Excessive half life
Phenytoin	18mg/kg at < 50mg/min	100mg 8hrly
Chlormethiazole	5–15ml/min to 100ml	0.1–1ml/min
Magnesium sulphate	20mmol over 10–20min	5–10mmol/h
Sodium valproate	400–800mg	
Clonazepam	1mg	1–2mg/h
Thiopentone	1–3mg/kg	Lowest possible dose

See also:
EEG / CFM monitoring, 130; Generalised seizures, 360; Pre-eclampsia & eclampsia, 478

Neuroprotective agents

Types

- Diuretics: e.g. mannitol, frusemide
- Steroids: e.g. dexamethasone
- Calcium antagonists: e.g. nimodipine
- Barbiturates: e.g. thiopentone

Uses

- Reduction of cerebral oedema (mannitol, frusemide, dexamethasone)
- Prevention of cerebral vasospasm (nimodipine)
- Reduction of cerebral metabolic rate (thiopentone)

Routes

- IV

Notes

Cerebral protection requires generalised sedation and abolition of seizures to reduce cerebral metabolic rate, cerebral oedema and neuronal damage during ischaemia and reperfusion.

Mannitol reduces cerebral interstitial water by the osmotic load. The effect is transient and at its best where the blood brain barrier is intact. The interstitial water is mainly reduced in normal areas of brain and this may accentuate cerebral shift. Repeated doses accumulate in the interstitium and may eventually increase oedema formation; mannitol should only be given 4–5 times in 48h. In addition to the osmotic effect there is some evidence of cerebral vasoconstriction due to a reduction in blood viscosity and free radical scavenging.

The loop diuretic effect of frusemide encourages salt and water loss. There may also be a reduction of CSF chloride transport reducing the formation of CSF.

Dexamethasone reduces oedema around space occupying lesions such as tumours. Steroids are not useful in head injury or after a cerebrovascular accident. It should be noted that steroids encourage salt water retention and they must be withdrawn slowly to avoid rebound oedema.

Nimodipine is used to prevent cerebral vasospasm during recovery from cerebrovascular insults. As a calcium channel blocker it also prevents calcium ingress during neuronal injury. This calcium ingress is associated with cell death. It is commonly used in the management of subarachnoid haemorrhage for 5–14 days.

Thiopentone reduces cerebral metabolism thus prolonging the time that the brain may sustain an ischaemic insult. However, it also reduces cerebral blood flow although blood flow is redistributed preferentially to ischaemic areas. Thiopentone acutely reduces intracranial pressure and this is probably the main cerebroprotective effect. Seizure control is a further benefit. Despite these effects, barbiturate coma has not been shown to improve outcome in cerebral insults of various causes.

Drug dosages

	Bolus	Infusion
Mannitol	20–40g 6hrly	
Frusemide		1–5mg/h
Dexamethasone	4mg 6hrly	
Nimodipine		0.5–2.0mg/h
Thiopentone	1–3mg/kg	Lowest possible dose

233

See also:
Intracranial pressure monitoring, 126; Jugular venous bulb saturation, 128;
EEG / CFM monitoring, 130; Other neurological monitoring, 132; Basic
resuscitation, 258; Generalised seizures, 360; Intracranial haemorrhage, 364;
Subarachnoid haemorrhage, 366; Raised intracranial pressure, 368; Head injury 1,
462; Head injury 2, 464

Haematological Drugs

235

Anticoagulants

Types

- Heparin
- Low molecular weight (LMW) heparin
- Anticoagulant prostanoids: e.g. epoprostenol, alprostadil
- Sodium citrate
- Warfarin

Modes of action

- Heparin potentiates naturally occurring AT-III, reduces the adhesion of platelets to injured arterial walls, binds to platelets and promotes *in vitro* aggregation.
- LMW heparin appears to specifically influence factor Xa activity; its simpler pharmacokinetics allow for a smaller (two thirds) dose to be administered to the same effect.
- The effects of the prostanoids depend on the balance between thromboxane (TXA_2) and epoprostenol (PGI_2). At a wounded endothelial surface the effects of TXA_2 predominate, allowing platelet activation, aggregation and plugging of the vessel wall. There is also local vasoconstriction to reduce blood flow into the wounded area. If PGI_2 is infused into an extracorporeal circuit the opposite effect is achieved since TXA_2 levels are very low.
- Sodium citrate chelates ionised calcium.
- Warfarin produces a controlled deficiency of vitamin K dependent coagulation factors (II, VII, IX and X).

Uses

- Maintenance of an extracorporeal circulation
- Treatment of thromboembolism
- Prevention of thromboembolism

Routes

- IV (heparins, anticoagulant prostanoids, sodium citrate)
- SC (heparins)
- PO (warfarin)

Side effects

- Bleeding
- Hypotension (anticoagulant prostanoids)
- Heparin induced thrombocytopenia
- Hypocalcaemia and hypernatraemia (sodium citrate)

Notes

Alprostadil has similar effects to epoprostanil but is less potent. It is also metabolised in the lungs so that systemic vasodilatation effects should be minimal. This may be an important advantage in the shocked patient.

For extracorporeal use citrate has advantages over heparin in that it has no known anti-platelet activity, is readily filtered by a haemofilter (reducing systemic anticoagulation), and is overwhelmed and neutralised when returned to central venous blood.

Warfarin is given orally and requires 48–72h to develop its effect.

Drug Dosages

Heparin
Dose requirement is variable to produce an APTT of 1.5–3 times control. This usually requires 500–2000IU/h with an initial loading dose of 3000–5000IU.

Low molecular weight heparin
For deep vein thrombosis prophylaxis give 2500IU 12hrly subcutaneously. For anticoagulation of an extracorporeal circuit a bolus of 35IU/kg is given intravenously followed by an infusion of 13IU/kg. The dose is adjusted to maintain anti-factor Xa activity at 0.5–1IU/ml (or 0.2–0.4IU/ml if there is a high risk of haemorrhage).

Anticoagulant prostaglandins
Usual to infuse 2.5–10ng/kg/min. If used for an extracorporeal circulation the infusion should be started 30min prior to commencement.

Sodium citrate
Infused at 5mmol per litre of extracorporeal blood flow

Warfarin
Start at 10mg/day orally for 2 days then 1–6mg/day according to INR. For DVT prophylaxis, pulmonary embolus, mitral stenosis, atrial fibrillation and tissue valve replacements the INR should be maintained between 2 and 3. For recurrent DVT or pulmonary embolus and mechanical valve replacements the INR should be kept between 3 and 4.5.

237

Thrombolytics

Types
- Alteplase (rt-PA)
- Anistreplase (APSAC)
- Streptokinase
- Urokinase

Modes of action
Activate plasminogen to form plasmin which degrades fibrin

Uses
- Life-threatening venous thrombosis
- Life-threatening pulmonary embolus,
- Acute myocardial infarction
- To unblock indwelling vascular access catheters.

Routes
- IV

Side effects
- Bleeding, particularly from invasive procedures
- Hypotension and arrhythmias
- Embolisation from pre-existing clot as it is broken down
- Anaphylactoid reactions (anistreplase, streptokinase, urokinase)

Contraindications (absolute)
- Cerebrovascular accident in last 2months
- Active bleeding in last 10 days
- Pregnancy
- Recent peptic ulceration
- Recent surgery

Contraindications (relative)
- Systolic BP > 200mmHg
- Aortic dissection
- Proliferative diabetic retinopathy

Notes
In acute myocardial infarction they are of most value when used within 12h of the onset. They may require adjuvant therapy (e.g. aspirin with streptokinase or heparin with rt-PA) to maximise the effect in acute myocardial infarction.

rt-PA is said to be clot selective and is therefore useful where a need for invasive procedures has been identified.

Streptokinase is the usual first line thrombolytic in acute myocardial infarction since it is cheaper and there is no additional benefit with the others.

Anaphylactoid reactions to streptokinase are not uncommon, particularly in those who have had streptococcal infections. Patients should not be exposed twice between 5 days and 1 year of receiving the last dose.

Drug dosages

Alteplase (rt-PA) — the dose schedule for acute myocardial infarction is 10mg in 1–2min, 50mg in 1h and 40mg over 2h intravenously.

Anistreplase — single intravenous injection of 30u over 4–5min.

Streptokinase — in acute myocardial infarction (1.5mu over 60min).
— in severe venous thrombosis (250 000u over 30min followed by 100 000u/h for 24–72h).

Urokinase — for unblocking indwelling vascular catheters 5 000–37 500iu are instilled.
— for thromboembolic disease 4400iu/kg is given over 10min followed by 4400iu/kg/h for 12–24h.

239

See also:
Coagulation monitoring, 146; Coagulants & antifibrinolytics, 242; Hypotension, 300; Tachyarrhythmias, 304; Bradyarrhythmias, 306; Acute myocardial infarction, 308; Anaphylactoid reactions, 492

Blood products

Types
- Plasma: e.g. fresh frozen plasma
- Platelets
- Concentrates of coagulation factors: e.g. cryoprecipitate, factor VIII concentrate, factor IX complex

Uses
- Vitamin K deficiency (fresh frozen plasma, factor IX complex)
- Haemophilia (cryoprecipitate)
- von Willebrand's disease (cryoprecipitate)
- Fibrinogen deficiency (cryoprecipitate)
- Christmas disease (factor IX complex)

Routes
- IV

Notes
A unit (150ml) of fresh frozen plasma is usually collected from one donor and contains all coagulation factors including 200u factor VIII, 200u factor IX and 400mg fibrinogen. Fresh frozen plasma is stored at $-30°C$ and should be infused within 2h once defrosted.

Platelet concentrates are viable for 3 days when stored at room temperature. If they are refrigerated viability decreases. They must be infused quickly via a short giving set with no filter. Indications for platelet concentrates include platelet count $< 10 \times 10^9/L$, platelet count $< 50 \times 10^9/L$ with spontaneous bleeding or to cover invasive procedures, and spontaneous bleeding with platelet dysfunction. They are less useful in conditions associated with immune platelet destruction (e.g. ITP).

A 15ml vial of cryoprecipitate contains 100u factor VIII, 250mg fibrinogen, factor XIII and von Willebrand factor and is stored at $-30°C$. In haemophilia, cryoprecipitate is given to achieve a factor VIII level $> 30\%$ of normal.

Factor VIII concentrate contains 300u factor VIII per vial. In severe haemorrhage due to haemophilia 10–15u/kg are given 12hrly.

Factor IX complex is rich in factors II, IX and X. It is formed from pooled plasma so fresh frozen plasma is preferred.

241

Coagulants & antifibrinolytics

Types
- Vitamin K
- Protamine
- Tranexamic acid

Uses
- To reverse a prolonged prothrombin time, e.g. malabsorption, oral anticoagulant therapy, β lactam antibiotics or critical illness (vitamin K)
- To reverse the effects of heparin (protamine)
- Bleeding from raw surfaces, e.g. prostatectomy, dental extraction (tranexamic acid)
- Bleeding from thrombolytics (tranexamic acid)

Routes
- IV (vitamin K, protamine, tranexamic acid)
- PO (vitamin K, tranexamic acid)

Notes
The effects of vitamin K are prolonged so it should be avoided where patients are dependent on oral anticoagulant therapy. A dose of 10mg is given orally or by slow intravenous injection daily. In life threatening haemorrhage 5–10mg is given by slow intravenous injection with other coagulation factor concentrates. If INR > 7 or in less severe haemorrhage 0.5–2mg may be given by slow intravenous injection with minimum lasting effect on oral anticoagulant therapy.

Protamine has an anticoagulant effect of its own in high doses. Protamine 1mg neutralises 100iu unfractionated heparin if given within 15min. Less is required if given later since heparin is excreted rapidly. Protamine should be given by slow intravenous injection according to the APTT. Total dose should not exceed 50mg. Protamine injection may cause severe hypotension

Tranexamic acid has an antifibrinolytic effect by antagonising plasminogen. The usual dose is 1–1.5g 6–12hrly orally or by slow intravenous injection.

243

Aprotinin

The role of serine protease inhibitors in coagulation and anticoagulation is complicated due to their effects at various points in the coagulation pathway. Aprotinin is a naturally occurring, non-specific serine protease inhibitor with an elimination half life of about 2h. Prevention of systemic bleeding with aprotinin does not promote coagulation within the extracorporeal circulation and may even contribute to the maintenance of extracorporeal anticoagulation.

Modes of action

The effects of aprotinin on the coagulation cascade are dependent on the circulating plasma concentrations (expressed as kallikrein inactivation units—kIU/ml) since the affinity of aprotinin for plasmin is significantly greater than that for plasma kallikrein. At a plasma level of 125kIU/ml aprotinin inhibits fibrinolysis and complement activation. Inhibition of plasma kallikrein requires higher doses to provide plasma levels of 250–500kIU/ml.

- Plasma kallikrein inhibition—reduces blood coagulation mediated via contact with anionic surfaces and, in the critically ill patient, improve circulatory stability via reduced kinin activation.
- Prevention of inappropriate platelet activation.—neutrophil activation (complement or kallikrein mediated) causes a secondary activation of platelets. Important in this platelet—neutrophil interaction is the release of Cathepsin G by neutrophil degranulation. It has been demonstrated recently that aprotinin can significantly inhibit the platelet activation due to purified Cathepsin G, this mechanism forming a direct inhibition of inappropriate neutrophil mediated platelet activation.

Uses

- The main role of aprotinin in the management of the extracorporeal circulation has been to prevent bleeding associated with heparinisation. High dose aprotinin given during cardiopulmonary bypass procedures has been shown to reduce post-operative blood loss dramatically.
- More recently, the same dose regimen of aprotinin has been used to arrest bleeding associated with prolonged extracorporeal CO_2 removal.

Drug dosages

Aprotinin—loading dose of 2×10^6kIU followed by $500\,000$kIU/h

245

See also:

Non-ventilatory respiratory support, 26; Haemo(dia)filtration 1, 54;
Haemo(dia)filtration 2, 56; Anticoagulants, 236; Post-operative intensive care,
510

Miscellaneous Drugs

Antimicrobials

Types

- Penicillins: e.g. benzylpenicillin, flucloxacillin, azlocillin, piperacillin, ampicillin
- Cephalosporins: e.g. cefotaxime, ceftazidime, cefuroxime
- Carbapenems: e.g. imipenem, meropenem
- Aminoglycosides: e.g. gentamicin, amikacin, netilmicin, tobramycin
- Other antibacterials: e.g. erythromycin, clindamycin, metronidazole, ciprofloxacin, co-trimoxazole, rifampicin, teicoplanin, vancomycin
- Antifungals: e.g. amphotericin, flucytosine, fluconazole
- Antivirals: e.g. acyclovir

Uses

- Treatment of infection.
- Prophylaxis against infection, e.g. peri-operatively
- Local choice of antimicrobial varies. However, as a guide, the following choices are common:
  - Pneumonia (hospital acquired)—ceftazidime or ciprofloxacin or meropenem
  - Pneumonia (community acquired)—cefuroxime + erythromycin
  - Systemic sepsis—cefuroxime + gentamicin (+ metronidazole if anaerobes likely)

Routes

Generally IV in critically ill patients.

Side-effects

- Hypersensitivity reactions (all)
- Seizures (high dose penicillins, high dose metronidazole, ciprofloxacin)
- Gastrointestinal disturbance (cephalosporins, erythromycin, clindamycin, teicoplanin, vancomycin, co-trimoxazole, rifampicin, metronidazole, ciprofloxacin, amphotericin, flucytosine)
- Vestibular damage (aminoglycosides)
- Renal failure (aminoglycosides, teicoplanin, vancomycin, ciprofloxacin, rifampicin, amphotericin, acyclovir)
- Erythema multiforme (co-trimoxazole)
- Leucopenia (co-trimoxazole, metronidazole, teicoplanin, ciprofloxacin, flucytosine, acyclovir)
- Peripheral neuropathy (metronidazole)

Notes

Antimicrobials should be chosen according to microbial sensitivities, usually based on advice from the microbiology laboratory.

Appropriate empiric therapy for serious infections should be determined by likely organisms taking into account known community and hospital infection and resistance patterns.

Up to 10% of penicillin allergic patients are also cephalosporin allergic.

Drug dosages (intravenous)

Benzylpenicillin	1.2g 6hrly (2hrly for pneumococcal pneumonia)
Flucloxacillin	500mg-2g 6hrly
Azlocillin	2–5g 8hrly
Piperacillin	4g 6hrly
Ampicillin	500mg-1g 6hrly
Cefotaxime	1–4g 8hrly
Ceftazidime	2g 8hrly
Cefuroxime	750mg-1.5g 8hrly
Gentamicin	1.5mg/kg stat then by levels (usually 80mg 8hrly)
Amikacin	7.5mg/kg stat then by levels (usually 500mg 12hrly)
Netilmicin	5–7.5mg/kg stat then by levels (usually 150mg 8hrly)
Tobramycin	5mg/kg stat then by levels (usually 100mg 8hrly)
Erythromycin	500mg-1g 6–12hrly
Metronidazole	500mg 8hrly or 1g 12hrly PR
Clindamycin	300–600mg 6hrly
Ciprofloxacin	200–400mg 12hrly
Co-trimoxazole	960mg12hrly in *Pneumocystis carinii* pneumonia
Imipenem	250mg-1g 6–8hrly
Meropenem	500mg-1g 8hrly
Rifampicin	600mg daily
Teicoplanin	400mg 12hrly for 3 doses then 400mg daily
Vancomycin	500mg 6hrly (monitor levels)
Amphotericin	250µg-1mg/kg daily
Flucytosine	25–50mg/kg 6hrly
Fluconazole	200–400mg daily
Acyclovir	10mg/kg 8hrly

Most antimicrobials need dose adjustment for renal or hepatic failure

249

Common choices for specific organisms

Staph aureus	flucloxacillin
Multi-resistant *Staph aureus*	teicoplanin, vancomycin
Strep pneumoniae	cefuroxime, benzylpenicillin
N meningitidis	cefuroxime, benzylpenicillin
H influenzae	cefuroxime, cefotaxime
E coli	cefotaxime, ceftazidime, ciprofloxacin, gentamicin, imipenem, meropenem
Klebsiella spp	cefotaxime, ceftazidime, ciprofloxacin, gentamicin, imipenem, meropenem
Ps aeruginosa	azlocillin, ceftazidime, ciprofloxacin, gentamicin, imipenem, meropenem, piperacillin

Steroids

Uses

- Anti-inflammatory—in the critically ill steroids are usually given in high dose for their anti-inflammatory effect, e.g. asthma, allergic and anaphylactoid reactions, vasculitic disorders, rheumatoid arthritis, inflammatory bowel disease, neoplasm-related cerebral oedema, the fibroproliferative phase of ARDS, pneumococcal meningitis, pneumocystis pneumonia, laryngeal oedema (e.g. after repeated intubation) and after spinal cord injury. Effect is unproved in cerebral oedema following head injury or cardio-respiratory arrest and is deleterious in cerebral malaria.
- Multi-centre trials have not shown efficacy in sepsis though there may be possible benefit in subgroups with (i) depressed adrenal function (subnormal Synacthen response, despite 'normal' plasma cortisol levels) and (ii) profound hypotension as steroids have also been shown to reduce nitric oxide production.
- Replacement therapy is needed for patients with Addison's disease and after adrenalectomy or pituitary surgery. In the longer term, fludrocortisone is usually required in addition for its mineralo-corticoid sodium-retaining effect. Higher replacement doses are needed in chronic steroid takers (i.e. > 2 weeks within the last year) undergoing a stress, e.g. surgery, infection.
- Immunosuppressive—after organ transplantation

Side-effects / complications

- Sodium and water retention (especially with mineralocorticoids)
- Hypoadrenal crisis if stopped abruptly after prolonged treatment
- Immunosuppressive—possibly increased infection risk *(q.v.)*
- Neutrophilia
- Impaired glucose tolerance/diabetes mellitus
- Hypokalaemic alkalosis
- Osteoporosis, proximal myopathy (long-term use)
- Increased susceptibility to peptic ulcer disease

Notes

The perceived heightened risk of systemic infection may be exaggerated. Chronic steroid users generally appear no more affected than the general population; studies in ARDS and sepsis revealed no greater incidence of infection post-steroid administration. Oral fungal infection is relatively common with inhaled steroids but systemic and pulmonary fungal infection is predominantly seen in the severely immunocompromised (e.g. AIDS, post-chemotherapy) and not those taking high-dose steroids alone.

The choice of corticosteroid for short-term anti-inflammatory effect is probably irrelevant provided the dose is sufficient. Chronic hydrocortisone should be avoided for anti-inflammatory use because of its mineralocorticoid effect but is appropriate for adrenal replacement.

Prednisone and cortisone are inactive until metabolised by the liver to prednisolone and hydrocortisone respectively; their use should be avoided.

Glucocorticoids antagonise the effects of anticholinesterase drugs. Steroids are not likely to cause critical illness myopathy.

Relative potency and activity

Drug	Gluco-corticoid activity	Mineralo-corticoid activity	Equivalent anti-inflammatory dose (mg)
Cortisone	+ +	+ +	25
Dexamethasone	+ + + +	−	0.75
Hydrocortisone	+ +	+ +	20
Methylprednisolone	+ + +	+	4
Prednisolone	+ + +	+	5
Prednisone	+ + +	+	5
Fludrocortisone	+	+ + + +	—

Drug dosages

Drug	Replacement dose	Anti-inflammatory dose
Dexamethasone	—	4–20mg tds IV
Hydrocortisone	20–30mg daily	100–200mg qds IV
Methylprednisolone	—	500mg-1g IV daily
Prednisolone	2.5–15mg mane	40–60mg od PO
Fludrocortisone	0.05–0.3mg daily	—

Weaning

Acute use (< 3–4 days) can stop immediately
Short-term use (≥3–4 days) wean over 2–5 days
Medium-term use (weeks) wean over 1–2 weeks
Long-term use (months/years) wean slowly (months to years)

251

Prostaglandins

Types
- Epoprostenol (prostacyclin, PGI_2)
- Alprostadil (PGE_1)

Modes of action
- Stimulate adenyl cyclase thus increasing platelet cAMP concentration; this inhibits phospholipase and cycloxygenase and thus reduces platelet aggregation (epoprostenol is the most potent inhibitor known)
- Reduces platelet procoagulant activity and release of heparin neutralising factor
- May have a fibrinolytic effect
- Pulmonary and systemic vasodilation by relaxation of vascular smooth muscle

Uses
- Anticoagulation, particularly for extracorporeal circuits, either as a substitute or in addition to heparin
- Pulmonary hypertension
- Microvascular hypoperfusion (including digital vasculitis)
- Haemolytic uraemic syndrome
- Acute respiratory failure (by inhalation)

Side-effect & complications
- Hypotension
- Bleeding (particularly cannula sites)
- Flushing, headache

Notes

Epoprostenol is active on both pulmonary and systemic circulations.

Although alprostadil is claimed to be metabolised in the lung and have only pulmonary vasodilating effects, falls in systemic blood pressure are not uncommonly seen, especially if metabolism is incomplete. Effects last up to 30 min following discontinuation of the drug.

Avoid extravasation into peripheral tissues as the solution has a high pH.

Recent studies have shown improvement in gas exchange by selective pulmonary vasodilatation following inhalation of epoprostenol at doses of 10–15ng/kg/min. The efficacy appears similar to that of nitric oxide inhalation but is not as rapid.

Prostaglandins may potentiate the effect of heparin.

Drug dosages

| Epoprostenol | 2–20ng/kg/min |
| Alprostadil | 2–20ng/kg/min |

Novel therapies in sepsis

Greater understanding of the pathophysiology of sepsis has stimulated development and investigation of various agents which modulate different components of the inflammatory response. These drugs have been targeted at triggers (e.g. endotoxin), cytokines (e.g. tumour necrosis factor, interleukin-1,), and effector cells and their products (e.g. neutrophils, free oxygen radicals, nitric oxide) or aim to boost a general anti-inflammatory response (e.g. steroids). An increasing area of research is in replacement or augmentation of endogenous anti-inflammatory systems e.g. antithrombin-III, interleukin-10, as there is an increasing realisation of the degree of disruption and imbalance between pro- and anti-inflammatory substances.

Unfortunately, due to deficiencies in trial design and size, choice of appropriate patient, timing of drug administration, dosage, and lack of standardisation of concurrent therapies, no multi-centre trial has shown conclusive benefit on an intention-to-treat basis. Promising results from post-hoc subgroup analysis and from tightly controlled small patient studies have not been reproduced. Concern over cost has highlighted the potential budgetary implications of any successful therapy though, in terms of life years, the cost–benefit will be relatively cheap.

Uses
- Sepsis
- Multiple-organ dysfunction

Drugs investigated in multi-centre studies

- Methylprednisolone
- Polyclonal immunoglobulin
- Anti-endotoxin antibody (HA-1A, E5)
- Anti-tumour necrosis factor antibody
- Tumour necrosis factor soluble receptor antibody
- Interleukin-1 receptor antagonist
- Platelet activating factor antagonists
- Bradykinin antagonists
- Naloxone
- Ibuprofen
- n-acetyl cysteine
- Prostaglandin E_1
- L-N-mono-methyl-arginine (L-NMMA)
- Antithrombin III

255

See also:
Systemic inflammatory response, 488; Sepsis / infection, 490

Resuscitation

Basic resuscitation

In any severe cardiorespiratory disturbance the order of priority should be to secure the airway, maintain respiration (i.e. manual ventilation if necessary), restore the circulation (with external cardiac massage if necessary) and consider mechanical ventilation. Initial assessment of the patient should include patency of the airway, palpation of the pulses, measurement of blood pressure, presumptive diagnosis and consideration of treatment of the cause.

Airway protection

The airway should be opened by lifting the jaw forward and tilting the forehead. The mouth and pharynx should be cleared by suction and loose fitting dentures removed. If necessary an oropharyngeal (Guedel) airway may be inserted.

Manual ventilation

Once the airway is protected the patient who is not breathing requires manual ventilation with a self inflating bag and mask (Ambu bag). Oxygen should be delivered in maximum concentration (FIO_2 1.0 for manual ventilation, FIO_2 0.6–1.0 for spontaneously breathing patients). If the patient breathes inadequately (poor arterial saturation, hypercapnia, rapid shallow breathing) ventilatory support should continue.

Circulation

If pulses are not palpable or are weak, or if the patient has a severe bradycardia external cardiac massage is required and treatment should continue as for a cardiac arrest. Hypotension should be treated initially with a fluid challenge although life-threatening hypotension may require blind treatment with adrenaline 0.05–0.2mg increments intravenously at 1–2min intervals until a satisfactory blood pressure is restored. Such treatment should not be prolonged without circulatory monitoring to ensure adequacy of cardiac output as well as correction of hypotension.

Venous access

Venous access must be secured early during basic resuscitation. Large bore cannulae are necessary, e.g. 14G. In cases of haemorrhage at least two cannulae are required. Small peripheral veins should be avoided; forearm flexure veins are appropriate if nowhere else is available. In very difficult patients a Seldinger approach to the femoral vein or a central neck vein may be appropriate. The latter has the advantage of providing central venous monitoring.

See also:

Cardiac arrest

As with basic resuscitation the order of priority is airway, breathing and circulation followed by drug treatment. If the cardiac arrest is witnessed a precordial thump may revert ventricular tachycardia or ventricular fibrillation. Initial management of the airway and respiration is as for basic resuscitation. When intubation is attempted it should be effected after adequate pre-oxygenation and quickly to avoid hypoxaemia. If intubation is difficult, maintain manual ventilation with an Ambu bag, mask and 100% oxygen.

Cardiac massage

External cardiac massage provides minimal circulatory support during cardiac arrest. A compression rate of 80–100/min is likely to provide the optimum blood flow during cardiac massage with a manual breath from an assistant for every 5 compressions. Avoid massage during manual inspiration if the patient is not intubated (to avoid gastric dilatation); otherwise cardiac massage is more effective if not synchronised to respiration.

Defibrillation

Defibrillation should be performed urgently if VT or VF cannot be excluded. It is important to restart cardiac massage immediately after defibrillation without waiting for the ECG to recover. Cerebral damage continues while there is no blood flow.

Drugs

Few drugs are necessary for first line cardiac arrest management. Drugs should be given via a large vein since vasoconstriction and poor flow create delay in injections given via small peripheral veins reaching the central circulation. Access should be secured early during the resuscitation; if venous access cannot be secured double or triple doses of drugs may be given via the endotracheal tube.

Adrenaline

The α constrictor effects predominate during cardiac arrest such that adrenaline helps to maintain aortic diastolic blood pressure and therefore coronary and cerebral perfusion. Adrenaline should be given irrespective of rhythm at 1mg (10ml of 1:10 000 solution) every 10 CPR sequences.

Atropine

A single 3mg dose is given early in asystole.

Calcium chloride

Used in electromechanical dissociation if there is hyperkalaemia, hypocalcaemia or calcium antagonist use. A dose of 10ml of a 10% solution is usual. The main disadvantage of calcium is the reduction of reperfusion of ischaemic brain and promotion of cytosolic calcium accumulation during cell death.

Sodium bicarbonate

Only used if resuscitation is prolonged to correct temporarily a potentially lethal pH. A dose of 50ml of 8.4% solution is given. The main disadvantage is that intracellular and respiratory acidosis are exacerbated unless ventilation is increased and the cause of the metabolic acidosis is not corrected.

261

Fluid challenge

Hypovolaemia must be treated urgently to avoid the serious complication of organ failure. An adequate circulating volume must be provided before considering other methods of circulatory support. Clinical signs of hypovolaemia (reduced skin turgor, low CVP, oliguria, tachycardia and hypotension) are late indicators. Lifting the legs of a supine patient and watching for an improvement in the circulation is a useful indicator of hypovolaemia. A high index of suspicion must be maintained; a normal heart rate, blood pressure and CVP do not exclude hypovolaemia and the CVP is particularly unreliable in pulmonary vascular disease, right ventricular disease, isolated left ventricular failure and valvular heart disease. The absolute CVP or PAWP are also difficult to interpret since peripheral venoconstriction may maintain CVP despite hypovolaemia; indeed, CVP may fall in response to fluid. The response to a fluid challenge is the safest method of assessment.

Choice of fluid

The aim of a fluid challenge is to produce a significant (200ml) and rapid increase in plasma volume. Colloid fluids are ideal; a gelatin solution is recommended for short term plasma volume expansion in simple hypovolaemia and hydroxyethyl starch where there is a probability of capillary leak. Packed red cells have a high haematocrit and do not adequately expand the plasma volume. Crystalloid fluids are rapidly lost from the circulation and do not give a reliable increase in plasma volume.

Assessing the response to a fluid challenge

Ideally, the response of CVP, or stroke volume and PAWP, should be monitored during a fluid challenge. Fluid challenges should be repeated while the response suggests continuing hypovolaemia. However, if such monitoring is not available it is reasonable to assess the clinical response to up to two fluid challenges (200ml each).

CVP response
The change in CVP after a 200ml fluid challenge depends on the starting blood volume (Figure). A 3mmHg rise in CVP represents a significant increase and is probably indicative of an adequate circulating volume. However, a positive response may sometimes occur in the vasoconstricted patient with a lower blood volume. It is important to assess the clinical response in addition; if inadequate it is appropriate to monitor stroke volume and PAWP before further fluid challenges or considering further circulatory support.

Stroke volume and PAWP response
In the inadequately filled left ventricle a fluid challenge will increase the stroke volume. Failure to increase the stroke volume with a fluid challenge may represent an inadequate challenge, particularly if the PAWP fails to rise significantly (3mmHg). This indicates that cardiac filling was inadequate and the fluid challenge should be repeated. Such a response may also be seen in right heart failure, pericardial tamponade and mitral stenosis. It is important to monitor stroke volume rather than cardiac output during a fluid challenge. If the heart rate falls appropriately in response to a fluid challenge the cardiac output may not increase despite an increase in stroke volume.

CVP and stroke volume response to fluid challenge

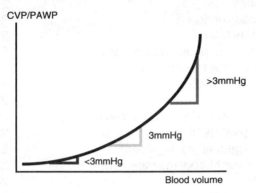

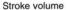

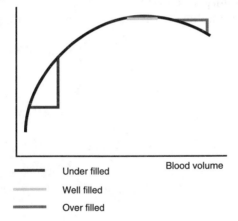

263

Respiratory Disorders

Dyspnoea

Defined as difficulty in breathing. The respiratory rate may be increased or decreased though the respiratory effort is usually increased with the use of accessory muscles. The patient may show signs of progressive fatigue and impaired gas exchange.

Commoner ICU causes

Respiratory	respiratory failure
Circulatory	heart failure, hypoperfusion, pulmonary embolus, severe anaemia
Metabolic	acidosis
Central	stimulants, e.g. aspirin
Anaphylactic	upper airway obstruction, bronchospasm
Psychogenic	hysterical

Principles of management

1 O_2 therapy to maintain SaO_2 (ideally $> 90\text{--}95\%$)
2 Correct abnormality where possible
3 Support therapy until recovery
   — mechanical, e.g. positive pressure ventilation, CPAP
   — pharmacological treatment, e.g. bronchodilators, vasodilators
4 Relieve anxiety

A psychogenic cause of dyspnoea is only made after exclusion of other treatable causes.
   Dual coexisting pathologies should be considered, e.g. chest infection and hypovolaemia.

267

Airway obstruction

Causes
- In the lumen, e.g. foreign body, blood clot, vomitus, sputum plug
- In the wall, e.g. epiglottitis, laryngeal oedema, neoplasm
- Outside the wall, e.g. trauma (facial, neck), thyroid mass

Presentation
- In spontaneously breathing patient: stridor, dyspnoea, fatigue, cyanosis
- In ventilated patient (intraluminal obstruction): raised airway pressures, decreased tidal volume, hypoxaemia, hypercapnia

Diagnosis
- Chest and lateral neck X-ray
- Fibreoptic laryngoscopy/bronchoscopy
- CT scan

Management
Presentation outside ICU/operating theatre:
1 High FIO_2
2 If collapsed or in extremis: immediate orotracheal intubation. If impossible, emergency cricothyroidotomy or tracheostomy.
3 If symptomatic but not in extremis: consider cause and treat as appropriate, e.g. fibreoptic or rigid bronchoscopy for removal of foreign body, laser treatment for neoplasm, surgery for thyroid mass, elective orotracheal intubation or tracheostomy.
4 With acute epiglottitis, the use of a tongue depressor or nasendoscopy may precipitate complete obstruction so should be undertaken in an operating theatre ready to perform emergency tracheostomy. The responsible organism is usually *Haemophilus influenzae* and early treatment with chloramphenicol should be begun. Acute epiglottitis is recognised in adults, even those of advanced age.
5 Consider Heliox (79%He/21%O_2) alone or as a supplement to oxygen to reduce viscosity and improve airflow.

Presentation within ICU/operating theatre
1 If intubated:
   - High FIO_2
   - Pass suction catheter down the ET tube, assess ease of passage and the contents suctioned. If the tube is patent, attempt repeated suction interspersed with 5ml boluses of 0.9% saline. Urgent fibreoptic bronchoscopy may be necessary for diagnosis and, if possible, removal of a foreign body. If this cannot be removed by fibreoptic bronchoscopy, urgent rigid bronchoscopy should be performed by an experienced operator. If the ET tube is obstructed, remove, oxygenate by mask then reintubate.
2 If not intubated:
   - As for out-of-ICU presentation.

- If recently extubated, consider laryngeal oedema. Post-extubation laryngeal oedema is unpredictable though occurs more commonly after prolonged or repeated intubation; the incidence may be reduced by proper tethering of the endotracheal tube and prevention of excessive coughing. If diagnosed (by nasendoscopy), dexamethasone 4mg × 3 doses over 24h may reduce the swelling though re-intubation is often necessary in the interim.

269

Respiratory failure

Defined as impaired pulmonary gas exchange leading to hypoxaemia and/or hypercapnia.

Commoner ICU causes

Central	Cerebrovascular accident, drugs (e.g. opiates, sedatives), raised intracranial pressure, trauma
Brainstem/spinal cord	trauma (at or above phrenic level), tetanus, Pickwickian syndrome, motor neurone disease
Neuropathy	Guillain–Barré, critical illness polyneuropathy
Neuromuscular	muscle relaxants, organophosphorus poisoning, myasthenia gravis
Chest wall/muscular	flail chest, heart failure, myopathy (including critical illness & disuse myopathy)
Airways	upper airways obstruction, airway disruption, asthma, anaphylaxis
Parenchymal	pneumonia, ARDS, fibrosis, pulmonary oedema
Extra-pulmonary	pneumothorax, pleural effusion, haemothorax
Circulatory	pulmonary embolus, heart failure, Eisenmenger intra-cardiac shunt

Types of respiratory failure

Type I: Hypoxaemic—often parenchymal in origin
Type II: Hypoxaemic, hypercapnic—often mechanical in origin

Principles of management

1 Ensure SaO_2 compatible with survival (i.e. > 80%, preferably > 90–95%)
2 Correct abnormality where possible, e.g. drain pneumothorax, relieve/bypass obstruction.
3 Support therapy until recovery
   - positive pressure ventilation
   - non-invasive respiratory support
   - pharmacological treatment, e.g. bronchodilators, antibiotics, opiate antagonists, respiratory stimulants
   - general measures, e.g. hydration, airway humidification, removal of secretions, physiotherapy, bronchoscopy
4 Unless the patient is symptomatic (e.g. drowsy, dyspnoeic), the $PaCO_2$ may be left elevated to minimise ventilator trauma (permissive hypercapnia) or if chronically hypercapnic (Type II respiratory failure).

See also:
Oxygen therapy, 2; Ventilatory support—indications, 4; Continuous positive airway pressure, 22; Non-invasive respiratory support, 24; Endotracheal intubation, 28; Pulse oximetry, 86; Blood gas analysis, 94; Opioid analgesics, 222; Sedatives, 226; Respiratory stimulants, 178; Basic resuscitation, 258; Dyspnoea, 266; Acute weakness, 356; Intracranial haemorrhage, 364; Subarachnoid haemorrhage, 366; Guillain– Barr[3] syndrome, 370; Myasthenia gravis, 372; Poisoning—general principles,438; Sedative poisoning, 444; Multiple trauma 1, 458; Multiple trauma 2, 460; Head injury 1, 462; Head injury 2, 464; Spinal cord injury, 466; Systemic inflammatory response, 488; Pain, 496; Post-operative intensive care, 510; HIV related disease, 512

Atelectasis and pulmonary collapse

A collapsed lobe or segment is usually visible on a chest X-ray. Macroatelectasis is also evident as volume loss. In microatelectasis the chest X-ray may be normal but A-aDO$_2$ will be high. Atelectasis reduces lung compliance and PaO$_2$, and increases work of breathing. This may result in poor gas exchange, increased airway pressures, reduced tidal volume and, if severe, circulatory collapse.

Causes

- Collapsed lobe/segment—bronchial obstruction (e.g. sputum retention, foreign body, blood clot, vomitus, misplaced endotracheal tube)
- Macroatelectasis—air space compression by heavy, oedematous lung tissue, external compression (e.g. pleural effusion, haemothorax), sputum retention
- Microatelectasis—inadequate depth of respiration, nitrogen washout by 100% oxygen with subsequent absorption of oxygen occurring at a rate greater than replenishment.

Sputum retention

Excess mucus (sputum) normally stimulates coughing. If ciliary clearance is reduced (e.g. smoking, sedatives) or mucus volume is excessive (e.g. asthma, bronchiectasis, cystic fibrosis, chronic bronchitis) sputum retention may occur. Sputum retention may also be the result of inadequate coughing (e.g. chronic obstructive lung disease, pain, neuromuscular disease) or increased mucus viscosity (e.g. hypovolaemia, inadequate humidification of inspired gas).

Preventive measures

- Sputum hydration—maintenance of systemic hydration and humidification of inspired gases (e.g. nebulized saline/bronchodilators, heated water bath, heat moisture exchanging filter).
- Cough—requires inspiration to near total lung capacity, glottic closure, contraction of abdominal muscles and rapid opening of the glottis. Dynamic compression of the airways and high velocity expiration expels secretions. The process is limited if total lung capacity is reduced, abdominal muscles are weak, pain limits contraction or small airways collapse on expiration. It is usual to flex the abdomen on coughing and this should be simulated in supine patients by drawing the knees up. This also limits pain in patients with an upper abdominal wound.
- Physiotherapy—postural drainage, percussion and vibration, hyperinflation, intermittent positive pressure breathing, incentive spirometry or manual hyperinflation.
- Maintenance of lung volumes—increased V$_T$, CPAP, PEEP, positioning to reduce compression of lung tissue by oedema.

Management

Specific management depends on the cause and should be corrective. All measures taken for prevention should continue. If there is lobar or segmental collapse with obstruction of proximal airways, bronchoscopy may be useful to allow directed suction, foreign body removal and saline instillation. Patients with high FIO$_2$ may deteriorate due to the effects of excessive lavage or suction reducing minute ventilation.

See also:
  Oxygen therapy, 2; Ventilatory support—indications, 4; IPPV—complications of ventilation, 12; Endotracheal intubation, 28; Minitracheotomy, 32; Bronchoscopy, 38; Chest physiotherapy, 40; Blood gas analysis, 94; Bronchodilators, 176; Chronic airflow limitation, 274; Post-operative intensive care, 510; Acute chest infection 1, 276; Acute chest infection 2, 278; Asthma—general management, 284; Asthma—ventilatory management, 286

Chronic airflow limitation

Many patients requiring ICU admission for a community-acquired pneumonia have chronic respiratory failure. An acute exacerbation (which may or may not be infection-related) results in decompensation and symptomatic deterioration. Infections resulting in acute exacerbations include viruses, *Haemophilus influenzae*, *Klebsiella* and *Staph. aureus* in addition to *Strep. pneumoniae*, *Mycoplasma pneumoniae* and *Legionella pneumophila*. Otherwise, patients with coincidental chronic airflow limitation (CAL) are admitted for other reasons or as a prophylactic measure in view of their limited respiratory function, e.g. for elective postoperative ventilation.

Problems in managing CAL patients on the ICU

- Disability due to chronic ill health
- Fatigue, muscle weakness and decreased physiological reserve leading to earlier need for ventilatory support, increased difficulty in weaning, and greater physical dependency on support therapies
- Psychological dependency on support therapies
- More prone to pneumothoraces
- Usually have greater levels of sputum production
- Right ventricular dysfunction (cor pulmonale)

Notes

- Decisions on whether or not to intubate should be made in consultation with the family, the patient (if appropriate), and a respiratory physician with knowledge of the patient. The patient should be given the benefit of the doubt and intubated in an acute situation where a precise history and quality of life is not known.
- Trials of non-invasive ventilatory support $\pm$ respiratory stimulants such as doxepram have shown considerable success in avoiding intubation and mechanical ventilation.
- Accept lower target levels of PaO_2.
- Accept higher target levels of $PaCO_2$ if patient is known or suspected to have chronic CO_2 retention on the basis of elevated plasma bicarbonate levels on admission to hospital.

Weaning the patient with CAL

- An early trial of extubation may be worthwhile before the patient becomes ventilator-dependent.
- Weaning may be a lengthy procedure.
- Provide plentiful encouragement and psychological support. Setting daily targets and early mobilisation may be advantageous.
- Do not tire by prolonged spontaneous breathing. Consider gradually increasing periods of spontaneous breathing interspersed by periods of rest. Ensure a good night's sleep.
- Use patient appearance and lack of symptoms (e.g. tachypnoea, fatigue) rather than specific blood gas values to judge the duration of spontaneous breathing.
- Early tracheostomy may benefit when difficulty in weaning is expected.
- The patient may cope better with a tracheostomy mask than CPAP.
- Addition of extrinsic PEEP or CPAP may prevent early airways closure and thus reduce the work of breathing. However, this should be done with caution because of the risk of increased air trapping.
- Consider heart failure as an occasional cause of difficulty in weaning.

275

Acute chest infection 1

Patients may present to intensive care as a result of an acute chest infection or may develop infection as a complication of intensive care management. Typical features include fever, cough, purulent sputum production, breathlessness, pleuritic pain and bronchial breathing. Urgent investigation includes arterial gases, chest X-ray, blood count and cultures of blood and sputum. In community acquired pneumonia acute phase antibody titres should be taken.

Diagnosis and initial antimicrobial treatment

Basic resuscitation is required if there is cardiorespiratory compromise. Appropriate treatment of the infection depends on chest X-ray and culture findings although empiric 'best guess' antibiotic treatment may be started before culture results are available. Treatment includes physiotherapy and methods to aid sputum clearance.

Clear chest X-ray

Acute bronchitis is associated with cough, mucoid sputum and wheeze. In previously healthy patients a viral aetiology is most likely and there is often an upper respiratory prodrome. Symptomatic relief is usually all that is required. Likely organisms in acute on chronic bronchitis include *Strep pneumoniae, H influenzae or Staph aureus*. Appropriate antibiotics include cefuroxime or ampicillin and flucloxacillin. Viral pneumonia may be confused by the presence of bacteria in the sputum but secondary bacterial infection is common.

Pulmonary cavitation on chest X-ray

Cavitation should alert one to the possibility of anaerobic infection (sputum is often foul smelling). *Staph aureus, K pneumoniae* or tuberculosis are also associated with cavitation. Appropriate antibiotics include metronidazole or clindamycin for anaerobic infection, flucloxacillin for *Staph aureus* and ceftazidime and gentamicin for *K pneumoniae*. A foreign body or pulmonary infarct should also be considered where there is a single abscess.

Consolidation on chest X-ray

The recent history is important for deciding the cause of a pneumonia:

- Hospital acquired pneumonia—enteric (Gram negative) organisms treated with ceftazidime and gentamicin, *Staph aureus* treated with flucloxacillin (or teicoplanin / vancomycin if multi-resistant).
- Recent aspiration—anaerobic or Gram negative infection treated with clindamycin or cefuroxime and metronidazole.
- Community acquired pneumonia in a previously healthy individual—*Strep pneumoniae* (often lobar, acute onset) or atypical pneumonia (insidious onset, known community outbreaks, renal failure and electrolyte disturbance in Legionnaire's disease). Appropriate antibiotic therapy is cefuroxime and erythromycin.
- Pneumonia complicating influenza—*Staph aureus* treated with flucloxacillin. Both *Staph aureus* and *H influenzae* are common in those debilitated by chronic disease (e.g. alcoholism, diabetes, chronic airflow limitation or the elderly).
- Immunosuppressed—opportunistic infections (e.g. tuberculosis, *Pneumocystis carinii*, Herpes viruses, CMV or fungi).

Antimicrobial treatment

Drug	Dose	Organism
Acyclovir	10mg/kg 8hrly IV	Herpes viruses
Amphotericin B	250mg–1g 6hrly IV	Fungi
Ampicillin	500mg–1g 6hrly IV	*H influenzae*
		Gram negative spp
Benzylpenicillin	1.2g 2–6hrly IV	*Strep pneumoniae*
Ceftazidime	2g 8hrly IV	*K pneumoniae*
		Ps aeruginosa
		Gram negative spp
Cefuroxime	750mg–1.5g 8hrly IV	*Strep pneumoniae*
		H influenzae
		Gram negative spp
Clindamycin	300–600mg 6hrly IV	Anaerobes
		Gram negative spp
Cotrimoxazole	120mg/kg/day IV	*Pneumocystis carinii*
Erythromycin	1g 6–12hrly	Atypical pneumonia
	(500mg 6hrly PO if less severe)	*Strep pneumoniae*
Flucloxacillin	2g 6hrly iv	*Staph aureus*
	(500mg–1g 6hrly PO if less severe)	
Ganciclovir	5mg/kg 12hrly iv (over 1h)	CMV
Gentamicin	1.5mg/kg stat IV	*K pneumoniae,*
	(thereafter by levels—	*Ps aeruginosa*
	usually 80mg 8hrly)	Gram negative spp
Metronidazole	500mg 8hrly IV or 1g 12hrly PR	Anaerobes
Teicoplanin	400mg 12hrly for 3 doses then 400mg daily	multi-resistant *Staph aureus*
Vancomycin	500mg 6hrly (monitor levels)	multi-resistant *Staph aureus*

See also:

Acute chest infection 2

Laboratory diagnosis
The following samples are required for laboratory diagnosis:
- Sputum (e.g. cough specimen, endotracheal tube aspirate, protected brush specimen, bronchoalveolar lavage specimen)
- Blood cultures
- Serology (in community acquired pneumonia)
- Urine for antigen tests (if Legionella or Candida suspected)

In severe pneumonia blind antibiotic therapy should not be withheld while awaiting results. Specimens should, however, be taken before starting antibiotics.

Microbiological yield is usually very low, especially if antibiotic therapy has started before sampling.

Where cultures are positive there is often multiple growth. Separating pathogenic organisms from colonising organisms may be difficult.

In hospital acquired pneumonia known nosocomial pathogens are the likely source.

Continuing treatment

Antibiotics should be adjusted according to sensitivities once available. Failure to respond to treatment in 72h should prompt consideration of infections more common in the immunocompromised.

Hospital acquired pneumonia requires treatment with appropriate antibiotics for 24h after symptoms subside (usually 3–5 days). After this period cultures should be repeated (off antibiotics if there has been improvement).

In atypical or pneumococcal pneumonia 10–14 days antibiotic treatment is usual.

279

See also:
   Bacteriology, 148; Virology, serology & assays, 150; Antimicrobials, 248; Acute
chest infection 1, 276

Adult respiratory distress syndrome 1

ARDS is the respiratory component of multiple organ dysfunction. It may be predominant in the clinical picture or be of lesser clinical importance in relation to dysfunction of other organ systems.

Aetiology

As part of the exaggerated inflammatory response following a major exogenous insult which may be either direct (e.g. chest trauma, inhalation injury) or distant (e.g. peritonitis, major haemorrhage, burns). Histology reveals aggregation and activation of neutrophils and platelets, patchy endothelial and alveolar disruption, interstitial oedema and fibrosis. The acute phase is characterised by increased capillary permeability and the fibroproliferative phase (after 7 days) by a predominant fibrotic reaction.

Definitions (Am J Respir Crit Care Med 1994; 149: 818–24)

Acute lung injury (ALI)
$PaO_2/FIO_2 \leqslant 300mmHg$ (40kPa)
- Regardless of level of PEEP
- With bilateral infiltrates on chest X-ray
- With pulmonary artery wedge pressure $<18mmHg$
Adult respiratory distress syndrome (ARDS)
As above but $PaO_2/FIO_2 \leqslant 200mmHg$ (26.7kPa)

Prognosis

Prognosis depends in part on the underlying insult, the presence of other organ dysfunctions and the age and chronic health of the patient. Predominant single-organ ARDS carries a mortality of 30–50%; there does appear to have been some improvement in the last few years.

Survivors following predominant single-organ ARDS often have few (if any) long-term sequelae. Some deterioration on lung function testing is usually detectable but this rarely impacts upon quality of life.

See also:
   Adult respiratory distress syndrome 2, 282; Inhalation injury, 294; Multiple
trauma 1 , 458; Multiple trauma 2, 460; Sepsis / infection, 490; Systemic
inflammatory response, 488

Adult respiratory distress syndrome 2

General management

1 Remove the cause whenever possible, e.g. drain pus, antibiotic therapy, fix long bone fracture.
2 Sedate with an opiate-benzodiazepine combination as mechanical ventilation is likely to be prolonged. Doses should be kept to the lowest possible but consistent with adequate sedation.
3 Muscle relaxation by continuous infusion is indicated in severe ARDS to improve chest wall compliance and gas exchange.
4 Haemodynamic manipulation with either fluid, vasodilators, vasopressors, diuretics and/or inotropes may improve oxygenation. This may be achieved by either increasing cardiac output and thus mixed venous saturation in low output states, or by decreasing cardiac output thereby lengthening pulmonary transit times in high output states. Care should be taken not to compromise the circulation.

Respiratory management

1 Maintain adequate gas exchange with increased FIO_2 and, depending on severity, either non-invasive respiratory support (e.g. CPAP) or positive pressure ventilation. Specific modes may be utilised, especially pressure controlled inverse ratio ventilation. While general agreement exists for minimising V_T ($\leqslant 10$ml/kg) and peak inspiratory pressures (< 35–40cmH$_2$O) if possible, there is no consensus regarding the upper desired level of FIO_2 and PEEP. The current European view favours the use of higher FIO_2 (up to 1.0) while a common US approach is to keep the $FIO_2 \leqslant 0.60$ but to maintain SaO_2 with higher levels of PEEP.
2 Non-ventilatory respiratory support techniques such as $ECCO_2R$ can be used in severe ARDS but have yet to show convincing benefit over conventional ventilatory techniques.
3 Blood gas values should be aimed at maintaining survival without striving to achieve normality. Permissive hypercapnia, where $PaCO_2$ values are allowed to rise, sometimes above 10 kPa, has been associated with outcome benefit. Acceptable levels of SaO_2 are controversial; in general, values $\geqslant 90$–95% are targeted but in severe ARDS this may be relaxed to 80–85%.
4 Patient positioning may provide improvements in gas exchange. This includes kinetic therapy using special rotational beds, and prone positioning with the patient being turned frequently through 180°.
5 Inhaled nitric oxide or epoprostenol improves gas exchange in some 50% of patients though any outcome effect remains to be proved.
6 High dose steroids commenced at 7–10 days (during the proliferative phase) are beneficial in 50–60% of patients.
7 Surfactant therapy is currently not indicated for adult RDS.
8 Ventilator trauma is ubiquitous. Multiple pneumothoraces are common and may require multiple chest drains. They may be difficult to diagnose by X-ray and, despite the attendant risks, CT scanning may reveal undiagnosed pneumothoraces and aid drain placement.

See also:

Asthma—general management

Pathophysiology

Acute bronchospasm and mucus plugging, often secondary to an insult such as infection. The patient may progress to fatigue, respiratory failure and collapse. The onset may develop slowly over days or occur rapidly within minutes to hours.

Clinical features

- Dyspnoea, wheeze (expiratory ± inspiratory), difficulty in talking, use of accessory respiratory muscles, fatigue, agitation, cyanosis, coma, collapse.
- Pulsus paradoxus is a poor indication of severity; a fatiguing patient cannot generate significant respiratory swings in intrathoracic pressure.
- A 'silent' chest is also a late sign and suggests severely limited airflow.
- Pneumothorax and lung / lobar collapse.

Management of asthma

Asthmatics must be managed in a well-monitored area. If clinical features are severe, they should be admitted to an intensive care unit where rapid institution of mechanical ventilation is available. Monitoring should comprise, as a minimum, pulse oximetry, continuous ECG, regular blood pressure measurement and blood gas analysis. If severe, an intra-arterial cannula ± central venous access should be inserted.

1. High FIO_2 ($\geqslant 0.60$) to maintain $SpO_2 \geqslant 95\%$.
2. Nebulised β_2-agonist (e.g. salbutamol)- may be repeated every 2–4h or, in severe attacks, administered continuously.
3. IV steroids for 24h then oral prednisolone. Nebulised ipratropium bromide may give additional benefit.
4. IV aminophylline. Check levels at 18–24h and adjust dose as necessary to lie within the therapeutic range.
5. Exclude pneumothorax and lung/Lobar collapse.
6. Ensure adequate hydration and fluid replacement.
7. Commence antibiotic therapy (cefuroxime ± erythromycin) if strong evidence of bacterial chest infection. Green sputum does not necessarily indicate a bacterial infection.
8. If no response to above measures or in extremis consider:
   - IV salbutamol infusion
   - Adrenaline SC or by nebulizer
   - Mechanical ventilation

Indications for mechanical ventilation.

- Increasing fatigue
- Respiratory failure—rising $PaCO_2$, falling PaO_2
- Cardiovascular collapse

Facilitating endotracheal intubation

Summon senior assistance. Pre-oxygenate with 100% O_2. Perform rapid sequence induction with suxamethonium and etomidate or ketamine. 'Breathing down' with an inhalational anaesthetic (e.g. isoflurane) before intubation should only be attempted by an experienced clinician.

Drug dosage

Adrenaline	0.5ml 1:1000 solution SC or
	2ml 1:10000 solution by nebulizer
Aminophylline	6mg/kg loading dose over 15–20min (if not already on theophyllines), then 0.5mg/kg/h infusion.
	(0.8mg/kg/h in smokers, chronic bronchitics, children)
Hydrocortisone	100–200mg qds
Ipratropium bromide	250–500µg qds by nebulizer
Prednisolone	40–60mg od initially
Salbutamol	2.5–5mg by nebulizer
	5–20µg/min by IV infusion

285

See also:

Oxygen therapy, 2; Ventilatory support—indications, 4; Endotracheal intubation, 28; Pulse oximetry, 86; Blood gas analysis, 94; Arterial cannulation, 106; Central venous catheter—use, 108; Bacteriology, 148; Bronchodilators, 176; Sedatives, 226; Muscle relaxants, 228; Steroids, 250; Dyspnoea, 266; Asthma—ventilatory management, 286; Anaphylactoid reactions, 492

Asthma—ventilatory management

Early period

1 Initially give low V_T (5ml/kg) breaths at low rate (5–10/min) to assess degree of bronchospasm and air trapping. Slowly increase V_T (to 10ml/kg) ± increase rate, taking care to avoid significant air trapping and high inspiratory pressures. Low rates with prolonged I:E ratio (e.g. 1:1) may be advantageous. Avoid very short expiratory time. Do not strive to achieve normocapnia.

2 Administer muscle relaxants for a minimum 2–4h, until severe bronchospasm has abated and gas exchange improved. Although atracurium causes histamine release it does not appear to worsen bronchospasm.

3 Sedate with either standard medication or with agents such as ketamine or isoflurane which have bronchodilating properties. Ketamine given alone may cause hallucinations while isoflurane carries a theoretical risk of fluoride toxicity.

4 If significant air trapping remains, consider ventilator disconnection and forced manual chest compressions every 10–15min.

5 If severe bronchospasm persists, consider injecting 1–2ml of 1:10000 adrenaline down ET tube. Repeat at 5min intervals as necessary.

Maintenance

1 Ensure adequate rehydration

2 Generous humidification should be given to loosen mucus plugs. Use a heat-moisture exchanger plus either hourly 0.9% saline nebulizers or instillation of 5ml 0.9% saline down the tube.

3 Physiotherapy assists mobilisation of secretions and removal of mucus plugs. Hyperventilation should be avoided.

4 With improvement, gradually normalise ventilator settings (V_T, rate, I:E ratio) to achieve normocapnia before allowing patient to waken and breathe spontaneously.

5 Consider pneumothorax or lung/Lobar collapse if acute deterioration occurs.

6 If mucus plugging constitutes a major problem, instillation of a mucolytic (N-acetyl cysteine) may be considered though this may induce further bronchospasm. Bronchoscopic removal of plugs should only be performed by an experienced operator.

Assessment of air trapping (intrinsic PEEP, PEEPi)

- Measure PEEPi by pressing end-expiratory hold button of ventilator
- No pause between expiratory and inspiratory sounds
- Disconnection of ventilator and timing of expiratory wheeze
- An increasing $PaCO_2$ may respond to reductions in minute volume which will lower the level of intrinsic PEEP.

Weaning

- Bronchospasm may increase on lightening sedation due to awareness of ET tube and increased coughing.
- May need trial of extubation while still on high FIO_2
- Consider extubation under inhalational anaesthesia
- Space out intervals between β_2-agonist nebulizers. Convert other anti-asthmatic drugs to oral medication. Theophylline dose should be adjusted to ensure therapeutic levels.

Pneumothorax

Significant collection of air in the pleural space that may occur spontaneously, following trauma (including iatrogenic), asthma, chronic lung disease, and is a common sequelum of ventilator trauma.

Clinical features

- May be asymptomatic.
- Dyspnoea, pain.
- Decreased breath sounds, hyper-resonant, asymmetric chest expansion—may be difficult to assess in a ventilated patient.
- Respiratory failure and deterioration in gas exchange.
- Increasing airway pressures and difficulty to ventilate.
- Cardiovascular deterioration with mediastinal shift (tension).

Diagnosis

- Chest X-ray—most easily seen on erect views where absent lung markings are seen lateral to a well-defined lung border. However, ventilated patients are often imaged in a supine position; pneumothorax may be easily missed as it may be lying anterior to normal lung giving the misleading appearance of lung markings on the radiograph. Supine pneumothorax should be considered if the following are seen:
- Hyperlucent lung field compared to the contralateral side
- Loss of clarity of the diaphragm outline
- 'Deep sulcus' sign, giving the appearance of an inverted diaphragm
- A particular clear part of the cardiac contour
  A lateral film may help. Tension pneumothorax results in marked mediastinal shift away from the affected side.
- Ultrasound—may be helpful but is highly operator dependent
- CT scan—very sensitive and may be useful in difficult situations, e.g. ARDS, and to direct drainage of localised pneumothorax

Pneumothorax must be distinguished from bullae, especially in those with long-standing emphysema; inadvertent drainage of a bulla may lead to a bronchopleural fistula. Assistance should be sought from a radiologist.

Management

1. Increase FIO_2 if hypoxaemic.
2. If life-threatening with circulatory collapse perform needle aspiration of the affected side followed by formal chest drain insertion.
3. Repeated needle aspiration may be sufficient in spontaneously breathing patients without respiratory failure; however, it is not recommended if the patient is ventilated.
4. Chest drain insertion. This may need to be done under ultrasound or CT guidance if localised due to surrounding lung fibrosis.

A small pneumothorax (< 10% hemithorax) may be left undrained but prompt action should be instituted if cardiorespiratory deterioration occurs. Patients should not be transferred between hospitals, particularly by air, with an undrained pneumothorax.

Bronchopleural fistula

Denoted by continual drainage of air. Usually responds to conservative treatment with continual application of 5 kPa negative pressure; this may take weeks to resolve. For severe leak and/or compromised ventilation, high frequency jet ventilation and/or a double lumen endobronchial tube may be considered. Surgical intervention is rarely necessary.

Chest X-ray appearance in pneumothorax

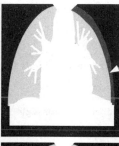

rim of air on erect X-ray

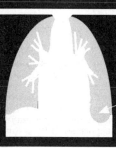

reverse sulcus sign of supine pneumothorax

289

Haemothorax

Usually secondary to chest trauma or following a procedure, e.g. cardiac surgery, chest drain insertion, central venous catheter insertion. Spontaneous haemothorax is very rare, even in patients with clotting disorders.

Clinical features

- Stony dullness.
- Decreased breath sounds.
- Hypovolaemia and deterioration in gas exchange (if large).

Diagnosis

- Erect chest X-ray—blunting of hemidiaphragm and progressive loss of basal lung field
- Supine chest X-ray—increased opacity of affected hemithorax plus decreased clarity of cardiac contour on that side.
- Large-bore needle aspiration to confirm presence of blood. A small-bore needle may be unable to aspirate a haemothorax if it has clotted.

Management

1 If small, observe with serial X-rays and monitor for signs of cardiorespiratory deterioration.
2 Ensure any coagulopathy is corrected by administration of fresh frozen plasma and/or platelets as indicated.
3 Ensure that cross-matched blood is available for urgent transfusion if necessary.
4 If significant in size or patient becomes symptomatic, insert large bore chest drain, e.g. size 28Fr. The drain should be directed postero-inferiorly toward the dependent area of lung and placed on 5kPa suction.
5 If drainage exceeds 1000ml or > 200ml/h for 3–4h despite correcting any coagulopathy, contact thoracic surgeon.
6 Drains inserted for a haemothorax with no pneumothorax may be removed after 1–2 days if no further bleeding occurs. IPPV is not a contraindication to removal in this case.

Perforation of an intercostal vessel during chest drain insertion may cause considerable bleeding into the pleura. If deep tension sutures around the chest drain fail to stem blood loss, remove the chest drain and insert a Foley urethral catheter through the hole. Inflate the balloon and apply traction on the catheter to tamponade the bleeding vessel. If these measures fail, contact a thoracic surgeon.

291

See also:
   Chest drain insertion, 34; Blood transfusion, 172; Blood products, 240;
Pneumothorax, 288; Bleeding disorders, 382

Haemoptysis

- May range from a few specks of blood in expectorated sputum to massive pulmonary haemorrhage.
- More likely to disrupt gas exchange before life-threatening hypovolaemia ensues.
- May be a presenting feature of a patient admitted to intensive care or may result from critical illness and its treatment.

Causes

Massive haemoptysis
- Disruption of a bronchial artery by acute inflammation or invasion (e.g. pulmonary neoplasm, trauma, cavitating TB, bronchiectasis, lung abscess and aspergilloma).
- Rupture of arteriovenous malformations and bronchovascular fistulae.
- Pulmonary infarction secondary to prolonged pulmonary artery catheter wedging or pulmonary artery rupture.

Minor haemoptysis
- Intrapulmonary inflammation or infarction (e.g. pulmonary embolus)
- Endotracheal tube trauma (e.g. mucosal erosion, balloon necrosis, trauma from the tube tip, trauma to a tracheostomy stoma, trauma from suction catheters).
- Tissue breakdown in critically ill patients (e.g. tissue hypoperfusion, coagulopathy, poor nutritional state, sepsis and hypoxaemia.)

Investigation and assessment

Urgent assessment of cardiorespiratory function and cardiorespiratory monitoring are required. Massive haemoptysis may require resuscitation and urgent intubation. The diagnosis may be suggested by the history and a chest X-ray may identify a cavitating lesion. Lower lobe shadowing on a chest X-ray may be the result of overspill of blood from elsewhere in the bronchial tree. Early surgical intervention should be prompted by a changing air-fluid level, persistent opacification of a previous cavity or a mobile intracavitory mass. Early bronchoscopy may identify the source of haemoptysis, although only while bleeding is active. Blood in multiple bronchial orifices may be confusing but saline lavage may leave the source visible. Rigid bronchoscopy is useful in massive haemoptysis allowing oxygenation and wide bore suction.

Management

- Basic resuscitation (high FIO_2, endotracheal intubation and blood transfusion) is urgent if there is cardiorespiratory compromise.
- Correction of coagulopathy is a priority.
- Bronchoscopy allows direct instillation of 1 in 200 000 adrenaline if the source of haemorrhage can be found or, alternatively, endobronchial tamponade with a balloon catheter.
- In cases of severe haemorrhage from one lung a double lumen endotracheal tube may prevent some overspill to the other lung while definitive treatment is organised.
- Definitive treatment may include radiological bronchial artery embolisation or surgical resection.
- Induced hypotension may be useful in bronchial artery haemorrhage.
- In cases of pulmonary artery haemorrhage PEEP may be used with mechanical ventilation to reduce pulmonary bleeding.

293

Inhalation injury

Causes include smoke, steam, noxious gases and aspiration of gastric contents.

Clinical features

- dyspnoea, coughing
- stridor (if upper airway obstruction)
- bronchospasm
- signs of lung/Lobar collapse (especially with aspiration)
- signs of respiratory failure
- cherry-red skin colour (carbon monoxide)
- agitation, coma
- ARDS (late)

General principles of management

1 100% O_2.
2 Early intubation if upper airway compromised or threatened.
3 Early bronchoscopy if inhalation of soot, debris, vomit suspected.

Specific conditions

Smoke inhalation

- Smoke rarely causes thermal injury beyond the level of bronchi as it has a low specific heat content. However, soot is a major irritant to the upper airways and can produce very rapid and marked inflammation.
- Urgent laryngoscopy should be performed if soot is present in the nares, mouth or pharynx.
- If soot is seen or the larynx appears inflamed, perform early endotracheal intubation. As the upper airway can obstruct within minutes it is advisable to intubate as a prophylactic measure rather than as an emergency where it may prove impossible.
- After intubation, perform urgent bronchoscopy with bronchial toilet using warmed 0.9% saline to remove as much soot as possible.
- Commence benzylpenicillin 1.2g qds IV.
- Specific treatment for poisons contained within smoke (e.g. carbon monoxide, cyanide)

Steam inhalation

- Consider early/prophylactic intubation.
- Steam has a much higher heat content than smoke and can cause injury to the whole respiratory tract.
- Consider early bronchoscopy and lavage with cool 0.9% saline.

Aspiration of gastric contents

- Early bronchoscopy and physiotherapy to remove as much particulate and liquid matter as possible.
- Either cefuroxime plus metronidazole, or clindamycin for 3–5 days.
- Steroid therapy has no benefit.

Pulmonary embolus

Aetiology

- Usually arises from a deep vein thrombosis in femoral or pelvic veins. The risk increases after prolonged immobilisation and with polycythaemia or hyperviscosity disorders.
- Amniotic fluid embolus
- Fat embolus after pelvic or long bone trauma
- Right heart source, e.g. mural thrombus

Clinical features

- Pleuritic-type chest pain, dyspnoea, $\pm$ haemoptysis.
- The patient with a major embolus will prefer to lie flat. Dyspnoea improves due to increased venous return and right heart loading.
- Deterioration in gas exchange—may find a low PaO_2, low or high $PaCO_2$ and a metabolic acidosis. However, these findings are inconsistent and non-diagnostic.
- Cardiovascular collapse.
- Chest X-ray: may be normal but a massive embolus may produce decreased vascular markings (pulmonary oligaemia) in one hemithorax $\pm$ a bulging pulmonary hilum. A wedge-shaped peripheral pulmonary infarct may be seen after a few days following a smaller embolus.
- ECG: acute right ventricular strain, i.e. $S_1Q_3T_3$, tachycardia, right axis deviation, right bundle branch block, P pulmonale.
- Echocardiogram: may reveal evidence of pulmonary hypertension and acute right ventricular strain.
- D-dimers—though a raised level is non-diagnostic, a normal value carries a high probability of exclusion of a pulmonary embolus.

Definitive diagnosis

- CT scan—the investigation of choice for major embolus.
- Pulmonary angiography.
- Ventilation–perfusion scanning—the degree of certainty is reduced if the area of non-perfused lung corresponds to any chest X-ray abnormality.
- Fat globules or foetal cells in pulmonary artery blood are diagnostic of fat and amniotic fluid embolus respectively.

General management

1 FIO_2 0.6–1.0 to maintain SaO_2 $\geqslant$ 90–95%
2 Lie patient flat.
3 Fluid challenge to optimise right heart filling.
4 Adrenaline infusion if circulation still compromised.
5 Mechanical ventilation may be necessary if the patient is tiring and/or to maintain adequate oxygenation. However, gas exchange may worsen due to loss of preferential shunting and decreases in cardiac output.

Management of blood clot embolus

Start anticoagulation with heparin. Consider thrombolysis if there is a major embolus and embolectomy if patient remains moribund. Otherwise, at 24–48h commence warfarinisation regimen.

Management of fat embolus

Other than general measures including oxygenation, fluid resuscitation and right heart loading, treatment remains controversial. Some authorities advocate steroids, others heparinisation while others suggest that no specific therapy is required.

Thrombolytic regimens

rt-PA—(100mg over 90min) should be given followed by a heparin infusion (24–36 000 units/day) to maintain the partial thromboplastin time at 2–3 × normal. This is the treatment of choice if surgery or angiography is contemplated,.

Streptokinase (500 000 units as a loading dose over 30min followed by 100 000 units/h for 24h).

NB—Central venous catheters should be inserted pre-thrombolysis.

297

Cardiovascular Disorders

Hypotension

The overall principle in the management of hypotension is to maintain the minimum mean arterial pressure that will ensure adequate tissue perfusion. A normal blood pressure does not guarantee an adequate cardiac output and circulatory support should aim to achieve adequate blood flow as well as adequate pressure. However, when the patient is in extremis the first line treatment options should include external cardiac massage and adrenaline 0.05–0.2mg intravenous boluses (1mg in cardiac arrest).

Assessment of hypotension

Hypotension requires treatment if the mean BP < 60mmHg (higher if the patient was previously hypertensive) with signs of poor tissue perfusion (e.g. oliguria, confusion, altered consciousness, cool peripheries, metabolic acidosis). Specific treatment should be considered for haemorrhage, acute myocardial infarction, arrhythmias, pulmonary embolus, cardiac tamponade, pneumothorax, anaphylaxis, diarrhoea and vomiting, ketoacidosis, hypoadrenalism, hypopituitarism and poisoning.

Initial treatment of hypotension

Most cases of hypotension require fluid as first line management to confirm an adequate circulating volume. Exceptions may include acute heart failure, arrhythmias, cardiac tamponade and pneumothorax. In cases of haemorrhage blood should be used as soon as it is available; if life threatening, group specific or O negative blood should be used urgently.

Pharmacological treatment

If hypotension persists after an adequate circulating volume has been restored the appropriate choice of drug treatment depends on whether there is myocardial failure (signs of low cardiac output or known measured low stroke volume) or peripheral vascular failure (warm, vasodilated periphery or measured normal stroke volume). A low stroke volume should be treated with an inotropic agent (e.g. adrenaline, dobutamine) and peripheral vascular failure with a vasopressor agent (e.g. noradrenaline).

Inotropic support

Adrenaline (started at 0.2μg/kg/min) or dobutamine (started at 5μg/kg/min) should be titrated against stroke volume if it is monitored. Most hypotensive patients requiring inotropes should have a pulmonary artery catheter inserted. The alternative is to titrate against blood pressure but there is a danger of producing inappropriate vasoconstriction. Dobutamine is safer in this respect but has the disadvantage of producing inappropriate vasodilatation in some patients.

Vasopressors

Once hypovolaemia has been corrected, noradrenaline (started at 0.05μg/kg/min) should be titrated against mean BP. In most patients, with a previously normal blood pressure, 60mmHg is an adequate target but may need to be higher to ensure organ perfusion in the elderly and those with previous hypertension. Noradrenaline may reduce cardiac output. This effect should be monitored and corrected by adjustment of dose.

301

See also:
Intra-aortic balloon counterpulsation, 50; Blood pressure monitoring, 104;
Arterial Cannulation, 106; Pulmonary artery catheter—use, 112; Pulmonary artery
catheter—insertion, 114; Cardiac output—thermodilution, 116; Cardiac output—
other invasive, 118; Cardiac output—non-invasive, 120; Colloids, 170; Blood
transfusion, 172; Inotropes, 184; Vasopressors, 188; Antiarrhythmics, 192; Basic
resuscitation, 258; Cardiac arrest, 260; Fluid challenge, 262; Pneumothorax, 288;
Haemothorax, 290; Pulmonary embolus, 296; Tachyarrhythmias, 304;
Bradyarrhythmias, 306; Acute myocardial infarction, 308; Heart failure—
assessment, 312; Heart failure—management, 314; Vomiting / gastric stasis, 326;
Diarrhoea, 328; Upper gastrointestinal haemorrhage, 332; Bleeding varices, 334;
Abdominal sepsis, 340; Pancreatitis, 342; Oliguria, 318; Agitation / confusion,
358; Metabolic acidosis, 420; Diabetic ketoacidosis, 428; Hypoadrenal crisis, 434;
Poisoning—general principles, 438; Multiple trauma 1, 458; Multiple trauma 2,
460; Burns—fluid management, 468; Burns—general management, 470; Post-
partum haemorrhage, 482; Systemic inflammatory response, 488; Pyrexia, 500;
Hyperthermia, 502

Hypertension

Often defined in adult patients as a diastolic pressure > 95mmHg and a systolic pressure > 180mmHg.

Common causes in intensive care

- Idiopathic/essential
- Agitation/pain
- Excessive vasoconstriction, e.g. cold, vasopressor drugs
- Head injury, raised intracranial pressure, cerebrovascular accidents
- Drug-related, e.g. excess vasopressor dosage, MAOI + tyramine-containing foods, Ecstasy reaction, abrupt clonidine withdrawal
- Endocrine, e.g. phaeochromocytoma (rare)
- Renal failure, renal artery stenosis (rare)
- Dissecting aneurysm, aortic coarctation
- Vasculitis, e.g. polyarteritis nodosa, thrombotic thrombocytopenic purpura
- (Pre-)eclampsia
- Spurious—underdamped transducer system leading to spuriously elevated systolic pressures

Agitation and/or pain should always be considered as a cause of a raised blood pressure in the paralysed but (partially) aware ICU patient.

Aortic coarctation may present acutely in adulthood as symptomatic hypertension.

Indications for urgency of treatment

Hypertensive encephalopathy, heart failure, eclampsia and acute dissecting aneurysm are the prime indications for rapid and aggressive albeit controlled reduction of blood pressure.

In other conditions, especially chronic hypertension and following acute neurological events, e.g. head injury, cerebrovascular accidents, a precipitate reduction in blood pressure may adversely affect perfusion leading to further deterioration. Hypertension post-cerebral event is not usually treated unless very high, e.g. mean BP > 140–150mmHg, systolic BP > 220–230mmHg. In this instance, controlled and partial reduction is mandatory, e.g. with a sodium nitroprusside infusion under continuous invasive monitoring. In the presence of a raised ICP (if measured), a cerebral perfusion pressure ⩾ 70mmHg is usually targeted.

Particularly in post-operative patients, non-pharmacological measures are often effective in reducing BP, e.g. warming, calming, treating hypovolaemia.

Sublingual nifedipine or intravenous hydrallazine may sometimes produce precipitate falls in BP. Use cautiously and start with low doses.

Hypertensive crisis

This occurs when the patient becomes symptomatic (increasing drowsiness, seizures, papilloedema, retinopathy) in the presence of elevated systemic pressures. The diastolic BP usually exceeds 120–130mmHg and the mean BP > 140–150mmHg, although encephalopathy can occur at lower pressures.

Principles of management

1 Adequate monitoring (invasive BP, ECG, CVP, CO, urine output...)
2 Consider pain, hypovolaemia and agitation, especially if paralysed.
3 Consider specific treatment as appropriate, e.g. phaeochromo-cytoma, thyroid crisis, aortic dissection, inflammatory vasculitis
4 Slow intravenous infusion of nitrate. Glyceryl trinitrate or isosor-bide dinitrate are usually given first before considering sodium nitroprusside. Other options include labetalol or esmolol infusions, hydrallazine (IV or IM), nifedipine (SL or PO).
5 Aim to reduce to mildly hypertensive levels unless dissecting aneurysm where systolic BP should be lowered < 100–110mmHg. After certain types of surgery (e.g. cardiac, aortic), control of systolic blood pressure < 100–120mmHg may be requested to reduce risk of bleeding.
6 Longer term treatment, e.g. an oral ACE inhibitor, should be instituted with caution, starting at low doses.

See also:
IPPV—failure to tolerate ventilation Blood pressure monitoring, 104; Intracranial pressure monitoring, 126; Hypotensive agents, 190; Intracranial haemorrhage, 364; Subarachnoid haemorrhage, 366; Head injury 1, 462; Head injury 2, 464; Pre-eclampsia & eclampsia, 478

Tachyarrhythmias

If pulses are not palpable or there is severe hypotension, a tachyarrhythmia requires cardiac massage and urgent DC cardioversion. Otherwise, the initial treatment prior to diagnosis includes correction of hypoxaemia and potassium to ensure a plasma $K^+ > 4.5$mmol/L.

Causes of tachyarrhythmias

Where possible the cause of a tachyarrhythmia should be treated. Common causes for which specific treatment may be required include hypovolaemia, hypotension (may also be due to the arrhythmia), acute myocardial infarction, pain, anaemia, hypercapnia, fever, anxiety, thyrotoxicosis and digoxin toxicity.

Diagnosis of tachyarrhythmias

Broad complex tachycardia
Regular complexes with AV dissociation (fusion beats, capture beats, QRS > 140msec, axis < −30°, concordance) suggest ventricular tachycardia. If there is no AV dissociation the arrhythmia is probably supraventricular with aberrant conduction; adenosine may be used as a diagnostic test since SVT may respond and VT will not. Irregular broad complexes are probably atrial fibrillation with aberration. Torsades de pointes is a form of ventricular tachycardia with a variable axis.

Narrow complex tachycardia
The absence of P waves suggests atrial fibrillation. A P wave rate > 150 is suggestive of SVT whereas slower P wave rates may represent a sinus tachycardia or atrial flutter with block. The P waves are abnormal (flutter waves) in atrial flutter and QRS complexes may be irregular if the block is variable. Extremely fast SVT may be due to a re-entry pathway with retrograde conduction and premature ectopic atrial excitation. In Wolff–Parkinson–White syndrome the re-entry pathway inserts below the His bundle allowing rapid AV conduction and re-entry tachyarrhythmias. This may be diagnosed by a short PR interval and a delta wave.

Treatment of tachyarrhythmias

Ventricular tachycardia
Lignocaine, amiodarone or magnesium form the mainstay of drug treatment. Overdrive pacing may be used if a pacing wire is *in situ*, capturing the ventricle at a pacing rate higher than the arrhythmia and gradually reducing the pacing rate. Torsades de pointes may be exacerbated by antiarrhythmics so magnesium or overdrive pacing are safest.

Supraventricular tachycardia and atrial flutter
Carotid sinus massage may be used in patients with no risk of calcified atheromatous carotid deposits. Amiodarone, adenosine or magnesium are usually the most useful drugs in the critically ill. Verapamil may be used if complexes are narrow (no risk of misdiagnosed ventricular tachycardia) although it and other AV node blockers should be avoided in re-entry tachycardias.

Atrial fibrillation
Acute or paroxysmal atrial fibrillation should be treated as for supraventricular tachycardia. Digoxin is more useful for chronic atrial fibrillation and does not prevent paroxysmal episodes.

Drug doses and cautions

Adenosine   3mg IV as a rapid bolus. If no response in 1min give 6mg followed by 12mg.

Verapamil   2.5mg IV slowly. If no response repeat to a maximum of 20mg. An intravenous infusion of 1–10mg may be used. 10ml CaCl 10% should be available to treat hypotension associated with verapamil. Verapamil should be avoided in re-entry tachyarrhythmias since ventricular response may increase. Life-threatening hypotension may occur in misdiagnosed ventricular tachycardia and life threatening bradycardia may occur if the patient has been β blocked.

Lignocaine   1mg/kg intravenously as a bolus followed by an infusion of 2–4mg/min.

Amiodarone   5mg/kg over 20min then infused at up to 15mg/kg/24h in 5% glucose via a central vein. Avoid with other class III agents (e.g. sotalol) since QT interval may be severely prolonged.

Magnesium   20mmol $MgSO_4$ over 2–3h. In an emergency it may be given over 5min

305

See also:
    Defibrillation, 44; ECG monitoring, 102; Antiarrhythmics, 192; Basic resuscitation, 258; Cardiac arrest, 260; Fluid challenge, 262; Respiratory failure, 270; Hypotension, 300; Acute myocardial infarction, 308; Hyperkalaemia, 406; Hypokalaemia, 408; Thyroid emergencies, 432; Tricyclic antidepressant poisoning, 446; Anaemia, 386; Pain, 496; Pyrexia, 500

Bradyarrhythmias

If peripheral pulses are not palpable a bradyarrhythmia requires external cardiac massage and treatment as for asystole. For asymptomatic bradycardia treatment may not be required other than close monitoring and correction of the cause. The exception to this is higher degrees of heart block occurring after an acute anterior myocardial infarction where pacing may be required prophylactically.

Causes of bradyarrhythmias

Where possible the cause of a bradyarrhythmia should be treated. Common causes for which specific treatment may be required include hypovolaemia, hypotension (may also be due to the arrhythmia), acute myocardial infarction, digoxin toxicity, β blocker toxicity, hyperkalaemia, hypothyroidism, hypopituitarism and raised intracranial pressure. Digoxin toxicity may require treatment with anti-digoxin antibodies.

Diagnosis of bradyarrhythmias

Sinus bradycardia
Slow ventricular rate with normal P waves, normal PR interval and 1:1 AV conduction.

Heart block
Normal P waves, a prolonged PR interval and 1:1 AV conduction suggest 1° heart block. In 2° heart block the ventricles fail to respond to atrial contraction intermittently. This may be associated with regular P waves and an increasing PR interval until ventricular depolarisation fails (Mobitz I or Wenkebach) or a normal PR interval with regular failed ventricular depolarisation (Mobitz II). In the latter case the AV conduction ratio may be 2:1 to 5:1. In 3° heart block there is complete AV dissociation with a slow, idioventricular rate.

Absent P wave bradycardia

Absent P waves may represent slow atrial fibrillation or sino-atrial dysfunction. In the latter case there will be a slow, idioventricular rate.

Treatment of bradyarrhythmias

Hypoxaemia must be corrected in all symptomatic bradycardias. First line drug treatment is usually atropine 0.3mg intravenously. If the arrhythmia fails to respond, 0.6mg followed by 1.0mg atropine may be given. An isoprenaline infusion (1–10μg/min) may be used to maintain an adequate ventricular rate. Failure to respond to drugs requires temporary pacing. This may be accomplished rapidly with an external system if there is haemodynamic compromise or transvenously. Other indications for temporary pacing are shown in the table. Higher degrees of heart block after an anterior myocardial infarction will usually require permanent pacing.

Indications for temporary pacing

Persistent symptomatic bradycardia
Blackouts associated with
   3° heart block
   2° heart block
   RBBB and left posterior hemiblock
Cardiovascular collapse
Inferior myocardial infarction with symptomatic 3° heart block
Anterior myocardial infarction with
   3° heart block
   RBBB and left posterior hemiblock
   Alternating RBBB and LBBB

See also:
Temporary internal pacing, 46; External pacing, 48; ECG monitoring, 102; Chronotropes, 194; Basic resuscitation, 258; Cardiac arrest, 260; Acute myocardial infarction, 308; Thyroid emergencies, 432; Hypothermia, 498

Acute myocardial infarction

Principles of management of the uncomplicated patient

- Oxygen—FIO_2 0.6–1.0 to maintain SpO_2 at 100%
- Good venous access
- Continuous ECG monitoring
- Adequate pain relief
- Early thrombolysis plus aspirin. (Heparin if using rt-PA)
- Early β-blockade
- Gradual mobilisation

Complications

- Cardiopulmonary arrest
- Continuing chest pain—may be ischaemic or pericarditic in origin
- Pump failure
- Hypotension—apart from cardiogenic shock consider hypovolaemia (e.g. post-diuretics) and a thrombolysis reaction
- Tachyarrhythmias/bradyarrhythmias
- Valve dysfunction—predominantly mitral
- Pericardial tamponade (rare)
- Ventricular septal defect (unusual, often presents 2–5 days post-infarct)
- Complications of thrombolytic therapy—arrhythmias, bleeding, anaphylactoid reaction

Management of the complicated patient

General

- Oxygen—FIO_2 0.6–1.0 to maintain SpO_2 at 100%
- Appropriate and prompt monitoring and investigations as indicated, e.g. echocardiogram, pulmonary artery catheter, angiography, ECG
- Early thrombolysis should still be given however rt-PA followed by heparin should be given in preference to streptokinase if invasive procedures and/or surgery are contemplated.
- Arterial or central venous cannulation should not be delayed if clinically indicated. These procedures should be performed by an experienced operator to minimise the risk of bleeding. The subclavian route should be avoided.
- Angioplasty or revascularization surgery is beneficial if performed early. The cardiologist should be informed promptly if a patient is admitted in pump failure, continuing pain, or valvular dysfunction.

Specific

- Cardiopulmonary arrest—cardiopulmonary resuscitation
- Continuing chest pain
- If ischaemic—iv nitrate and heparin infusions, calcium antagonist and β-blocker (unless contraindicated); consider angiography.
- If pericarditic—consider non-steroidal anti-inflammatory agent
- Management of heart failure
- Tachyarrhythmia—antiarrhythmics, synchronised DC cardioversion
- Bradycardias—chronotrope, consider temporary pacing
- Valve dysfunction—heart failure management; consider surgery
- Pericardial tamponade—pericardial aspiration
- Ventricular septal defect—heart failure management, consider surgery
- Thrombolysis complications

Drug dosage

Diamorphine	2.5mg IV. Repeat prn + anti-emetic
Streptokinase	1.5million units in 100ml 0.9% saline IV over 1h
rt-PA (alteplase)	100mg IV over 90min (15mg bolus, then 50mg over 30min, then 35mg over 60min
APSAC	30 units IV over 5min
Aspirin	150mg PO od
Atenolol	50mg PO od (increase to 100mg od if not hypotensive and HR exceeds 70 bpm) or 5mg slow IV bolus
Propranolol	0–40mg PO qds (titrate to HR of 60 bpm)
Isosorbide dinitrate	2–40mg/h IV
Glyceryl trinitrate	10–200µg/min IV or 0.5–1mg SL
Diltiazem	60mg PO tds
Nifedipine	5–10mg sublingual or PO tds
Atropine	0.3mg IV. Repeat to maximum of 2mg
Isoprenaline	1–4µg/min. Titrate to clinical effect.
Lignocaine	1mg/kg slow IV bolus then 2–4mg/min
Amiodarone	5mg/kg over 20min then infused up to 15mg/kg/day in 5% glucose via central vein. (In emergency give 150–300mg in 10–20ml 5% glucose over 3min)

309

Angina

Ischaemic or, rarely, spasmodic constriction of coronary arteries resulting in pain, usually precordial, pressing or crushing, and with or without radiation to jaw, neck or arms. The sedated, ventilated patient will not usually complain of pain but signs of discomfort may be apparent, e.g. sweating, hypertension, tachycardia. The ECG should be regularly scrutinised for ST segment and/or T wave changes.

Unstable angina encompasses a spectrum of syndromes between stable angina and myocardial infarction. Anginal attacks may be increased in frequency and/or severity, persist longer, respond less to nitrates, and occur at rest or after minimal exertion.

Pathophysiology

- Myocardial oxygen supply–demand imbalance usually due to coronary artery atheroma ± disruption of plaque or new non-occlusive thrombus formation. Spasm (Prinzmetal angina) is uncommon.
- Vasopressor drugs may compromise myocardial perfusion by further constricting an already stenosed vessel.
- Vasodilator drugs may also compromise myocardial perfusion by a 'coronary steal' phenomenon where blood flow is re-distributed away from stenosed vessels.

Diagnosis

- Symptoms, especially chest pain but also non-specific, e.g. sweating
- ECG changes—ST segment elevation/depression, T wave inversion
- No rise in cardiac enzymes
- Dyskinetic areas of myocardium may be seen by echocardiography or angiography

Treatment

- Ensure adequate oxygenation
- Correct hypotension and tissue hypoperfusion
- Consider drug causes, e.g. vasopressors
- Glyceryl trinitrate 0.5mg SL, or nitrolingual spray (0.4–0.8mg) repeated as necessary
- If symptoms are severe and/or persisting, maintain bed rest
- Aspirin 75mg od PO should be prescribed unless contraindicated.
- If symptoms or ST-segment changes persist despite optimal pharmacological intervention, inform cardiologist with a view to angiography and possible angioplasty or surgery.

For continuing angina:
- IV nitrate infusion, e.g. glyceryl trinitrate, isosorbide trinitrate
- Consider calcium antagonist, e.g. diltiazem
- Consider β-blocker (unless contraindicated), e.g. propranolol, atenolol
- Heparinisation (unless contraindicated)
- If symptoms/signs persist, consider angiography with view to angioplasty or surgery

See also:
ECG monitoring, 102; Blood pressure monitoring, 104; Central venous
catheter—use, 108; Central venous catheter—insertion, 110; Vasodilators, 186;
Acute myocardial infarction, 308; Heart failure—assessment Heart failure—
management, 314; Pain, 496

Heart failure—assessment

Impaired ability of the heart to supply adequate oxygen and nutrients to meet the demands of the body's metabolising tissues.

Major causes

- Myocardial infarction/ischaemia
- Drugs e.g. β-blockers
- Tachy- or bradyarrhythmias
- Valve dysfunction
- Septal defect
- Cardiomyopathy/myocarditis
- Pericardial tamponade

Clinical features

Decreased forward flow leading to poor tissue perfusion
- Muscle fatigue leading ultimately to hypercapnia and collapse
- Confusion, agitation, drowsiness, coma
- Oliguria
- Increasing metabolic acidosis and dyspnoea
- ECG changes due to poor myocardial perfusion
- Arterial hypoxaemia

Increased venous congestion secondary to right heart failure
- peripheral oedema
- Hepatic congestion
- Splanchnic ischaemia
- Raised intracranial pressure

Increased pulmonary hydrostatic pressure secondary to left heart failure
- Pulmonary oedema, dyspnoea
- Hypoxaemia

Investigations

Test	Diagnosis
ECG	myocardial ischaemia/infarction, arrhythmias
Chest X-ray	with left heart failure: pulmonary oedema (interstitial perihilar ('bat's wing') shadowing, upper lobe blood diversion, Kerley B lines, pleural effusion) ± cardiomegaly
Pulmonary artery catheter	low cardiac output and stroke volume, low mixed venous oxygen saturation (< 60%), raised PAWP (with left heart failure), raised RAP (with right heart failure), V waves with mitral or tricuspid regurgitation
Blood gases	low SaO_2, variable $PaCO_2$, base deficit > 2mmol/L
Echocardiogram	poor myocardial contractility, pericardial effusion, valve stenosis/incompetence

Notes

Peripheral oedema implies total body salt and water retention but not necessarily intravascular fluid overload.

Heart failure—management

Basic measures

1 Determine likely cause and treat as appropriate, e.g. antiarrhythmic.
2 Oxygen—FIO_2 0.6–1.0 to maintain SpO_2 at 100%
3 GTN spray SL then commence iv nitrate infusion titrated rapidly until good clinical effect. Beware hypotension which, at low dosage, is suggestive of left ventricular underfilling, e.g. hypovolaemia, tamponade, mitral stenosis, pulmonary embolus.
4 If patient agitated or in pain, give diamorphine IV.
5 Consider early CPAP and/or IPPV (+ PEEP) to reduce work of breathing and provide good oxygenation. Cardiac output will often improve in this condition. Do not delay until the patient is in extremis.
6 Frusemide is rarely needed as first-line therapy unless intravascular fluid overload is causative. Initial symptomatic relief is provided by its prompt vasodilating action; however, subsequent diuresis may result in marked hypovolaemia leading to compensatory vasoconstriction, increased cardiac work and worsening myocardial function. Diuretics may be indicated for acute-on-chronic failure, especially if the patient is on long-term diuretic therapy but should not be used if the patient is hypovolaemic. If frusemide is required, start at low doses then reassess.

Directed management

1 Adequate monitoring (usually pulmonary artery catheterisation) and investigation (echocardiography).
2 If evidence exists for hypovolaemia, give 100–200ml colloid fluid challenges to achieve optimal stroke volume.
3 If vasoconstriction persists (SVR > 1400dyn·sec·cm^{-5}), titrate nitrate infusion further to optimise stroke volume and, ideally, reduce SVR < 1300dyn·sec·cm^{-5}. If hypovolaemia is suspected (i.e. stroke volume falls), fluid challenges should be given to re-optimise the stroke volume. After 24 hours of nitrate infusion, commence ACE inhibition, initially at low dose but rapidly increased to appropriate long-term doses.
4 Inotropes are indicated if evidence of tissue hypoperfusion, hypotension or vasoconstriction persists despite optimal fluid loading and nitrate dosing. Consider either adrenaline or dobutamine; while adrenaline may sometimes cause excessive constriction, dobutamine may excessively vasodilate.
5 Intra-aortic balloon counterpulsation augments cardiac output, reduces cardiac work and improves coronary artery perfusion.
6 Angioplasty or surgical revascularization have been shown to be beneficial if performed early after myocardial infarction. Surgery may also be necessary for mechanical defects, e.g. acute mitral regurgitation.

Treatment end-points

1 BP and cardiac output adequate to maintain organ perfusion (e.g. no oliguria, confusion, dyspnoea nor metabolic acidosis). A mean BP of 60mmHg is usually sufficient but may need to be higher, especially if pre-morbid blood pressures are high.
2 A mixed venous oxygen saturation $\geqslant 60\%$. Excessive inotrope dosage should be avoided as myocardial oxygen demand is increased.

Drug dosage

glyceryl trinitrate	2–40mg/h IV or 0.4–0.8mg by SL spray
isosorbide dinitrate	2–40mg/h IV
sodium nitroprusside	20–400µg/min IV
captopril	6.25mg PO test dose increasing to 25mg tds
enalapril	2.5mg PO test dose increasing to 40mg od
lisinopril	2.5mg PO test dose increasing to 40mg od
adrenaline	infusion starting from 0.05µg/kg/min
dobutamine	2.5–25µg/kg/min IV
dopexamine	0.5–6µg/kg/min IV
milrinone	loading dose of 50µg/kg IV over 10min followed by infusion from 0.375–0.75µg/kg/min.
enoximone	loading dose of 0.5–1mg/kg IV over 10min followed by infusion from 5–20µg/kg/min.
diamorphine	2.5mg IV. Repeat every 5min as necessary
frusemide	10–20mg IV bolus. Repeat or increase as necessary

Renal Disorders

Oliguria

Defined as a urine output <0.5ml/kg/h and caused by:

- Post-renal—urinary tract obstruction, e.g. blocked catheter, ureteric trauma, prostatism, raised intra-abdominal pressure, blood clot, bladder tumour
- Renal—established acute renal failure, acute tubular necrosis, glomerulonephritis
- Pre-renal—hypovolaemia, low cardiac output, hypotension, inadequate renal blood flow.

Obstruction and pre-renal causes of oliguria must be excluded before resorting to diuretics.

Urinary tract obstruction

A full bladder should be excluded by palpation. Ensure a patent catheter is present. If obstruction is due to blood clot the bladder should be irrigated. If obstruction is suspected higher in the renal tract an ultrasound scan is required for diagnosis and possible urological intervention (e.g. nephrostomies). Raised intra-abdominal pressure may cause oliguria by impeding renal venous drainage (particularly if >20mmHg). Relief of the high pressure often promotes a diuresis.

Hypovolaemia

Once renal tract obstruction has been excluded it is mandatory to correct hypovolaemia by fluid challenge. Oliguria in hypovolaemic patients may be physiological or may be due to a reduced renal blood flow.

Inadequate renal blood flow and / or pressure

If cardiac output remains low despite correction of hypovolaemia correction with vasodilators and/or inotropes will be necessary. If the blood pressure remains low after improving the cardiac output vasopressors may be needed to achieve a mean blood pressure of at least 60mmHg. In elderly patients and others with pre-existing hypertension a higher mean blood pressure may be necessary to maintain urine output.

Persistent oliguria

Attempts to increase urine output with diuretics may follow the above measures if oliguria persists. Frusemide and/or low dose dopamine (1.0–2.5µg/kg/min IV) are the usual first-line agents. Frusemide is given in a dose of 5–10mg intravenously with higher increments at 30min intervals to a maximum of 250mg. Higher doses may be needed if the patient has previously received diuretic therapy or a low dose infusion may be started (1–5mg/h IV). Mannitol (20g intravenously) may be considered although failure to promote a diuresis may increase oedema formation. Failure to re-establish urine output may require renal support in the form of dialysis or haemofiltration. There is no point in continuing diuretic therapy if it is not effective; loop diuretics in particular may be nephrotoxic. Indications for renal support include fluid overload, hyperkalaemia, metabolic acidosis, creation of space for nutrition or drugs, persistent renal failure with rising urea and creatinine, and symptomatic uraemia.

Biochemical Assessment

	Pre-renal cause	Renal cause
Urine osmolality (mOsm/kg)	> 500	< 400
Urine Na (mmol/L)	< 20	> 40
Urine : Plasma creatinine	> 40	< 20
Fractional Na excretion[*]	< 1	> 2

$$* \ 100 \times \frac{\text{urine plasma Na}}{\text{urine plasma creatinine}}$$

Acute renal failure—diagnosis

Renal failure is defined as renal function inadequate to clear the waste products of metabolism despite absence or correction of haemodynamic or mechanical causes. Renal failure is suggested by:

- uraemic symptoms (drowsiness, nausea, hiccough, twitching)
- Raised plasma creatinine ($>200\mu mol/L$)
- Hyperkalaemia
- Hyponatraemia
- Metabolic acidosis.

Persistent oliguria may be a feature of acute renal failure but non-oliguric renal failure is not uncommon; 2–3L of poor quality urine per day may occur despite an inadequate glomerular filtration rate. The prognosis is better if urine output is maintained. Clinical features may suggest the cause of renal failure and dictate further investigation. Acute tubular necrosis is the commonest cause of renal failure in critically ill patients (e.g. following hypovolaemia, sepsis, extensive burns, acute pancreatitis) but other causes must be borne in mind. Anaemia implies chronic renal failure.

Post-operative renal failure

Usually due to acute tubular necrosis; risk factors include hypovolaemia, haemodynamic instability (particularly hypotension), major abdominal surgery in those >50 years, major surgery in jaundiced patients and biliary and other sepsis. Surgical procedures (particularly gynaecological) may be complicated by damage to the lower urinary tract with an obstructive nephropathy. Abdominal aortic aneurysm surgery may be associated with renal arterial disruption and should be investigated urgently with renography and possible arteriography or re-exploration.

Other causes

- Nephrotoxins—may cause renal failure via acute tubular necrosis, interstitial nephritis or renal tubular obstruction. All potential nephrotoxins should be withdrawn.
- Rhabdomyolysis—myoglobinuria and raised CPK in patients who have suffered a crush injury, coma or seizures are suggestive.
- Glomerular disease—the presence of red cell casts, haematuria, proteinuria and systemic features (e.g. hypertension, purpura, arthralgia, vasculitis) are all suggestive of glomerular disease. A renal biopsy or specific blood tests (e.g. Goodpasture's syndrome, vasculitis) are required to confirm the diagnosis and appropriate treatment.
- Haemolytic uraemic syndrome—suggested by haemolysis, uraemia, thrombocytopenia and neurological abnormalities.
- Crystal nephropathy—suggested by the presence of crystals in the urinary sediment. Microscopic examination of the crystals confirms the diagnosis (e.g. urate, oxalate). Release of purines and urate cause acute renal failure in the tumour lysis syndrome.
- Renovascular disorders—loss of vascular supply may be diagnosed by renography. Complete loss of arterial supply may occur in abdominal trauma or aortic disease (particularly dissection). More commonly, the arterial supply is partially compromised (e.g. renal artery stenosis) and blood flow is further reduced by haemodynamic instability or locally via drug therapy (e.g. NSAIDs, ACE inhibitors). Renal vein obstruction may be due to thrombosis or external compression (e.g. raised intra-abdominal pressure).

Nephrotoxins

The following are some common nephrotoxins:

Allopurinol	Aminoglycosides
Amphotericin	Cephalosporins
Dextran 40	Frusemide
Heavy metals	Herbal medicines
Narcotics	NSAIDs
Organic solvents	Paraquat
Penicillins	Pentamidine
Phenytoin	Radiographic contrast
Sulphonamides	Tetracyclines
Thiazides	Vancomycin

32

Acute renal failure—management

Identification and correction of reversible causes of renal failure is necessary. All cases require careful attention to fluid management and nutritional support. Early use of dialysis and/or filtration techniques may improve outcome and allow normal fluid and nutritional intake.

Urinary tract obstruction

Lower urinary tract obstruction requires the insertion of a urinary catheter (suprapubic if there is urethral disruption) to allow urinary tract decompression. Ureteric obstruction requires urinary tract decompression by nephrostomy or stent. A massive diuresis is common after urinary tract decompression so it is important to ensure an adequate circulating volume.

Haemodynamic management

Pre-renal failure is reversible before acute tubular necrosis becomes established. Careful fluid management to ensure an adequate circulating volume and any necessary inotrope or vasopressor support may establish a diuresis. If oliguria persists after pre-renal factors have been corrected, the use of diuretics may establish a diuresis. The circulating volume must be corrected first.

Metabolic management

Hyperkalaemia may be life threatening (> 6.5mmol/L or ECG changes) and may be prevented by potassium restriction, early dialysis or haemo(dia)filtration. Hypocalcaemia and hyponatraemia are best treated with dialysis and/or haemo(dia)filtration although calcium supplementation may be used. Hyponatraemia is usually due to water excess although salt losing nephropathies (acute tubular necrosis, other renal tubular disorders) may require sodium chloride supplements. Hyperphosphataemia may be treated with dialysis, filtration or aluminium hydroxide orally. Metabolic acidosis (not due to tissue hypoperfusion) may be corrected with dialysis, filtration or 1.26% sodium bicarbonate infusion.

Nephrotoxins and crystal nephropathies

All nephrotoxic agents should be withheld if possible. All necessary drugs should have their dosage modified according to the GFR. In some cases urinary excretion of nephrotoxins and crystals may be encouraged by urinary alkalinisation to maintain their solubility with an induced diuresis (rhabdomyolysis, acidic crystals). Dialysis may also be useful.

Glomerular disease

Immunosuppressive therapy may be useful after diagnosis has been confirmed. Dialysis is often required for the more severe forms of glomerulonephritis despite steroid responsiveness.

Renal replacement therapy

Continuous haemofiltration forms the mainstay of replacement therapy in critically ill patients who often cannot tolerate haemodialysis due to haemodynamic instability. Peritoneal dialysis is not commonly used. Acute renal failure in the critically ill usually recovers within 1–6 weeks; permanent renal failure is rare.

Urgent treatment of hyperkalaemia

- 10–20ml calcium chloride 10% by slow intravenous injection
- 50ml 8.4% sodium bicarbonate intravenously repeated prn
- Glucose (50g) and insulin (10–20iu) intravenously with careful blood glucose monitoring
- Urgent haemodialysis

Indications for dialysis or haemo(dia)filtration

Fluid excess (e.g. pulmonary oedema)
Hyperkalaemia ($>6.0mmol/L$)
Metabolic acidosis ($pH < 7.2$) due to renal failure
Clearance of dialysable nephrotoxins and other drugs
Creatinine rising $>100\mu mol/L/day$
Creatinine $>300–600\mu mol/L$
Urea rising $>16–20mmol/L/day$
To create space for nutrition or drugs

32

Gastrointestinal Disorders

Vomiting / gastric stasis

While vomiting *per se* is relatively rare in the ICU patient, large volume gastric aspirates are commonplace and probably represent the major reason for failure of enteral nutrition.

Ileus

Ileus affects the stomach more frequently than the rest of the GI tract. Abdominal surgery, drugs (particularly opiates), gut dysfunction as a component of multi-organ dysfunction, hypoperfusion and prolonged starvation may all contribute to gastric ileus. Early and continued use of the bowel for feeding appears to maintain forward propulsive action. Management consists of treating the cause where possible, the use of motility stimulants such as metoclopramide, cisapride or erythromycin and, in resistant cases, bypassing the stomach with a nasoduodenal/ nasojejunal tube or a jejunostomy.

Upper bowel obstruction

Relatively unusual; apart from primary surgical causes such as neoplasm or adhesions, the predominant cause in the ICU is gastric outlet obstruction. This may be related to long-standing peptic ulcer disease or may occur in the short term from pyloric and/or duodenal swelling consequent to gastritis or duodenitis. This can be diagnosed endoscopically and treated by bowel rest plus an H_2 antagonist, proton pump inhibitor or sucralfate.

Gastric irritation

Drugs or chemicals—either accidental or adverse reaction (e.g. steroids, aspirin), intentional (e.g. alcohol, bleach) or therapeutic (e.g. ipecacuanaha syrup) may induce vomiting. Treatment, where appropriate, may comprise (i) removal of the cause, (ii) dilution with copious amounts of fluid (iii) neutralisation with alkali and/or H_2 antagonist or proton pump inhibitor and (iv) administration of antiemetic (e.g. metoclopramide).

Neurological

Stimulation of the emetic centre may follow any neurological event (e.g. trauma, CVA), drug therapy (e.g. chemotherapy), pain and metabolic disturbances. Management is by treating the cause where possible and by judicious use of anti-emetics, initially metoclopramide or prochlorperazine. Consider ondansetron if these are unsuccessful.

See also:
Enteral nutrition, 72; Electrolytes (Na^+, K^+, Cl^-, HCO_3^-), 138; Opioid analgesics, 222; Anti-emetics, 212; Gut motility agents, 214; Bowel perforation and obstruction, 336; Intracranial haemorrhage, 364; Subarachnoid haemorrhage, 366; Raised intracranial pressure, 368; Electrolyte management, 400; Poisoning—general principles, 438

Diarrhoea

The definition of diarrhoea in the ICU patient is problematic as the amount of stool passed daily is difficult to measure. Frequency and consistency may also vary significantly. Loose/watery and frequent ($\geq 4 \times$ day) stool will often require investigation and/or treatment.

Commoner ICU causes

- Infection—*Clostridium difficile*, gastroenteritis (e.g. *Salmonella, Shigella*), rarer tropical causes (e.g. cholera, dysentry, giardiasis, tropical sprue)
- Drugs, e.g. antibiotics, laxatives
- Gastrointestinal—feed (e.g. lactose intolerance), coeliac disease, other malabsorption syndromes, inflammatory bowel disease, diverticulitis, pelvic abscess, bowel obstruction with overflow

Enteral feed is often implicated but rarely causative.

For bloody diarrhoea consider infection, ischaemic or inflammatory bowel disease.

Diagnosis

- Rectal examination to rule out impaction with overflow. Consider sigmoidoscopy if colitis or *C. difficile* suspected (pseudomembrane seen).
- Stool sent to laboratory for MC & S, *C. difficile* toxin.
- Fat estimation (malabsorption) is rarely necessary in the ICU patient.
- If ischaemic or inflammatory bowel disease suspected, perform supine abdominal X-ray and inspect for dilated loops of bowel (n.b. toxic megacolon), thickened walls (increased separation between loops) and 'thumbprinting' (suggestive of mucosal oedema). Fluid levels seen on erect or lateral abdominal X-ray may be seen in diarrhoea or paralytic ileus and do not necessarily indicate obstruction.
- If abscess suspected, perform ultrasonography or CT scan.

Management

1 Treat cause where possible e.g. for *C. difficile,* metronidazole plus cholesytramine (binds the toxin)
2 Consider temporary (12–24h) cessation of enteral feed if very severe. Consider change in feed if appropriate e.g. coeliac disease, lactose intolerance.
3 Consider stopping antibiotics.
4 Give anti-diarrhoeal if infection excluded
5 Careful attention to fluid and electrolyte balance (in particular Na^+, K^+, Mg^{2+})
6 Request surgical opinion if infarcted or inflamed bowel or abscess suspected.

329

See also:
Enteral nutrition, 72; Antidiarrhoeals, 216; Abdominal sepsis, 342

Failure to open bowels

Commoner ICU causes

- Prolonged ileus/decreased gut motility (e.g. opiates, post-surgery)
- Lack of enteral nutrition
- Bowel obstruction—this is a relatively uncommon secondary event and is mainly seen postoperatively, either after a curative procedure or with development of adhesions

Management

1 Clinically exclude obstruction and confirm presence of stool per rectum.
2 Ensure adequate hydration.
3 Anti-constipation therapy may be given, usually starting with laxatives (e.g. lactulose or, for more urgent response, magnesium sulphate), then proceeding to glycerine suppositories and, finally, enemata if gentler measures prove unsuccessful.
4 Consider reducing/stopping dose of opiate if possible.

See also:
Anti-constipation agents, 218; Bowel perforation and obstruction, 336

Upper gastrointestinal haemorrhage

Causes
- peptic ulceration
- oesophagitis/gastritis/duodenitis
- varices
- Mallory-Weiss lower oesophageal tear
- neoplasms

Pathophysiology

Peptic ulceration is related to protective barrier loss leading to acid or biliary damage of the underlying mucosa and submucosa. Barrier loss occurs secondary to critical illness, alcohol, drugs, e.g. nonsteroidals, poisons including corrosives. Direct damage, especially at the lower oesophagus, may occur from feeding tubes. Mucosal damage ('stress ulcers') may also occur as a consequence of tissue hypoperfusion. Gastric hypersecretion is uncommon in critically ill patients; indeed, gastric acid content and secretion is often reduced.

Prophylaxis
- Small-bore feeding tubes.
- Nasogastric enteral nutrition (nasojejunal and parenteral feeding has also been shown to reduce the incidence of stress ulcer bleeding).
- Adequate tissue perfusion (flow and pressure).
- The role of prophylactic drug therapy including H_2 antagonists, proton pump inhibitors and sucralfate is controversial. Evidence suggests that enteral nutrition alone is as effective and there are claims that loss of the acid environment in the stomach predisposes the patient to nosocomial infection. Patients at highest risk are those requiring prolonged mechanical ventilation or with a concurrent coagulopathy.

Treatment of major haemorrhage
- Fluid resuscitation with colloid and blood with blood products as appropriate to correct any coagulopathy. Maintain haemoglobin > 10g/dl and have adequate cross-matched blood available should further large haemorrhages occur.
- If possible, discontinue any on-going anticoagulation, e.g. heparin
- Urgent diagnostic fibreoptic endoscopy. Local injection of adrenaline into bleeding peptic ulcer base or sclerosing agent into bleeding varices may arrest or prevent further bleeding.
- If oesophageal varices are known or highly suspected, consider Sengstaken-type tube for severe haemorrhage. Remember that sources of bleeding other than varices may be present, e.g. peptic ulcer.
- For peptic ulceration and generalised inflammation commence H_2 antagonist or proton pump inhibitor. Give intravenously to ensure effect. Enteral antacid may also be beneficial.
- Surgery is rarely necessary but should be considered if bleeding continues, e.g. > 6–10 unit transfusion requirement. Inform surgeon promptly of any patient with major bleeding.

333

Bleeding varices

Varices develop following a prolonged period of portal hypertension, usually related to liver cirrhosis. Approximately one third will bleed. They are commonly found in the lower oesophagus but occasionally in the stomach or duodenum. Torrential haemorrhage may occur. Approximately 50% of patients will die within 6 weeks of presentation of their first variceal bleed; each subsequent bleed carries a 30% mortality.

Management

1 If airway and/or breathing are compromised, perform endotracheal intubation and institute mechanical ventilation. This facilitates Sengstaken-type tube placement and endoscopy though may be associated with severe hypotension secondary to covert hypovolaemia. If possible, ensure adequate intravascular filling before intubation.

2 Fluid resuscitation with colloid and blood with blood products as appropriate to correct any coagulopathy. Ensure good venous access (at least two 14G cannulae). Group-specific or O-negative blood may be needed for emergency use. Maintain haemoglobin > 10g/dl and have at least 4 units of cross-matched blood available for urgent transfusion. There is a theoretical risk that over-transfusion may precipitate further bleeding by raising portal venous pressure. Pulmonary artery catheterisation should be considered if the patient remains haemodynamically unstable or there is a history of heart disease.

3 If bleeding is torrential, insert a Sengstaken-type tube.

4 If bleeding is not massive, placement of a large-bore nasogastric tube facilitates drainage of blood, lessens the risk of aspiration and can be used to assess continuing blood loss.

5 Perform urgent fibreoptic endoscopy to exclude other sources of bleeding. This also permits local injection of sclerosing agent or variceal ligation. Bleeding is arrested in up to 90% of cases. Endoscopy may be impossible in the short-term if bleeding is too severe. It may have to be delayed for 6–24h until a period of tamponade by the Sengstaken-type tube has enabled some control of the bleeding.

6 If endoscopy or balloon tamponade is delayed, then either octreotide or vasopressin can be administered. Vasopressin controls bleeding in approximately 60% of cases and its efficacy appears to be enhanced by concurrent GTN. Octreotide is a somatostatin analogue but longer-acting than its parent compound; like somatostatin, it is at least as effective as vasopressin but without the side-effects.

7 If bleeding continues after prolonged balloon tamponade (2–3 days) and repeated endoscopy, consider transjugular intrahepatic portosystemic stented shunt (TIPSS). This can be performed quickly and carries a relatively low mortality compared to surgery although the risk of encephalopathy is increased.

8 The traditional alternative to TIPSS is oesophageal transection (now performed with a staple gun) with or without devascularization. Mortality in the acute situation is approximately 30%.

Drug dosages

octreotide	50µg bolus then 50µg/h infusion
vasopressin	20 units over 20min then 0.4 units/min infusion
	Also give glyceryl trinitrate 2–20mg/h to counteract myocardial and mesenteric ischaemia

335

Bowel perforation and obstruction

Patients with bowel perforation or obstruction may be admitted to the ICU after surgery, for pre-operative resuscitation and cardio-respiratory optimisation, or for conservative management. Although rarely occurring *de novo* in the ICU patient, these conditions may be difficult to diagnose because of sedation $\pm$ muscle relaxation. Consider when there is:

- abdominal pain, tenderness, peritonism
- abdominal distension
- agitation
- increased nasogastric aspirates, vomiting
- increasing metabolic acidosis
- signs of hypovolaemia or sepsis

A firm diagnosis is often not made until laparotomy although supine and either erect or lateral abdominal X-ray may reveal either free gas in the peritoneum (perforation) or dilated bowel loops with multiple fluid levels (obstruction). Ultrasound is usually unhelpful though faecal fluid may occasionally be aspirated from the peritoneum following perforation.

It may be difficult to distinguish bowel obstruction from a paralytic ileus as (i) bowel sounds may be present or absent in either and (ii) X-ray appearances may be similar.

Management

1 Correct fluid and electrolyte abnormalities. Resuscitation should be prompt and aggressive and usually consists of colloid replacement plus blood to maintain haemoglobin > 10g/dl. Inotropes or vasopressors may be required to restore an adequate circulation, particularly following perforation. Early insertion of a pulmonary artery catheter should be considered if circulatory status remains unstable or vasoactive drugs are required.

2 The surgeon should be informed at an early stage. A conservative approach may be adopted, e.g. with upper small bowel perforation; however, surgery is usually required for large bowel perforation. Small or large bowel obstruction may sometimes be managed conservatively as spontaneous resolution may occur, e.g. adhesions. Prompt surgical exploration should be encouraged if the patient shows signs of systemic toxicity.

3 Both conservative and post-operative management of perforation and obstruction usually require continuous nasogastric drainage to decompress the stomach, nil by mouth and parenteral nutrition.

4 Pain relief should not be withheld.

5 Broad spectrum antibiotic therapy should also be commenced for the treatment of bowel perforation after appropriate specimens have been taken for laboratory analysis. Therapy usually comprises aerobic and anaerobic Gram negative cover (e.g. 2nd or 3rd generation cephalosporin, quinolone or carbapenem, plus metronidazole $\pm$ aminoglycoside).

6 Post-operative management of bowel perforation may involve repeated laparotomies to exclude collections of pus and bowel ischaemia/infarction; surgery should be expedited if the patient's condition deteriorates. Alternatively, regular ultrasonic and/or CT examinations may be needed.

337

Lower intestinal bleeding & colitis

Causes of lower gastrointestinal bleeding

- Bowel ischaemia/infarction
- Inflammatory bowel disease (ulcerative colitis, Crohn's disease)
- Infection, e.g. *Shigella, Campylobacter,* amoebic dysentry
- Upper gastrointestinal source, e.g. peptic ulceration
- Angiodysplasia
- Neoplasm

Although relatively rare, massive lower gastrointestinal haemorrhage can be life-threatening.

Ischaemic / infarcted bowel

Can occur following prolonged hypoperfusion or, occasionally, secondary to a mesenteric embolus. It usually presents with severe abdominal pain, bloody diarrhoea and signs of systemic toxicity including a rapidly increasing metabolic acidosis. Plasma phosphate levels may also be elevated. X-ray appearances of thickened, oedematous bowel loops ('thumb-printing') with an increased distance between bowel loops is suggestive. Treatment is by restoration of tissue perfusion, blood transfusion to maintain haemoglobin > 10g/dl and, if clincal features fail to settle promptly, laparotomy with a view to bowel excision.

Inflammatory bowel disease

Presents with weight loss, abdominal pain and diarrhoea which usually contains blood. Complications of ulcerative colitis include perforation and toxic megacolon while complications of Crohn's disease include fistulae, abscesses and perforations.

Management involves:

1 Fluid and electrolyte replacement.
2 Blood transfusion to maintain haemoglobin > 10g/dL.
3 High dose steroids parenterally and, if distal bowel involvement, by enema.
4 Nutrition (often parenteral).
5 Regular surgical review. Surgery may be indicated if symptoms fail to settle after 5–7 days, for toxic megacolon, perforation, abscesses or obstruction.
6 Antidiarrhoeal drugs should be avoided.

Angiodysplasia

Usually presents as fresh bleeding per rectum which may be considerable. It is due to an arteriovenous malformation and commoner in the elderly. Surgery is often required if bleeding fails to settle on conservative management though localisation of the lesion may be difficult, necessitating extensive bowel resection. Localisation by angiography may be useful during active bleeding.

339

Abdominal sepsis

A common but difficult to diagnose condition in intensive care patients. A proportion of such patients are admitted following laparotomy but others may develop abdominal sepsis *de novo* or as a secondary complication following abdominal surgery, in particular after bowel resection. Sepsis may either be localised to an organ, e.g. cholecystitis, or the peritoneal cavity (abscess); alternatively, there may be a generalised peritonitis. Non-bowel infection or inflammation can present in a similar manner, e.g. pancreatitis, cholecystitis, gynaecological infection, pyelonephritis

Clinical features

- Non-specific signs including pyrexia (especially swinging), neutrophilia, falling platelet count, increasing metabolic acidosis, circulatory instability.
- Abdominal distension ± localised discomfort, peritonism
- Abdominal mass, e.g. gall bladder, pseudocyst, abscess
- Failure to tolerate enteral feed/Large nasogastric aspirates
- Pleural effusion (if subdiaphragmatic sepsis)
- Diarrhoea (if pelvic sepsis)

Diagnosis

- Ultrasound
- CT scan
- Laparotomy
- Gallium white cell scans are occasionally useful for identification of abscesses.

Samples should be taken for microbiological analysis from blood, urine, stool, abdominal drain fluid and vaginal discharge if present. A sample of pus is preferred to a swab. Hyperamylasaemia may suggest pancreatitis though amylase levels can also be elevated with other intra-abdominal pathologies.

Treatment

- Antibiotic therapy providing aerobic and anaerobic Gram negative cover (e.g. 2nd or 3rd generation cephalosporin, quinolone or carbapenem, plus metronidazole ± aminoglycoside). Treatment can be changed depending on culture results and patient response
- Ultrasonic or CT-guided drainage of pus
- Laparotomy with removal of pus, peritoneal lavage, etc...

A negative laparotomy should be viewed as a useful means of excluding intra-abdominal sepsis rather than an unnecessary procedure. Laparotomy should be encouraged if the patient's condition deteriorates and a high suspicion of abdominal pathology persists.

Cholecystitis, with or without (acalculous) the presence of gallstones, may present with signs of infection. There is a characteristic ultrasound appearance of an enlarged organ with a thickened, oedematous wall surrounded by fluid. Treatment may be conservative with antibiotics (as above) and percutaneous, ultrasound-guided drainage via a pigtail catheter. Cholecystectomy may be necessary in the acute situation, especially for acalculous cholecystitis.

See also:
 Enteral nutrition, 72; Parenteral nutrition, 74; Infection control, 78;
Bacteriology, 148; Colloids, 170; Inotropes, 184; Vasopressors, 188;
Antimicrobials, 248; Basic resuscitation, 258; Fluid challenge, 262; Bowel
perforation and obstruction, 336; Pancreatitis, 342; Systemic inflammatory
response, 488; Sepsis / infection, 490

Pancreatitis

Inflammation of the pancreas and surrounding retroperitoneal tissues. The appearance of the pancreas may range from mildly oedematous to haemorrhagic and narcotising. A pseudocyst may develop which can become infected and the bile duct may be obstructed causing biliary obstruction and jaundice. Though mortality is quoted at 5–10%, this is considerably higher in those requiring intensive care.

Causes
- Alcohol
- gallstones
- Miscellaneous, e.g. ischaemia, trauma, viral, hyperlipidaemia
- Part of the multiple organ failure syndrome

Diagnosis
- Non-specific features include central, severe abdominal pain, pyrexia, haemodynamic instability, vomiting, ileus. Discoloration around the umbilicus (Cullen's sign) or flanks (Grey Turner's sign) is rarely seen.
- Plasma enzymes—elevated levels of amylase (usually > 1000IU/ml) and pancreatic lipase are suggestive but non-specific. The levels may be normal, even in severe pancreatitis.
- Ultrasound
- CT scan
- Laparotomy

Complications
- Multi-organ dysfunction syndrome
- Infection/abscess formation
- Hypocalcaemia
- Diabetes mellitus

Management
- General measures including fluid resuscitation, blood transfusion to maintain haemoglobin > 10g/dL, respiratory support, analgesia, and anti-emetics. Routine antibiotics are of unproved benefit.
- Adequate monitoring should be instituted, including pulmonary artery catheterisation if cardiorespiratory instability is present.
- Patients are usually kept nil by mouth with continuous nasogastric drainage. Nutrition and vitamins are usually provided parenterally.
- If gallstone obstruction is the cause, this should be relieved either endoscopically or surgically.
- Hypocalcaemia, if symptomatic, should be treated by intermittent slow IV injection (or, occasionally, infusion) of 10% CaCl.
- Hyperglycaemia should be controlled by continuous IV insulin.
- No specific treatment is routinely used. PAF antagonists are currently being investigated in multi-centre trials. One centre has reported success with continuous drainage of lymph from the thoracic duct replaced fresh frozen plasma and albumin.
- The role of surgery remains controversial; many surgeons strongly advocate either conservative or aggressive, interventional approaches. The former may utilise percutaneous drainage of infected and/or necrotic debris while surgery frequently consists of regular (often daily) laparotomy with debridement of necrotic tissue and peritoneal lavage. Pseudocysts may resolve or require drainage either percutaneously or into the bowel.

Ranson's signs of severity in acute pancreatitis

On hospital admission:
- age > 55 years old
- blood glucose > 11mmol/L
- serum lactate dehydrogenase > 300U/L
- serum aspartate aminotransferase > 250U/L
- white blood count > 16000/mm^3

At 48h after admission:
- haematocrit fall > 10%
- blood urea nitrogen rise > 1mmol/L
- serum calcium < 2mmol/L
- PaO$_2$ < 8kPa
- arterial base deficit > 4mmol/L
- estimated fluid sequestration > 6000ml

343

Hepatic Disorders

Jaundice

Jaundice is a clinical diagnosis of yellow pigmentation of sclera and skin resulting from a raised plasma bilirubin. It is usually visible when the plasma bilirubin exceeds 30–40μmol/L.

Commoner causes seen in the ICU

- Pre-hepatic—intravascular haemolysis (e.g. drugs, malaria, haemolytic uraemic syndrome), Gilbert's syndrome.
- Hepatocellular—critical illness, viral (Hepatitis A, B, C, Epstein–Barr), alcohol, drugs (e.g. paracetamol, halothane), toxoplasmosis, leptospirosis.
- Cholestatic—critical illness, intrahepatic causes (e.g. drugs such as chlorpromazine, erythromycin and isoniazid, primary biliary cirrhosis), extrahepatic causes (e.g. biliary obstruction by gallstones, neoplasm, pancreatitis).

Diagnosis

- Urinalysis—unconjugated bilirubin does not appear in the urine.
- Measurement of conjugated and unconjugated bilirubin—conjugated bilirubin predominates in cholestatic jaundice, unconjugated bilirubin in pre-hepatic jaundice, and a mixed picture is often seen in hepatocellular jaundice.
- Plasma alkaline phosphatase is usually markedly elevated in obstructive jaundice while prothrombin times, aspartate transaminase and alanine aminotransferase are elevated in hepatocellular jaundice.
- Ultrasound or CT scan will diagnose extrahepatic biliary obstruction.

Management

1 Identify and treat cause. Where possible, discontinue any drug that could be implicated. If extrahepatic, consider percutaneous transhepatic drainage, bile duct stenting or, rarely, surgery.
2 Liver biopsy is rarely necessary in a jaundiced ICU patient unless the diagnosis is unknown and the possibility exists of liver involvement in the underlying pathology, e.g. malignancy.
3 Non-obstructive jaundice usually settles with conservative management as the patient recovers.
4 An antihistamine and topical Calamine lotion may provide symptomatic relief for pruritus if troublesome. Cholestyramine 4g tds PO may be helpful in obstructive jaundice.

See also:
Parenteral nutrition, 74; Infection control, 78; Liver function tests, 142; Acute
liver failure, 348; Chronic liver failure, 352; Haemolysis, 390; Systemic
inflammatory response, 488

Acute liver failure

Results from massive necrosis of liver cells leading to severe liver dysfunction and encephalopathy. Survival rates for liver failure with Grade 3 or 4 hepatic encephalopathy vary from 10–40% on medical therapy alone to 60–80% with orthotopic liver transplantation.

Major causes
- Alcohol
- Drugs, particularly paracetamol overdose
- Viral hepatitis, particularly hepatitis B, hepatitis C
- Poisons, e.g. carbon tetrachloride
- Acute decompensation of chronic liver disease, e.g. infection.

Diagnosis
- Should be considered in any patient presenting with jaundice, generalised bleeding, encephalopathy or marked hypoglycaemia.
- Abnormal liver function tests, in particular, prolonged international normalised ratio (INR) and hyperbilirubinaemia. In severe liver failure the plasma enzyme levels may not be elevated.

Management
- General measures include fluid resuscitation and blood transfusion to keep haemoglobin > 10g/dL. The circulation is usually hyperdynamic and dilated; vasopressors may be needed to maintain BP.
- Correction of coagulopathy is often withheld as this provides a good guide to recovery or the need for transplantation. Use of fresh frozen plasma is restricted to patients who are bleeding or are about to undergo an invasive procedure.
- Adequate monitoring should be instituted, including pulmonary artery catheterisation if cardiorespiratory instability is present.
- Mechanical ventilation may be necessary if the airway is unprotected or respiratory failure develops. Lung shunts are frequent.
- Infection is commonplace and is frequently either Gram positive or fungal. Clinical signs are often absent. Samples of blood, sputum, urine, wound sites, drain fluid, intravascular catheter sites and ascites should be sent for regular microbiological surveillance. Systemic antimicrobial therapy, with or without selective gut decontamination, has been shown to reduce the infection rate. Fungal infections are also well-recognised in conjunction with bacterial infection. Some Regional Liver Units give prophylactic anti-fungal therapy.
- Hypoglycaemia is a common occurrence. It should be frequently monitored and treated with either enteral (or parenteral) nutrition, or a 10–20% glucose infusion to maintain normoglycaemia.
- Renal failure occurs in 30–70% of cases and may necessitate renal replacement therapy. The incidence may be reduced by careful maintenance of intravascular volume.
- Upper gastrointestinal bleeding is more common due to the associated coagulopathy. Prophylactic H_2-blockers or proton pump inhibitors may be of benefit.
- N-acetylcysteine and/or epoprostenol improves O_2 consumption. Though tissue hypoxia may be reduced by these drugs, particularly when vasopressor drugs are needed, benefit remains unproved.
- Corticosteroids, prostaglandin E_1 and charcoal haemoperfusion have not been shown to have any outcome benefit.

See also:
Ventilatory support—indications, 4; Liver function tests, 142; Hepatic encephalopathy, 350; Paracetamol poisoning, 442

Hepatic encephalopathy

Grading

1 confused, altered mood
2 inappropriate, drowsy
3 stuporose but rousable, very confused, agitated
4 coma, unresponsive to painful stimuli

The risk of cerebral oedema is far higher at Grades 3 and 4 (50–85%) and is the leading cause of death. Suggestive signs include systemic hypertension, progressive heart rate slowing, and increasing muscle rigidity and occur at intracranial pressures > 30mmHg.

Management

- Correct/avoid potential aggravating factors, e.g. gut haemorrhage, over-sedation, hypoxia, hypoglycaemia, infection, electrolyte imbalance.
- Consider early intracranial pressure (ICP) monitoring. CT and clinical features correlate poorly with ICP though no controlled studies have yet been performed to show outcome benefit from ICP monitoring which carries its own complication rate (bleeding, infection).
- Maintain patient in slight head-up position (20–30°).
- Regular lactulose, e.g. 20–30ml qds PO, to achieve 2–3 bowel motions/day.
- Dietary restriction of protein.
- Hyperventilation to achieve a $PaCO_2$ of 3.5–4 kPa is often attempted but is frequently unsuccessful in achieving improvement. It may also compromise cerebral blood flow.
- Mannitol (0.5–1mg/kg over 20–30min) if serum osmolality < 320mOsmol/kg and either a raised ICP or clinical signs of cerebral oedema persist. If severe renal dysfunction is present, use renal replacement therapy in conjunction with mannitol.
- If no response to above, consider barbiturate administration, e.g. thiopentone infusion at 1–5mg/kg/h, ideally with ICP monitoring.
- If still no response, consider urgent liver transplantation.
- Exercise caution with concomitant drug usage.

Identification of patients unlikely to survive without transplantation

- Prothrombin time > 100sec

Or any three of the following:

- Age < 10 or > 40 years
- Aetiology is hepatitis C, halothane, or other drug reaction
- Duration of jaundice pre-encephalopathy > 2days
- Prothrombin time > 50sec
- Serum bilirubin > 225µmol/L

If paracetamol-induced:

- pH < 7.3 or prothrombin time > 100sec and creatinine > 200µmol/L plus Grade 3 or 4 encephalopathy.

As only 50–85% of patients identified as requiring transplantation will survive long enough to receive one, the Regional Liver Unit should be informed soon after diagnosis of all possible candidates.

351

Chronic liver failure

Patients admitted to intensive care with chronic liver failure may develop specific associated problems:

- Acute decompensation; this may be secondary to infection, sedation, hypovolaemia, hypotension, diuretics, gastrointestinal haemorrhage, excess dietary protein and electrolyte imbalance
- Infection; the patient may transmit infection, e.g. hepatitis A, B or C and, by being immunosuppressed, is also more prone to acquiring infections such as TB and fungi.
- Drug metabolism—as may drugs are all or part-metabolised by the liver and/or excreted into the bile, the drug action may be prolonged or slowed depending on whether the metabolites are active or not. In particular, sedatives may have a greatly prolonged duration of action.
- Portal hypertension—results in ascites, varices and splenomegaly. Ascites may produce diaphragmatic splinting and is at risk of becoming infected. Drainage may incur a considerable protein loss. Varices may bleed while splenomegaly may result in thrombocytopenia. Renal failure is also recognised due to high intra-abdominal pressure.
- Bleeding—an increased risk is present due to decreased production of clotting factors (II, VII, IX, X), varices and splenomegaly-related thrombocytopenia.
- Alcohol—the most frequent cause of cirrhosis in the western world, acute withdrawal may lead to delirium tremens with severe agitation, hallucinations, seizures and cardiovascular disturbances.
- $2°$ hyperaldosteronism—results in oliguria, salt and water retention.
- Increased tendency to jaundice, especially during critical illness.

Management

1 Ascites
   - Take specimens for microbiological analysis (including TB), protein and cytology. If WBC > 250 per high power field, give Gram negative antibiotic cover.
   - If present in large quantity, (i) decrease sodium and water intake, (ii) commence spironolactone PO (or potassium canrenoate IV) $\pm$ frusemide. Paracentesis $\pm$ colloid replacement, or ascitic reinfusion (if uninfected/non-pancreatitic in origin) may be considered, particularly if diaphragmatic splinting occurs.
2 Coagulopathy
   - Vitamin K 10mg/day slow IV bolus for 2–3 days
   - Fresh frozen plasma, platelets as necessary
3 Hypoglycaemia—should be prevented by adequate nutrition or a 10% or 20% glucose infusion
4 Adequate nutrition and vitamin supplementation
5 Acute decompensation—avoid any precipitating causes, e.g. infection, sedation, hypovolaemia, electrolyte imbalance.
6 Drug administration—review type and dose regularly.

353

Neurological Disorders

Acute weakness

Severe acute weakness may require urgent intubation and mechanical ventilation if the FVC < 1L or gas exchange deteriorates acutely.

Investigation

- Metabolic myopathies—exclude and treat hypophosphataemia, hypokalaemia, hypocalcaemia and hypomagnesaemia.
- Prolonged effects of muscle relaxants—a prolonged effect of suxamethonium will usually be clinically obvious and should prompt assessment of pseudocholinesterase levels. Suxamethonium effects will also be prolonged in myasthenics. Prolonged effects of non-depolarising muscle relaxants is suggested by a response to an anticholinesterase (neostigmine 0.5mg by slow IV bolus with an anticholinergic). This should not be attempted if paralysis is complete. Patients with myasthenia gravis will also respond.
- Guillain–Barré syndrome—a lumbar puncture should be performed to confirm raised CSF protein with normal cells. If these features are not found but suspicion is strong, nerve conduction studies may demonstrate segmental demyelination with slow conduction velocities.
- Myasthenia gravis—fatiguable weakness or ptosis suggests myasthenia gravis; response to IV edrophonium (Tensilon test) and a strongly positive acetylcholine receptor antibody titre confirm this diagnosis. A myasthenic syndrome associated with malignancy (Eaton–Lambert syndrome) involves pelvic and thigh muscles predominantly, tending to spare the ocular muscles.
- Other diagnoses are made largely on the basis of clinical suspicion and specific specialised tests.

General management

- FVC should be monitored 2–4hrly and intubation and mechanical ventilation should follow if FVC < 1L. Other indices of respiratory function are less sensitive. In particular, arterial blood gases may be maintained up to the point of respiratory arrest.
- Weak respiratory muscles lead to progressive basal atelectasis and sputum retention. Chest infection is a significant risk; regular chest physiotherapy with intermittent positive pressure breathing are required for prevention where mechanical ventilation is not necessary.
- Patients who are immobile are at risk of venous stasis and deep venous thrombosis. Prophylaxis with subcutaneous heparin is reasonable. Immobile patients also require attention to posture to prevent pressure sores and contractures.
- Weak bulbar muscles may compromise swallowing with consequent malnutrition or pulmonary aspiration. Enteral nutritional support via a nasogastric tube is necessary.
- In cases with coexistent autonomic neuropathy enteral nutrition may be impossible necessitating parenteral nutritional support. These patients may also suffer arrhythmias and hypotension requiring appropriate support.

Causes of severe weakness

Common in ICU
Metabolic myopathies
Prolonged effects of muscle relaxants
Critical illness neuropathy or myopathy
Guillain–Barré syndrome
Myasthenia gravis
Pontine CVA
Substance abuse (especially benzene ring compounds)

Uncommon in ICU
Chronic relapsing polyneuritis
Endocrine myopathies
Sarcoid neuropathy
Poliomyelitis
Diphtheria
Carcinomatous neuropathy
Porphyria
Botulism
Familial periodic paralysis
Multiple sclerosis
Lead poisoning
Organophosphorus poisoning

357

Agitation / confusion

In the ICU, agitation and/or confusion are predominantly related to sepsis, cerebral hypoperfusion or drugs/drug withdrawal. 'ICU psychosis', with loss of day-night rhythm and inability to sleep, is a common occurrence in the patient recovering from severe illness. Commoner ICU causes

- Infection—including generalised sepsis, chest, cannula sites, urinary tract. Cerebral infection such as meningitis, encephalitis are malaria are relatively rare but should always be considered.
- Drug-related—(i) adverse reaction (particularly affecting the elderly), e.g. sedatives, analgesics, diuretics; (ii) withdrawal e.g. sedatives, analgesics, ethanol; (iii) abuse, e.g. opiates, amphetamines, alcohol, hallucinogens.
- Metabolic—e.g. hypo- or hyperglycaemia, hypo- or hypernatraemia, hypercalcaemia, uraemia, hepatic encephalopathy, hypo- or hyperthermia, dehydration.
- Respiratory—infection, hypoxaemia, hypercapnia.
- Neurological—infection (meningo-encephalitis, malaria), post-head injury, space-occupying lesion (including haematoma), post-ictal, post-cardiac arrest.
- Cardiac—low output state, hypotension, endocarditis.
- Pain—full bladder (blocked Foley catheter), abdominal pain.
- Psychosis—'ICU psychosis', other psychiatric states.

Principles of management

1 Examine for signs of (i) infection (e.g. pyrexia, purulent sputum, catheter sites, neutrophilia, falling platelet count, chest X-ray, meningism . . .), (ii) cardiovascular instability (hypotension, increasing metabolic acidosis, oliguria, arrhythmias . . .), (iii) covert pain, particularly abdominal and lower limbs e.g. compartment syndrome, DVT), (iv) focal neurological signs (e.g. meningism, unequal pupils, hemiparesis), (v) respiratory failure (arterial blood gases), (vi) metabolic derangement (biochemical screen). If any of the above are found, treat as appropriate. Psychosis should not be assumed until treatable causes are excluded.

2 Reassure and calm the patient. Maintain quiet atmosphere and reduce noise levels. Attempt to restore day–night rhythm, e.g. by changing ambient lighting and use of oral hypnotic agents, e.g. temazepam, a tot of alcohol, chloral.

3 Consider starting, changing or increasing the dose of sedative or major tranquilliser to control agitation. If highly agitated and likely to endanger themselves, rapid short-term control can be achieved by a slow IV bolus of sedative. Consider propofol, a benzodiazepine, haloperidol, chlorpromazine or chlormethiazole in the smallest possible dose to achieve the desired effect; observe for hypotension, respiratory depression, arrhythmias and extra-pyramidal effects. Opiates may be needed, especially if pain or withdrawal is a factor. An ethanol infusion can be considered for delirium tremens resulting from alcohol withdrawal.

4 Sedation can be maintained by continuous infusion or intermittent injection, either regularly or as required. The less agitated patient may respond to IM injections of a major tranquilliser though these should be avoided with concurrent coagulopathy.

Drug dosages for severe agitation

- Chlorpromazine—12.5mg by slow iv bolus. Repeat, doubling dose, every 10–15minutes until effect. May need up to 100mg. For regular prescription, give qds.
- Haloperidol—2.5mg by slow IV bolus. Repeat, doubling dose, every 10–15 minutes until effect. For regular prescription, give qds.
- Midazolam/diazepam—2–5mg by slow iv bolus
- Propofol—30–100mg by slow IV bolus.
- Morphine—2.5–5mg by slow IV bolus
- Chlormethiazole—30–100ml over 10–15min then infusion thereafter if needed.

See also:

Generalised seizures

Control of seizures is necessary to prevent ischaemic brain damage, to reduce cerebral oxygen requirements and to reduce intracranial pressure. Where possible correct the cause and give specific treatment. A CT scan may be necessary to identify structural causes. Common causes include:

- hypoxaemia
- hypoglycaemia
- hypocalcaemia
- space occupying lesions
- metabolic and toxic disorders
- drug withdrawal, e.g. alcohol, benzodiazepines, anticonvulsants
- infection, especially meningoencephalitis
- trauma
- idiopathic epilepsy

Most seizures are self limiting, requiring no more than protection from injury (coma position, protect head and do not force anything into the mouth).

Specific treatment

- Hypoxaemia should be corrected with oxygen (FIO_2 0.6–1.0).
- Intubation and ventilation if the airway is unprotected or $SpO_2 < 90\%$.
- Blood glucose should be measured urgently and hypoglycaemia corrected with IV 50ml 50% glucose.
- Anticonvulsant levels should be corrected in known epileptics.
- Cerebral oedema should be managed with sedation, induced hypothermia, controlled hyperventilation and osmotic diuretics.
- In patients with a known tumour, arteritis or parasitic infection high dose dexamethasone may be given.
- Thiamine 100mg IV should be given to alcoholics.
- Consider surgery for space occupying lesions, e.g. blood clot, tumour.

Anticonvulsants

Anticonvulsants are necessary where there are repeated seizures, a single seizure lasts > 30min, or cyanosis is present.

- Diazepam is the usual first line treatment.
- Phenytoin: a loading dose should be given intravenously if the patient has not previously received phenytoin. Phenytoin may not provide immediate control of seizures within the first 24h.

If seizures continue appropriate anticonvulsants include:

- Diazepam given in increments to a maximum of 20mg.
- Chlormethiazole 0.8% by infusion
- Magnesium sulphate
- Clonazepam, which is particularly useful for myoclonic seizures.
- Thiopentone or propofol infusion in severe intractable epilepsy.

With all anticonvulsants care should be taken to avoid hypoventilation and respiratory failure. However, mechanical ventilation will certainly be required if thiopentone is used and probably to maintain oxygenation in cases of continued seizures.

Other supportive treatment

Muscle relaxants prevent muscular contraction during seizures but will not prevent continued seizures. They may be necessary to facilitate mechanical ventilation but continuous EEG monitoring should be used to judge seizure control. Correction of circulatory disturbance is required to maintain optimal cerebral blood flow.

Drug dosages

Diazepam	initially 2.5–5mg IV or PR. Further increments as necessary to a maximum of 20mg.
Phenytoin	loading dose 18mg/kg IV at a rate < 50mg/min with continuous ECG monitoring. Maintenance at 300mg/day IV, IM or PO adjusted according to levels.
Chlormethiazole	loading dose 40–100ml 0.8% solution IV over 10min then titrated to seizure control.
Magnesium sulphate	initially 20mmol over 3–5min followed by 5–10mmol/h by infusion as necessary.
Clonazepam	1mg/h IV
Thiopentone	1–3mg/kg IV followed by lowest dose to maintain control.
Propofol	0.5–2mg/kg IV followed by 1–3mg/kg/h

361

See also:

Ventilatory support—indications, 4; ECG monitoring, 102; EEG / CFM monitoring, 130; Calcium, magnesium & phosphate, 140; Toxicology, 152; Sedatives, 226; Muscle relaxants, 228; Anticonvulsants, 230; Steroids, 250; Basic resuscitation, 258; Respiratory failure, 270; Meningitis, 362; Intracranial haemorrhage, 364; Subarachnoid haemorrhage, 366; Raised intracranial pressure, 368; Hypomagnesaemia, 410; Hypocalcaemia, 414; Hypoglycaemia, 424; Poisoning—general principles, 438; Head injury 1, 462; Head injury 2, 464; Pre-eclampsia & eclampsia, 478

Meningitis

A life-threatening condition which demands prompt treatment. The classical presentation of meningism may be absent and a high index of suspicion should be held in any patient presenting with obtundation, agitation, seizures or neurological signs. Signs may be subtle or present insidiously in neutropenics and the elderly. Meningococcaemia presents with a prominent rash in 50% of cases while *Listeria monocytogenes* may cause seizures and focal neurological defects.

Diagnosis

- Diagnosis of bacterial meningitis is based on CSF examination. Lumbar puncture (LP) samples should be sent for urgent microscopy and culture, protein and glucose estimation (with concurrent plasma sample). Normal or lymphocytic CSF may be found in early pyogenic meningitis, especially *L. monocytogenes*; if indicated, repeat the LP.
- Raised intracranial pressure is a common accompaniment; unless confidently excluded, lumbar puncture (LP) should be delayed until after CT scanning. However, a normal CT scan does not completely exclude raised intracranial pressure.
- If delay is necessary, empiric antibiotic therapy should be commenced immediately after taking blood cultures. The choice should be based on the patient's age. CSF cultures are positive in 50% of those given antibiotics compared with 60–90% in untreated cases.
- CSF bacterial antigen testing is available for most infecting organisms; sensitivity varies from 50–100% while specificity is high.

Management

1 Antibiotic therapy for a minimum 10 days (see table opposite).
2 Dexamethasone 0.15mg/kg qds IV should be considered in high-risk categories, e.g. evidence of cerebral oedema or coma. This should be given with or just before the first dose of antibiotic.
3 General measures include attention to fluid and electrolyte replacement, adequate gas exchange, nutrition, and skin care.
4 Management of raised intracranial pressure if present.
5 Rifampicin should be given to all family and close social contacts of meningococcal (600mg bd PO for 2 days) and haemophilus (600mg od PO for 4 days) meningitis. The index case should also receive the appropriate dose before discharge home.

Aseptic meningitis

No organisms are identified by routine CSF analysis despite a high neutrophil and/or lymphocyte count. Causes include viruses (e.g. mumps, measles), Lyme disease, fungi, leptospirosis, listeriosis, brucellosis, atypical TB, sarcoidosis, SLE, and a partially treated bacterial meningitis.

Encephalitis

Presenting features include drowsiness, coma, agitation, pyrexia, seizures and focal signs; meningism need not necessarily be present.

Causes :
- bacterial (as for meningitis)
- viruses (in particular, herpes simplex and up to 14 days post-measles, chicken pox, mumps infection)

Herpes simplex classically affects the temporal lobe and can be diagnosed by EEG. Acyclovir 10mg/kg tds IV is given for 10 days.

Typical CSF values in meningitis

	Pyogenic	*Viral*	*Tuberculosis*
appearance	turbid	clear	fibrin web
predominant cell type	polymorphs	lymphocytes	lymphocytes
cell count/mm^3	> 1000	< 500	50–1500
protein (g/L)	> 1	0.5–1	1–5
CSF:blood glucose	< 60%	> 60%	< 60%

Organisms and empiric starting antibiotic therapy

Patients often affected	*Organism*	*Antibiotic & dosage regimen (alternatives in brackets)*
Young adults	*Neisseria meningitidis* (Meningococcus)	cefotaxime 50mg/kg IV 8hrly (benzylpenicillin 1.2g IV 2–4hrly) (chloramphenicol 12.5mg/kg IV 6hrly)
Older adults	*Streptococcus pneumoniae* (Pneumococcus)	cefotaxime 50mg/kg IV 8hrly (chloramphenicol 12.5mg/kg IV 6hrly)
Children	*Haemophilus influenzae*	cefotaxime 50mg/kg IV 8hrly (chloramphenicol 12.5mg/kg IV 6hrly)
Elderly, immuno-compromised	*Listeria monocytogenes*	ampicillin 1g IV 4–6hrly plus gentamicin 120mg IV stat, then 80mg 8–12hrly. (adjust by plasma levels)
	Mycobacterium tuberculosis	quadruple therapy (rifampicin/isoniazid/ethambutol/ pyrazinamide)
Immuno-compromised	*Cryptococcus neoformans*	amphotericin B starting at 250µg/kg iv od + flucytosine 50mg/kg IV 6hrly
	Staph. aureus	flucloxacillin 2g IV 6hrly

Rarer causes include leptospirosis and brucellosis; the CSF reveals no organisms but a high lymphocyte count is present. If indicated, send CSF for acid fast stain (TB) and India Ink stain (Cryptococcus).

363

See also:

Infection control, 78; Bacteriology, 148; Virology, serology & assays, 150; Antimicrobials, 248; Steroids, 250; Basic resuscitation, 258; Hypotension, 300; Generalised seizures, 360; Raised intracranial pressure, 368; Systemic inflammatory response, 488; syndrome Sepsis / infection, 490; Pyrexia, 500

Intracranial haemorrhage

Extradural haemorrhage

Usually presents acutely after head injury. Characterised by falling Glasgow Coma Score progressing to coma, focal signs (lateralising weakness or anaesthesia, pupillary signs), visual disturbances and seizures. Treatment by random burr holes has been supplanted by directed drainage following CT scan localisation.

A conservative approach may be adopted for small haematomata but increasing size (assessed by regular CT scanning or clinical deterioration) are indications for surgical drainage.

Subdural haemorrhage

Classically presents days to weeks following head trauma with a fluctuating level of consciousness (35%), agitation, confusion, seizures and signs of raised intracranial pressure, localising signs, or a slowly evolving stroke. Diagnosis is made by CT scan. Treatment is by surgical drainage.

Intracerebral haemorrhage

Causes include hypertension, neoplasm, vasculitis, coagulopathy and mycotic aneurysms associated with bacterial endocarditis.

Clinical features include sudden onset coma, drowsiness and/or neurological deficit. Headache usually occurs only with cortical and intraventricular haemorrhage. The rate of evolution depends on the site and size of the bleed. The area affected is the putamen (55%), thalamus (10%), cerebral cortex (15%), pons (10%) and cerebellum (10%).

Diagnosis

CT scan is the definitive test. A coagulation and vasculitis blood screen may be indicated. Angiography is indicated if surgical repair is contemplated though not for simple drainage of blood clot.

Treatment
- bed rest
- supportive (e.g. hydration, nutrition, analgesia, ventilatory support)
- physiotherapy
- blood pressure control (maintain systolic BP < 220–230mmHg)
- correct any coagulopathy
- control raised intracranial pressure
- surgery—contact Regional Centre, e.g. for evacuation of haematoma, repair/clipping of aneurysm
- steroid therapy is ineffective

Subarachnoid haemorrhage

Pathology
- In 15% no cause is found; of the remainder, 80% are due to a ruptured aneurysm, 5% to arteriovenous malformations and 15% follow trauma.
- The anterior part of the Circle of Willis is affected in 90–95% of subarachnoid haemorrhage (SAH) while 10–15% affect the vertebrobasilar system.
- There is a 30% risk of rebleeding for which the mortality is 40%. Those surviving a month have a 90% chance of surviving a year.
- Cerebral vasospasm occurs in 40–70% of patients at 4–12 days after the bleed. This is the most important cause of morbidity and mortality.
- Hydrocephalus, seizures, hyponatraemia and inappropriate ADH secretion are recognised complications.

Clinical features
- SAH may be preceded by a prodrome of headache, dizziness and vague neurological symptoms.
- Often there is rapid onset (minutes to hours) presentation including collapse, severe headache, ± meningism.
- Cranial nerve palsies, drowsiness and hemiplegia may also occur.

Diagnosis
Diagnosis is usually made by CT scan; if there is no evidence of raised intracranial pressure, a lumbar puncture may be performed revealing blood-stained CSF with xanthochromia.

Management
- Bed rest
- Maintain adequate hydration, nutrition, analgesia, sedation.
- Cerebral vasospasm is prevented by nimodipine infusion and maintenance of a full intravascular volume.
- Systemic hypertension should only be treated if severe (e.g. systolic pressure > 220–230mmHg) and prolonged.
- Surgery—the timing is controversial with either early or delayed (7–10 days) intervention being advocated. The Regional Neurosurgical Centre should be consulted for local policy.
- Antifibrinolytic therapy (e.g. tranexamic acid) reduces the incidence of rebleeding but has no beneficial effect on outcome.

Raised intracranial pressure

Clinical features
- Headache, vomiting
- Seizures, focal neurology, papilloedema
- Increasing blood pressure, bradycardia
- Agitation, increasing drowsiness, coma
- Slow deep breaths, Cheyne-Stokes breathing, apnoea
- Ipsilateral progressing to bilateral pupillary dilatation
- Decorticate progressing to decerebrate posturing

Diagnosis
- CT scan
- Intracranial pressure (ICP) measurement

Lumbar puncture should be avoided because of the risk of coning.
Neither CT scan nor absence of papilloedema will exclude a raised ICP.

Management
1. Bed rest, 20–30° head-up tilt, sedation, quiet environment, minimal suction and noise. If ventilated, short-acting sedation, e.g. propofol, may be useful to achieve rapid control and enable regular assessment of the underlying conscious level. The tape tethering the ET in place should not occlude jugular venous drainage.
2. Ventilate if GCS ⩽8, airway unprotected or excessively agitated.
3. Maintain $PaCO_2$ at 3.5–4 kPa and avoid rapid rises. CSF bicarbonate levels re-equilibrate within 4–6h, negating any benefit from hyperventilation.
4. If possible, monitor ICP. Aim to maintain mean systemic BP > 80–100mmHg, ICP < 20mmHg and cerebral perfusion pressure (= MAP-ICP) > 50–60mmHg. Vasopressor therapy may be needed. Do not treat systemic hypertension unless very high (e.g. systolic > 220–230mmHg).
5. Other monitoring techniques, e.g. jugular bulb venous saturation and lactate may be useful though do not detect regional ischaemia.
6. Give mannitol 0.5mg/kg over 15min. Repeat at 4hrly intervals depending on cerebral perfusion pressure (CPP) measurements and/or clinical signs of deterioration. Stop when plasma osmolality reaches 310–320mOsmol/kg.
7. Avoid severe alkalosis as cerebral vascular resistance rises and cerebral ischaemia increases.
8. Consider specific treatment, e.g. for meningoencephalitis, malaria, hepatic encephalopathy, surgery. Some neurosurgeons will decompress the cranium for generalised oedema by removing a skull flap. Seek local advice. Dexamethasone 4–16mg qds IV is beneficial for oedema surrounding a tumour and for herpes simplex encephalitis.

Acute deterioration/risk of imminent coning
1. Mechanically ventilate to $PaCO_2$ 3.0–3.5 kPa for 10–20min.
2. Give mannitol 0.5g/kg iv over 15min. Repeat 4hrly as necessary and stop when plasma osmolality > 310–320mOsmol/kg. Consider addition of frusemide.
3. If no response in ICP, CPP and/or clinical features, give thiopentone. (successful in 50% of resistant cases).
4. Consider repeat CT scan and refer for urgent surgery if a surgically-amenable space-occupying lesion is diagnosed.

Causes

- space-occupying lesion (e.g. neoplasm, blood clot, abscess)
- increased capillary permeability (e.g. trauma, infection, hepatic encephalopathy)
- cell death (e.g. post-arrest hypoxia)
- obstruction (e.g. hydrocephalus)

369

Guillain–Barré syndrome

Guillain–Barré syndrome is an immunologically mediated acute demyelinating polyradiculopathy. Viral infections and immunisations are common antecedents. The syndrome includes a progressive, areflexic motor weakness (often symmetrical, ascending and involving cranial nerves including facial, bulbar and extraocular weakness) with progression over a few days to a few weeks. There are often minor sensory disturbances (e.g. paraesthesiae). Autonomic dysfunction is not unusual. There is no increase in cell count on CSF examination but protein levels usually rise progressively (> 0.4g/L). Nerve conduction studies show slow conduction velocities with prolonged F waves. Other features include muscle tenderness and back pain. The major contributors to morbidity and mortality are respiratory muscle weakness and autonomic dysfunction (hypotension, hypertension, arrhythmias, ileus and urinary retention).

Differential diagnosis

Other causes of acute weakness must be excluded before a diagnosis of Guillain–Barré syndrome can be made.

Specific treatment

- Plasma exchange is effective in improving the rate of recovery if started within 7 days of the onset of symptoms. A total of 5×3000ml exchanges are made within the first week. Further plasma exchanges may be made if there is rapid and continued improvement. Fresh frozen plasma is not needed for replacement.
- Intravenous gammaglobulin (0.4g/kg/day for 5 days) is effective if started in the first 2 weeks after symptoms begin.
- Steroids have not been shown to be beneficial.

Supportive treatment

Respiratory care
Regular chest physiotherapy and spirometry are required. Mechanical ventilation is needed if FVC < 1L or $PaCO_2$ is raised. An early tracheostomy is useful since mechanical ventilation is likely to continue for several weeks. Patients with bulbar involvement or inadequate cough should have a tracheostomy even if spontaneous breathing continues.

Cardiovascular care
Continuous cardiovascular monitoring is required due to the effects of autonomic involvement. Arrhythmias are particularly likely with anaesthesia (especially with suxamethonium). Blood pressure responses are generally exaggerated with vasoactive drugs.

Nutritional support
Parenteral nutrition will be required in cases where there is ileus. Enteral nutrition is preferred, however, energy and fluid requirements are reduced in Guillain–Barré syndrome.

Analgesia
Analgesia is required for muscle, abdominal and back pain. Although NSAIDs may be useful opiates are often required.

Other support
Particular attention is required to pressure areas and deep vein thrombosis prophylaxis.

Myasthenia gravis

Myasthenia gravis is associated with painless weakness which is worse after exertion and deteriorates during stress, infection or trauma. Tendon reflexes are normal. It is an autoimmune disease associated with acetylcholine receptor and, rarely, anti-striated muscle antibodies.

There is also an association with other autoimmune diseases (e.g. thyroid disease, SLE, rheumatoid arthritis).

Younger (< 45years), predominantly female patients may have a thymoma which, if resected, may provide remission.

Severe weakness may be the result of a myasthenic or cholinergic crisis (e.g. sweating, salivation, lacrimation, colic, fasciculation, confusion, ataxia, small pupils, bradycardia, hypertension, seizures).

Diagnosis of myasthenia

Edrophonium is a short acting anticholinesterase used in the diagnosis of myasthenia in patients with no previous history of myasthenia gravis. In myasthenic patients with an acute deterioration the test may distinguish a myasthenic from a cholinergic crisis. In cholinergic crisis there is a possibility of further deterioration and atropine and facilities for urgent intubation and ventilation should be available. An initial dose of 2mg IV is given. If there are no cholinergic side effects a further 8mg may be given. A positive test is judged by improvement of weakness within 3min of injection. The test may be combined with objective assessment of respiratory function by measuring the FVC response or by assessing the response to repetitive stimulation with an EMG.

Maintenance treatment

Anticholinesterase drugs provide the mainstay of symptomatic treatment but steroids, immunosuppressives and plasma exchange may provide pharmacological remission.

Myasthenic crisis

New myasthenics may present in crisis and treatment should be started with steroids, azathioprine and pyridostigmine. Plasma exchange may be useful to reduce the antibody load. In known myasthenics an increased dose of pyridostigmine and steroids will be required. If the condition deteriorates drug therapy should be stopped; plasma exchange may be life saving. Anticholinesterases may produce improvement in some muscle groups and cholinergic deterioration in others due to differential sensitivity. As with any case of acute weakness mechanical ventilatory support is required if $FVC < 1L$ or the $PaCO_2$ is raised.

Cholinergic crisis

Cholinergic symptoms are usually at their most severe 2h after the last dose of anticholinesterase. It is common to give atropine prophylactically in the treatment of myasthenia which may mask some of the cholinergic symptoms. If a deterioration of myasthenia fails to respond to edrophonium all drugs should be stopped and atropine given (1mg IV every 30min to a maximum of 8mg). The edrophonium test should be repeated every 2h and anticholinesterases reintroduced when the test is positive. Mechanical ventilation is required if $FVC < 1L$ or the $PaCO_2$ is raised.

Drug dosages

Prednisolone	80mg/day orally
Azathioprine	2.5mg/kg/day orally
Pyridostigmine	60–180mg 6hrly orally
Atropine	0.6mg 6hrly orally

Drugs causing a deterioration in myasthenia

Aminoglycosides
Streptomycin
Tetracyclines
Local anaesthetics
Muscle relaxants
Opiates

373

See also:
  Ventilatory support—indications, 4; Endotracheal intubation, 28; Special
support surfaces, 82; Plasma exchange, 60; Pulmonary function tests, 90;
Steroids, 250; Respiratory failure, 270; Hypotension, 300; Tachyarrhythmias, 304;
Bradyarrhythmias, 306; Acute weakness, 356; Rheumatic disorders, 506;
Vasculitides, 508

ICU neuromuscular disorders

Neuromuscular disorders in the critically ill have long been recognised, particularly in those mechanically ventilated. First suspicions are often raised when patients fail to wean from mechanical ventilation or limb weakness is noted on stopping sedation. Disuse atrophy, catabolic states and drug therapy (e.g. high dose steroids, muscle relaxants) are probably responsible for some cases but do not explain all. A neuromyopathic component of multi-organ dysfunction syndrome may be implicated.

Critical illness neuropathy

Neurophysiological studies have demonstrated an acute idiopathic axonal degeneration in patients with a flaccid weakness following a prolonged period of intensive care. Nerve conduction velocities are normal indicating no demyelination. CSF is normal unlike Guillain–Barré syndrome. The neuropathy is self limiting but prolongs the recovery phase of critical illness. Recovery may take weeks to years. Pyridoxine (100–150mg daily PO) has been used in the treatment.

Critical illness myopathy

- Drug induced myopathy is not uncommon in critically ill patients.
- Steroid induced myopathy is less common as the indications for high dose steroids have been reduced.
- Muscle relaxants may have a prolonged effect and may be potentiated by β_2 agonists.
- Muscle histological studies have demonstrated abnormalities (fibre atrophy, mitochondrial defects, myopathy and necrosis) which could not be associated with steroid or muscle relaxant therapy.
- Myopathy may cause renal damage via myoglobinuria.
- Critical illness myopathy is associated with various forms of muscle degeneration but is usually self limiting.
- Recovery may take weeks to years.

See also:
   Ventilatory support—indications, 4; IPPV—assessment of weaning, 16;
Endotracheal intubation, 28; Special support surfaces, 82; Pulmonary function
tests, 90; Steroids, 250; Respiratory failure, 270; Acute weakness, 356; Guillain–
Barr³ syndrome, 370

Tetanus

The clinical syndrome caused by the exotoxin tetanospasmin from the anaerobe *Clostridium tetani* in contaminated or devitalised wounds. Tetanospasmin ascends intra-axonally in motor and autonomic nerves blocking the release of inhibitory neurotransmitters. The disease may be modified by previous immunisation such that milder or localised symptoms may occur with heavier toxin loads.

Clinical features

- Gradual onset of stiffness, dysphagia, muscle pain, hypertonia, rigidity and muscle spasm.
- Laryngospasm often follows dysphagia.
- Muscle spasm is often provoked by minor disturbance, e.g. laryngospasm may be provoked by swallowing.
- Onset of symptoms within 5 days of injury implies a heavy toxin load and severe disease.
- The disease is self limiting so treatment is supportive but may need to continue for several weeks.

Management of the wound

If a contaminated wound is present it should be debrided surgically to remove the source of the toxin. Benzylpenicillin 1.2g 6hrly and metronidazole 500mg 8hrly IV are appropriate antibiotics.

Passive immunisation

Human tetanus immunoglobulin 1000–1500 units IM may shorten the course of the disease by removing circulating toxin. Rapid fixation of the toxin to tissues limits the usefulness of this approach.

Mild tetanus

Patients with mild symptoms, no respiratory distress and a delayed onset of symptoms should be nursed in a quite environment with mild sedation to prevent tetanic spasms.

Severe tetanus

- Intubate and ventilate since asphyxia may occur due to prolonged respiratory muscle spasm.
- Sedation may be achieved with diazepam (20mg 4–6hrly NG and 5mg IV as necessary).
- Muscle rigidity is best treated with chlorpromazine 25–75mg 4hrly IV or NG with muscle relaxants if necessary.
- Autonomic hyper-reactivity is a feature (arrhythmias, hypotension, hypertension and myocardial ischaemia). It is minimised by sedation, anaesthesia and treated by atropine 1–20mg/h IV, propranolol 10mg 8hrly IV or NG and magnesium sulphate 20mmol/h IV.

Tetanus toxoid prophylaxis

The disease confers no immunity so patients must be immunised prior to hospital discharge.
- Last dose of tetanus toxoid <5 years   no further dose
- Last dose of tetanus toxoid <10 years   1 dose
- No previous immunisation   3 doses

See also:
  Ventilatory support—indications, 4; Sedatives, 226; Muscle relaxants, 228;
Antimicrobials, 248; Respiratory failure, 270; Hypotension, 300; Hypertension,
302; Tachyarrhythmias, 304; Bradyarrhythmias, 306

Botulism

An uncommon, lethal disease caused by the exotoxins of the anaerobe *Clostridium botulinum*. Botulism is most commonly a foodborne disease, especially associated with canned foods. It may be contracted by wound contamination with aquatic soils. The toxin is carried in the blood to cholinergic neuromuscular junctions where it binds irreversibly. Symptoms begin between 6h and 8 days after contamination and are more severe with earlier onset. Botulism is diagnosed by isolating *Clostridium botulinum* from the stool or by mouse bioassay (survival of immunised mice and death of non-immunised mice when infected serum is injected).

Clinical features

- Symptoms include gastrointestinal disturbance, sore throat, fatigue, dizziness, paraesthesiae, cranial involvement and a progressive, descending flaccid weakness.
- Parasympathetic symptoms are common.
- The disease is usually self limiting within several weeks.

Respiratory care

Regular spirometry and mechanical ventilation if FVC < 1L. Patients with bulbar palsy need intubation for airway protection.

Toxin removal

If there is no ileus the use of non-magnesium containing cathartics may remove the toxin load. Magnesium may enhance the effect of the toxin.

Antitoxin

May shorten the course of the disease if given early and the toxin type is known (seven have been identified). There is a high risk of anaphylactoid reactions.

Wound botulism

Surgical debridement and penicillin are the mainstay of treatment for contaminated wounds.

See also:
Ventilatory support—indications, 4; Antimicrobials, 248; Respiratory failure, 270; Bradyarrhythmias, 306; Anaphylactoid reactions, 492

Haematological Disorders

Bleeding disorders

A common problem in the critically ill, this may be due to (i) large vessel bleeding—usually 'surgical' or following a procedure (e.g. chest drain, tracheostomy, accidental arterial puncture, removal of intravenous or intra-arterial catheter); peptic ulcer bleeding is now relatively uncommon due to improved attention to perfusion and nutrition; (ii) around vascular catheter sites or from intubated/instrumented lumens and orifices—usually related to severe multisystem illness or excess anticoagulant therapy, including thrombolytics; (iii) small vessel bleeding, e.g. skin petechiae, gastric erosions—usually related to anticoagulation or severe generalised illness including disseminated intravascular coagulation.

A falling platelet count is often an early sign of sepsis and critical illness. Recovery of the count usually coincides with overall patient recovery.

Common ICU causes

- Decreased platelet production, e.g. sepsis- or drug-induced
- Decreased production of coagulation factors, e.g. liver failure
- Increased consumption, e.g. DIC, major trauma, bleeding, heparin-induced thrombocytopenia, anti-platelet antibodies, extracorporeal circuits
- Impaired or deranged platelet function
- Drugs, e.g. heparin, aspirin
- Decreased protease inhibitors, e.g. antithrombin III, protein S & protein C deficiency (following sepsis)

Principles of management

1 An International Normalised Ratio (INR) between 1.5–2.5 and/or platelet count of 20–40 $\times$ 10^9/L do not usually require correction if the patient is not bleeding or at high-risk e.g. active peptic ulcer, recent cerebral haemorrhage, undergoing an invasive procedure. 5–10 units of platelets will raise the count by only 10–20 $\times$ 10^9/L and the effect is transient ($<$24h). Treatment of symptomatic thrombocytopenia aims to increase the count $>$50 $\times$ 10^9/L. A target INR $<$1.5 is acceptable. Vitamin K is given for liver failure and considered with warfarin overdosage. 1mg Vitamin K will reverse warfarin effects within 12h while 10mg will saturate liver stores, preventing warfarin activity for some weeks. Fresh frozen plasma (FFP) is given for short-term control.

2 If bleeding and INR = 1.5–2, give 2–3 units FFP. If INR $>$2, give 4–6 units FFP. If not bleeding (or high-risk), generally only correct if INR $>$2.5–3. Repeat clotting screen 30–60min after infusion of FFP. Give further FFP if bleeding continues and/or INR $>$3.

3 For bleeding related to thrombolysis, (i) stop the drug infusion (ii) give either aprotinin 500 000 units over 10min, then 200 000 units over 4h or tranexamic acid 10mg/kg repeated 6–8hrly (iii) give 4 units FFP.

4 Cryoprecipitate is rarely needed. Consider when the thrombin time is elevated e.g. with DIC. Similarly, Factor VIII is generally used for haemophiliacs only.

5 If aspirin has been taken within past 1–2 weeks, platelet function may be deranged. Give fresh platelets, even though count may be adequate.

Management of major bleeding.

1 If external, direct occlusion/deep suture.
2 Urgent expert opinion—e.g. for surgery, endoscopy + injection, etc..
3 Correct coagulopathy.

Management of vascular catheter or percutaneous drain site bleeding

1 Direct pressure/occlusive dressing.
2 Correct coagulopathy; consider use of aprotinin or tranexamic acid.
3 Surgical intervention rarely necessary though perforation/Laceration of local artery/vein should be considered if bleeding fails to stop or becomes significant.

Clotting disorders

Uncommon as a secondary event in critically ill patients as they tend to be auto-anticoagulated. The risk of major venous thrombosis increases with long-term immobility and paralysis and in specific pro-thrombotic conditions such as pregnancy, thrombotic thrombocytopenic purpura, SLE (lupus anticoagulant), sickle cell crisis, hyperosmolar diabetic coma.

Disseminated intravascular coagulation is associated with microvascular clotting, a consumption coagulopathy and increased fibrinolysis.

Clotting of extracorporeal circuits, e.g. for renal replacement therapy may be due to (i) mechanical obstruction to flow, e.g. kinked catheter, (ii) inadequate anticoagulation or (iii) in severe illness, a decrease in endogenous anticoagulants (e.g. antithrombin III); this may result in circuit blockage despite a coexisting thrombocytopenia and/or coagulopathy.

Axillary vein or subclavian vein thrombosis may result from indwelling intravenous catheters.

Management

If patient is not auto-anticoagulated, prophylactic subcutaneous heparin (5000 U bd or tds) should be given for long-term immobility/paralysis and to high-risk patients (e.g. previous DVT, femoral fractures)

Full heparinisation (20–40 000 U/day) should be given for proven or highly suspected deep vein thrombosis. Partial thromboplastin times (PTT) should be checked regularly and maintained at approximately 2–3 × normal.

Intra-arterial clot can be treated with local infusion of thrombolytics, usually followed by heparinisation. Seek vascular surgical advice.

Axillary vein or subclavian vein thrombosis should be managed by elevation of the affected arm, e.g. in a Bradford sling, and heparinisation to maintain PTT at approximately 2–3 × normal.

Specific conditions may require specific therapies e.g. plasma exchange for SLE and TTP, whole blood exchange for sickle cell crisis.

Warfarinisation should generally be avoided until shortly before ICU discharge because of the risk of continued bleeding following routine invasive procedures such as central venous catheterisation.

Anaemia

Defined as a low haemoglobin due to a decreased red cell mass, it may also be 'physiological' due to dilution from an increased plasma volume, e.g. pregnancy, vasodilated states.

Major causes in the ICU patient

- Blood loss, e.g. haemorrhage, regular blood sampling
- Severe illness—analogous to the 'anaemia of chronic disease', there is decreased marrow production and, possibly, a decreased life-span.

Rarer causes include:

- Microcytic anaemia—predominantly iron deficiency
- Normocytic—
  - Chronic disease
  - Bone marrow failure (idiopathic, drugs, neoplasm, radiation)
  - Haemolysis
  - Renal failure
- Macrocytic—vitamin B_{12} and folate deficiency, alcoholism, cirrhosis, sideroblastic anaemia, hypothyroidism
- Congenital diseases—sickle cell, thalassaemia

Management

1 Treatment of the cause where possible
2 Blood transfusion—
  - The ideal haemoglobin level for optimal oxygen carriage and viscosity remains contentious. A commonly accepted target value is approximately 10g/dL.
  - Transfusion is usually given as packed cells with or without a small dose of frusemide to maintain fluid balance. This may need to be given rapidly during active blood loss or slowly for correction of a gradually falling haemoglobin level.
  - Rarely, patients admitted with a chronically low haemoglobin, e.g. <4–5g/dL, which often follows long term malnutrition or vitamin deficiency, will need a much slower elevation in haemoglobin level to avoid precipitating acute heart failure. An initial target of 7–8g/dL is often acceptable. Obviously, this may need to be altered in the light of any concurrent acute illness where elevation of oxygen delivery is deemed necessary.

See also:
Upper gastrointestinal endoscopy, 66; Nutrition—use and indications, 70; Full blood count, 144; Blood transfusion, 172; Acute renal failure—diagnosis, 320; Acute renal failure—management, 322; Upper gastrointestinal haemorrhage, 332; Bleeding varices, 334; Lower intestinal bleeding & colitis, 338; Bleeding disorders, 382; Sickle cell disease, 388; Haemolysis, 390; Post-partum haemorrhage, 482; Rheumatic disorders, 506; Post-operative intensive care, 510

Sickle cell disease

A chronic, hereditary disease almost entirely confined to the black population where the gene for Hb S is inherited from each parent. The red blood cells lack Hb A; when deprived of oxygen these cells assume sickle and other bizarre shapes resulting in erythrostasis, occlusion of blood vessels, thrombosis and tissue infarction. After stasis, cells released back into the circulation are more fragile and prone to haemolysis. Occasionally, there may also be bone marrow failure.

Chronic features

Patients with sickle cell disease are usually chronically anaemic (7–8g/dL) with a hyperdynamic circulation. Splenomegaly is common in youth but, with progressive episodes of infarction, splenic atrophy occurs leading to an increased risk of infection, particularly pneumococcal.

Chronic features include skin ulcers, renal failure, avascular bone necrosis (± supervening osteomyelitis, especially *Salmonella*), hepatomegaly, jaundice and cardiomyopathy. Sudden cardiac death is not uncommon, usually before the age of 30.

Sickle cell crises

Crises are precipitated by various triggers including hypoxaemia (e.g. air travel, anaesthesia), infection, cold, dehydration and emotional stress.

Thrombotic crisis
This occurs most frequently in the bones or joints but also affect chest and abdomen giving rise to severe pain. Occasionally, neurological symptoms (e.g. seizures, focal signs), haematuria or priapism may be present. Pulmonary crises are the commonest reason for ICU admission; secondary chest infection or ARDS may supervene, worsening hypoxaemia and further exacerbating the crisis.

Aplastic crisis
Related to parvovirus infection, it is suggested by worsening anaemia and a reduction in the normally elevated reticulocyte count (10–20%).

Haemolytic crisis
Intravascular haemolysis with haemoglobinuria, jaundice and renal failure sometimes occurs.

Sequestration crisis
Rapid hepatic and splenic enlargement due to red cell trapping with severe anaemia. This condition is particularly serious.

Management

Prophylaxis against crises includes avoidance of hypoxaemia and other known precipitating factors, prophylactic penicillin and pneumococcal vaccine, and exchange transfusions.
1 Painful crises usually require prompt opiate infusions. Although psychological dependence is high, analgesia should not be withheld.
2 Give oxygen at high FIO_2 to maintain SaO_2 at 100%.
3 Rehydrate with intravenous fluids and keep warm.
4 If infection is suspected, antibiotics should be given as indicated.
5 Transfuse blood if haemoglobin level drops or central nervous system or lung complications present.
6 Lower proportion of sickle cells to < 30% by exchange transfusion.
7 Mechanical ventilation may be necessary for chest crises.

See also:
Oxygen therapy, 2; Ventilatory support—indications, 4; Pulse oximetry, 86; Full blood count, 144; Bacteriology, 148; Acute chest infection 1, 276; Acute chest infection 2, 278; Adult respiratory distress syndrome 1, 280; Adult respiratory distress syndrome 2, 282; Acute renal failure—diagnosis, 320; Acute renal failure—management, 322; Jaundice, 346; Generalised seizures, 360; Anaemia, 386; Haemolysis, 390

Haemolysis

Shortening of erythrocyte lifespan below the expected 120 days. Marked intravascular haemolysis may lead to jaundice and haemoglobinuria.

Causes

- Blood transfusion reactions
- Haemolytic uraemic syndrome (microangiopathic haemolytic anaemia)
- Trauma (cardiac valve prosthesis)
- Malaria
- Sickle cell haemolytic crisis
- Drugs—e.g. high-dose penicillin, methyl dopa
- Autoimmune (cold- or warm antibody-mediated)—may be idiopathic or secondary, e.g. lymphoma, SLE, mycoplasma
- Glucose-6–phosphate dehydrogenase deficiency—oxidative crises occur following ingestion of fava beans, primaquine, sulphonamides leading to rapid onset anaemia and jaundice

Diagnosis

- Unconjugated hyperbilirubinaemia, increased urinary urobilinogen (increased RBC breakdown)
- Reticulocytosis (increased RBC production)
- Splenic hypertrophy (extravascular haemolysis)
- Methaemoglobinaemia, haemoglobinuria, free plasma haemoglobin (intravascular haemolysis), reduced serum haptoglobins
- RBC fragmentation (microangiopathic haemolytic anaemia)
- Coombs' test (immune-mediated haemolysis)
- Other (including haemoglobin electrophoresis, bone marrow biopsy)

Management

1 Identification and specific treatment of the cause where possible.
2 Blood transfusion to maintain haemoglobin > 10g/dL
3 Massive intravascular haemolysis may lead to acute renal failure. Maintain a good diuresis and haemo(dia)filter if necessary.

Platelet disorders

Thrombocytopenia

This is rarely symptomatic until the platelet count $< 50 \times 10^9$/L; spontaneous bleeding is much more likely when the count $< 20 \times 10^9$/L. Although bleeding is often minor, e.g. skin petechiae, oozing at intravascular catheter sites, it may occasionally be massive or life-threatening, e.g. haemoptysis, intra-cranial haemorrhage.

Causes
- Sepsis—in the ICU this is the commonest cause of a low platelet count is sepsis; indeed, this often provides a good barometer of either recovery or deterioration.
- Disseminated intravascular coagulation
- Drugs
  - Related to anti-platelet antibody production, e.g. heparin (heparin-induced thrombocytopenia syndrome, 'HITS'), sulphonamides, quinine
  - Resulting in bone marrow suppression, e.g. chemotherapy agents
  - Others, .e.g. aspirin, chlorpromazine, prochlorperazine, digoxin
- Following massive bleeding and multiple blood transfusions
- Bone marrow failure, e.g. tumour infiltration, drugs
- Splenomegaly
- Thrombotic thrombocytopenic purpura (TTP), haemolytic uraemic syndrome (HUS)
- Idiopathic thrombocytopenic purpura (ITP)
- Specific infections, e.g. measles, infectious mononucleosis, typhus
- Collagen vascular diseases, e.g. SLE

Management
1 Directed at the cause, e.g. antibiotics for sepsis, stopping offending drugs, plasma exchange for TTP, splenectomy and steroids for ITP.
2 Platelet support—
   - Generally given routinely (e.g. 6–10 units/day) when < 10–20×10^9/L
   - 6–10 units given if $< 50 \times 10^9$/L and either symptomatic or due to undergo surgery or another invasive procedure
3 Unless actively bleeding, platelet transfusions should be avoided in TTP or HUS.

Deranged platelet function

Function may be deranged albeit with normal counts, e.g. following aspirin within past 1–2 weeks, epoprostenol, uraemia. Fresh platelets may be required if the patient is symptomatic. In uraemia, one dose of vasopressin (20µg IV over 30min) may be useful before surgery.

Thrombocythaemia

A rare occurrence in ICU patients, platelet counts often exceed 800 $\times 10^9$/L.

Causes
Prolonged low-level bleeding, post-splenectomy, myeloproliferative disorders. Essential (idiopathic) thrombocythaemia is unusual.

Management
As the major risk is thrombosis, management is based upon mobilising the patient and administration of either prophylactic aspirin (150mg bd PO) or heparin (5000U 8–12hrly SC). Dipyridamole (300–600mg tds PO) is occasionally used.

393

Neutropenia

Neutropenia is defined as a neutrophil count $< 2 \times 10^9$/L. Life-threatening infections rarely develop below 1×10^9/L but are much more common at levels $< 0.5 \times 10^9$/L.

Absolute numbers of neutrophils are more relevant than percentage levels as the total white cell count may be either decreased, normal or increased.

Clinical features

- Usually asymptomatic until infection supervenes

Infections

- Initial infections are with common organisms such as pneumococci, staphylococci and coliforms.
- With recurrent infections or after repeated courses of antibiotics, more unusual and/or antibiotic-resistant organisms may be responsible, e.g. pseudomonas, fungi (particularly *Candida* and *Aspergillus* spp), pneumocystis, cytomegalovirus, TB.

Management

1 If no diagnosis has been made, urgent investigations including a bone marrow aspiration are indicated.
2 Any implicated drugs should be immediately discontinued.
3 If the neutrophil count falls below 1×10^9/L, the patient should be kept under protective isolation in a cubicle with strict infection control procedures. Consider laminar flow air conditioning if available.
4 Minimise invasive procedures.
5 Maintain good oral hygiene. Apply topical treatment as necessary, e.g. nystatin mouthwashes for oral fungal infection
6 Clotrimazole cream should be prescribed for fungal skin infection.
7 Antibiotic therapy
   - For suspected infection, antibiotic therapy should be aggressive, parenteral and, if no organism has been isolated, broad spectrum.
   - A high index of suspicion should be held for atypical infections such as fungi.
   - Although prophylactic broad-spectrum antibiotics are often prescribed for the neutropenic patient, this will encourage antibiotic resistance. An alternative approach is to maintain strict infection control with regular surveillance and to treat infections aggressively as indicated by likely sites and laboratory results. Local policy should be sought from microbiologists and haematologists.
   - Some centres use selective gut decontamination by topical and parenteral antibiotics to reduce the risk of acquired infection.
8 Avoid uncooked foods, e.g. salads (pseudomonas risk), and pepper (aspergillus risk).
9 Granulocyte-colony stimulating factor (G-CSF) is now frequently given to stimulate a bone marrow response.
10 Neutrophil infusions are short-lived, expensive and often induce a pyrexial response. Their role remains controversial.

Causes

- Systemic inflammation—resulting in margination and aggregation of neutrophils in vital organs, e.g. lung, liver, gut. Predominantly seen in the first 24h following severe infection or trauma, it is often a precursor of multiple organ dysfunction.
- Haemopoietic diseases, e.g. leukaemia, lymphoma, myeloma or as a consequence of chemotherapy or radiation
- Nutritional deficiencies, e.g. folate, vitamin B_{12}, malnutrition
- Adverse drug reaction, e.g. carbimazole, sulphonamides
- Part of the aplastic anaemia syndrome, e.g. idiopathic, drugs, infection
- Specific infections, e.g. brucellosis, typhoid, viral, protozoal
- Hypersplenism
- Anti-neutrophil antibodies, e.g. systemic lupus erythematosis

See also:
Infection control, 78; Full blood count, 144; Bacteriology, 148; Antimicrobials, 248; Sepsis / infection, 490

Leukaemia

Such patients may present acutely to an ICU with complications arising from either the disease or the therapy.

Complications arising from the disease

- Decreased resistance to infection
- Hyperviscosity syndrome—drowsiness, coma, focal neurological defects
- Central nervous system involvement
- Anaemia, thrombocytopenia, bleeding tendency, DIC

Complications arising from the therapy

- Tumour lysis syndrome—hyperkalaemia, hyperuricaemia and acute renal failure may follow rapid destruction of a large white cell mass.
- Neutropenia leading to immune compromise and an increased risk of infection
- Anaemia
- Thrombocytopenia leading to spontaneous bleeding, usually from intravascular catheter sites, skin, lung, gut and brain.
- Lung fibrosis, e.g. following radiotherapy, bleomycin
- Myocardial failure, e.g. following mitozantrone
- Graft versus host disease (GVHD)—features include mucositis, hepatitis, jaundice, diarrhoea, abdominal pain, rash and pneumonitis

Management

1 Tumour lysis syndrome can be prevented by adequate hydration, maintaining a good diuresis and administering allopurinol. Once established, haemo(dia)filtration and other measures to lower serum potassium levels may be necessary.
2 The raised white cell mass may be reduced by leucophoresis.
3 Frequent blood transfusions to maintain haemoglobin levels at 10g/dl
4 Platelet transfusions are required if counts remain $< 20 \times 10^9/L$, or if $< 50 \times 10^9/L$ and remaining symptomatic or undergoing an invasive procedure.
5 Give fresh frozen plasma and other blood products as needed.
6 Neutropenia management, including protective isolation, appropriate antibiotic therapy, $\pm$ granulocyte-colony stimulating factor.
7 GVHD is managed by supportive treatment and parenteral nutrition. Prostaglandin E_1 may be helpful.
8 Psychological support for both patient and family is vital.

Respiratory failure

1 Maintenance of gas exchange. Mortality is extremely high if mechanical ventilation is necessary. Non-invasive techniques including CPAP and BiPAP can prove highly effective in avoiding the need for intubation.
2 Where possible, treat the cause. Infection (including atypical organisms), fluid overload, ARDS and a pneumonitis/fibrosis secondary to chemo- or radiotherapy should be considered.

See also:
Ventilatory support—indications, 4; Continuous positive airway pressure, 22; Non-invasive respiratory support, 24; Adult respiratory distress syndrome 1, 280; Adult respiratory distress syndrome 2, 282; Heart failure—assessment, 312; Heart failure—management, 314; Acute renal failure—diagnosis, 320; Acute renal failure—management, 322; Diarrhoea, 328; Jaundice, 346; Anaemia, 386; Platelet disorders, 392; Neutropenia, 394; Hyperkalaemia, 406; Sepsis / infection, 490

Metabolic Disorders

Electrolyte management

A balance must be achieved between electrolyte intake and output. Consider:
- Altered intake
- Impaired renal excretion
- Increased body losses
- Body compartment redistribution (e.g. secondary hyperaldosteronism).

As well as Na^+ and K^+, also consider Mg^{2+}, Ca^{2+}, Cl^- and PO_4^{3-} balance.

Plasma electrolyte values are poorly reflective of whole body stores however excessively high or low plasma levels may induce symptoms and deleterious physiological and metabolic sequelae.

Water balance must also be taken into account; water depletion or excess repletion may respectively concentrate or dilute electrolyte levels.

The usual daily requirements of Na^+ and K^+ are 60–80mmol.

Gravitational peripheral oedema implies increased total body Na^+ and water though intravascular salt and water depletion may coexist.

Electrolyte losses

- Large nasogastric aspirate, vomiting Na^+, Cl^-
- Sweating Na^+, Cl^-
- Polyuria Na^+, Cl^-, K^+, Mg^{2+}
- Diarrhoea Na^+, Cl^-, K^+, Mg^{2+}
- Ascitic drainage Na^+, Cl^-, K^+

Principles of management

1 Establish sources and degree of fluid & electrolyte losses.
2 Assess patient for signs of (i) intravascular fluid depletion—hypotension (e.g. following changes in posture, PEEP, vasodilating drugs) oliguria, increasing metabolic acidosis, thirst (ii) total body NaCl and water overload—i.e. gravitational oedema
3 Measure urea, creatinine, osmolality & electrolyte content of plasma and urine.
4 As appropriate, either replace estimated fluid and electrolyte deficit or increase excretion (with diuretics, haemofiltration). For rate of fluid and specific electrolyte replacement see individual sections.

Hypernatraemia

Clinical features

Thirst, lethargy, coma, seizures, muscular tremor & rigidity, and an increased risk of intracranial haemorrhage. Thirst usually occurs when the plasma sodium rises 3–4mmol/L above normal. Lack of thirst is associated with central nervous system disease.

Treatment

Depends upon the cause, whether total body sodium stores are normal, low or elevated and whether body water is normal or low.

Rate of correction
- If hyperacute (< 12h), correction can be rapid.
- Otherwise, aim for gradual correction of plasma sodium levels (over 1–3 days), particularly in chronic cases (> 2 days' duration), to avoid cerebral oedema through sudden lowering of osmolality. A rate of plasma sodium lowering < 0.7mmol/h has been suggested.

Hypovolaemia
- If hypovolaemia is accompanied by haemodynamic alterations, use colloid initially to restore the circulation. Otherwise, use isotonic saline.
- Artificial colloid solutions consist of hydroxyethyl starches (e.g. Hespan, EloHAES) or gelatins (e.g. Gelofusin, Haemaccel) dissolved in isotonic saline.

Normal total body Na (water loss)
- Water replacement either PO (addition to enteral feed) or as 5% glucose IV. Up to 5L/day may be necessary.
- If cranial diabetes insipidus (CDI): restrict salt and give thiazide diuretics. Complete CDI will require desmopressin (10µg bd intranasal or 1–2µg bd IV) whereas partial CDI may require desmopressin but often responds to drugs that increase the rate of ADH secretion or end-organ responsiveness to ADH, e.g. chlorpropamide, hydrochlorthiazide
- If nephrogenic DI: manage by a low salt diet and thiazides. High dose desmopressin may be effective. Consider removal of causative agents, e.g. lithium, demeclocycline.

Low total body Na$^+$ (Na$^+$ and water losses)
- Treat hyperosmolar non-ketotic diabetic crisis, uraemia as appropriate.
- Otherwise consider 0.9% saline or hypotonic (0.45%) saline. Up to 6L/day may be needed.

Increased total body Na$^+$ (Na$^+$ gain)
- Water replacement either PO (addition to enteral feed) or as 5% glucose IV. Up to 5L/day may be necessary.
- In addition, frusemide 10–20mg IV prn may be necessary

Causes of hypernatraemia

Type	Aetiology	Urine
Low total body Na	Renal losses: diuretic excess, osmotic diuresis (glucose, urea, mannitol)	$[Na^+] > 20mmol/L$ iso- or hypotonic
	Extra-renal losses: excess sweating	$[Na^+] < 10mmol/L$ hypertonic
Normal total body Na	Renal losses: diabetes insipidus	$[Na^+]$ variable hypo-, iso- or hypertonic
	Extra-renal losses: respiratory and renal insensible losses	$[Na^+]$ variable hypertonic
Increased total body Na	Conn's syndrome, Cushing's syndrome, excess NaCl, hypertonic $NaHCO_3$	$[Na^+] > 20mmol/L$ iso- or hypertonic

Hyponatraemia

Clinical features
Nausea, vomiting, headache, fatigue, weakness, muscular twitching, obtundation, psychosis, seizures and coma. Symptoms depend on the rate as well as the magnitude of fall in the plasma $[Na^+]$.

Treatment
Rate and degree of correction
- In chronic hyponatraemia correction should not exceed 0.5mmol/L/h in the first 24h and 0.3mmol/L/h thereafter.
- In acute hyponatraemia the ideal rate of correction is controversial though elevations in $[Na^+]$ can be faster, but < 20mmol/L/day.
- A plasma Na^+ of 125–130mmol/L is a reasonable target for initial correction of both acute and chronic states. Attempts to achieve normo- or hypernatraemia rapidly should be avoided.
- Neurological complications, e.g. central pontine myelinolysis (CPM), are related to the degree of correction and (in chronic hyponatraemia) the rate. Premenopausal women are more prone to (CPM).

Extracellular fluid (ECF) volume excess
- If symptomatic (e.g. seizures, agitation), and not oedematous, 100ml aliquots of hypertonic (1.8%) saline can be given, checking plasma levels every 2–3h.
- If symptomatic and oedematous, consider frusemide (10–20mg IV bolus prn), mannitol (0.5g/kg IV over 15–20min), and replacement of urinary sodium losses with aliquots of hypertonic saline. Check plasma levels every 2–3h. Haemofiltration or dialysis may be necessary if renal failure is established.
- If not symptomatic, restrict water to 1–1.5L/day. If hyponatraemia persists, consider inappropriate ADH (SIADH) secretion.
- If SIADH likely, give isotonic saline and consider demeclocycline.
- If SIADH unlikely, consider frusemide (10–20mg IV bolus prn), mannitol (0.5g/kg IV over 15–20min), and replacement of urinary sodium losses with aliquots of hypertonic saline.
- Check plasma levels regularly. Haemofiltration or dialysis may be necessary if renal failure is established.

Extracellular fluid volume (ECF) depletion
- If symptomatic (e.g. seizures, agitation), give isotonic (0.9%) saline. Consider hypertonic (1.8%) saline.
- If not symptomatic, give isotonic (0.9%) saline.

General points
- Equations that calculate excess water are unreliable. It is safer to perform frequent estimations of plasma sodium levels.
- Hypertonic saline may be dangerous in the elderly and those with impaired cardiac function. An alternative is to use frusemide with replacement of urinary sodium (and potassium) losses each 2–3h. Thereafter simple water restriction is usually sufficient.
- Many patients achieve normonatraemia by spontaneous water diuresis.
- Use isotonic solutions for reconstituting drugs, parenteral nutrition, etc.
- Hyponatraemia may intensify the cardiac effects of hyperkalaemia.
- A true hyponatraemia may occur with a normal osmolality in the presence of abnormal solutes e.g. ethanol, ethylene glycol, glucose.

Causes of hyponatraemia

Type	Aetiology	Urine [Na+]
ECF volume depletion	Renal losses: diuretic excess, osmotic diuresis (glucose, urea, mannitol), renal tubular acidosis, salt-losing nephritis, mineralocorticoid deficiency	> 20mmol/L
	Extra-renal losses: vomiting, diarrhoea, burns, pancreatitis	< 10mmol/L
Modest ECF volume excess (no oedema)	water intoxication (n.b. post-operative, TURP syndrome), inappropriate ADH secretion, hypothyroidism, drugs (e.g. carbamazepine, chlorpropamide,), glucocorticoid deficiency, pain, emotion ...	> 20mmol/L
ECF volume excess (oedema)	acute and chronic renal failure	> 20mmol/L
	nephrotic syndrome, cirrhosis, heart failure	< 10mmol/L

Causes of inappropriate ADH secretion

- Neoplasm, e.g. lung, pancreas, lymphoma
- Most pulmonary lesions
- Most central nervous system lesions
- Surgical and emotional stress
- Glucocorticoid and thyroid deficiency
- Idiopathic
- Drugs, e.g. chlorpropamide, carbamazepine, narcotics

405

See also:

Haemo(dia)filtration 1, 54; Haemo(dia)filtration 2, 56; Enteral nutrition, 72; Parenteral nutrition, 74; Electrolytes (Na+, K+, Cl−, HCO$_3$−), 138; Urinalysis, 156; Crystalloids, 166; Colloids, 170; Diuretics, 200; Acute renal failure—diagnosis, 320; Acute renal failure—management, 322; Electrolyte management, 400; Hyperosmolar diabetic emergencies, 430; Diabetic ketoacidosis, 428

Hyperkalaemia

Plasma potassium depends on the balance between intake, excretion and the distribution of potassium across cell membranes. Excretion is normally controlled by the kidneys.

Causes

- Reduced renal excretion (e.g. chronic renal failure, adrenal insufficiency, diabetes, potassium sparing diuretics),
- Intracellular potassium release (e.g. acidosis, rapid transfusion of old blood, cell lysis including rhabdomyolysis, haemolysis and tumour lysis)
- Potassium poisoning.

Clinical features

Hyperkalaemia may cause dangerous arrhythmias including cardiac arrest. Arrhythmias are more closely related to the rate of rise of potassium than the absolute level. Clinical features such as paraesthesiae and areflexic weakness are not clearly related to the degree of hyperkalaemia but usually occur after ECG changes (tall 'T' waves, flat 'P' waves, prolonged PR interval and wide QRS).

Management

Potassium restriction is necessary for all cases and haemo(dia)filtration or haemodialysis may be needed for resistant cases.

Cardiac arrest associated with hyperkalaemia
Sodium bicarbonate (8.4%) 50–100ml should be given in addition to standard CPR and other treatment detailed below.

Potassium > 7mmol/L
Calcium chloride (10%) 10ml should be given urgently in addition to treatment detailed below. Although calcium chloride does not reduce the plasma potassium, it stabilises the myocardium against arrhythmias.

Clinical features of hyperkalaemia or potassium >6mmol/L with ECG changes
Glucose (50ml 50%) and soluble insulin (10iu) should be given IV over 20min. Blood glucose should be monitored every 15min and more glucose given if necessary. In addition calcium resonium 15g qds PO or 30g bd PR should be considered.

Potassium >5.3mmol/L
Consider calcium resonium 15g qds PO or 30g bd PR.

See also:
Haemo(dia)filtration 1, 54; Haemo(dia)filtration 2, 56; Enteral nutrition, 72;
Parenteral nutrition, 74; Electrolytes (Na^+, K^+, Cl^-, HCO_3^-), 138; Urinalysis, 156;
Crystalloids, 166; Diuretics, 200; Cardiac arrest, 260; Bradyarrhythmias, 306;
Acute renal failure—diagnosis, 320; Acute renal failure—management, 322;
Electrolyte management, 400

Hypokalaemia

Plasma potassium depends on the balance between intake, excretion and the distribution of potassium across cell membranes. Excretion is normally controlled by the kidneys.

Causes
- Inadequate intake
- Gastrointestinal losses (e.g. vomiting, diarrhoea, fistula losses)
- Renal losses (e.g. diabetic ketoacidosis, Conn's syndrome, secondary hyperaldosteronism, Cushing's syndrome, renal tubular acidosis, metabolic alkalosis, hypomagnesaemia, drugs including diuretics, steroids, theophyllines, β_2 stimulants and β lactam antibiotics)
- Haemofiltration losses
- Potassium transfer into cells (e.g. acute alkalosis, glucose infusion, insulin treatment, familial periodic paralysis).

Clinical features
- Arrhythmias (SVT, VT and Torsades de Pointes)
- ECG changes (ST depression, 'T' wave flattening, 'U' waves)
- Metabolic alkalosis
- Constipation
- Ileus
- Weakness

Management
- Wherever possible the cause of potassium loss should be treated.
- Potassium replacement should be intravenous with ECG monitoring when arrhythmias are present (20mmol over 30min, repeated according to levels).
- Slower intravenous replacement (20mmol over 1h) can be used when arrhythmias are absent.
- Oral supplementation (to a total intake of 80–120mmol/day, including nutritional input) can be given when there are no clinical features.

See also:
Haemo(dia)filtration 1, 54; Haemo(dia)filtration 2, 56; Enteral nutrition, 72; Parenteral nutrition, 74; Electrolytes (Na^+, K^+, Cl^-, HCO_3^-), 138; Urinalysis, 156; Crystalloids, 166; Bronchodilators, 176; Diuretics, 200; Steroids, 250; Cardiac arrest, 260; Tachyarrhythmias, 304; Acute renal failure—diagnosis, 320; Acute renal failure—management, 322; Electrolyte management, 400; Diabetic ketoacidosis, 428

Hypomagnesaemia

Causes

- excess loss, e.g. diuretics, other causes of polyuria (including poorly controlled diabetes mellitus), severe diarrhoea, prolonged vomiting, large nasogastric aspirates,
- inadequate intake, e.g. starvation, parenteral nutrition, alcoholism, malabsorption syndromes

Clinical features

Magnesium is primarily an intracellular ion involved in production and utilisation of energy stores and in the mediation of nerve transmission. Low plasma levels, which do not necessarily reflect either intracellular or whole body stores, may thus be associated with features related to these functions:

- Confusion, irritability
- Seizures
- Muscle weakness, lethargy
- Arrhythmias
- Symptoms related to hypocalcaemia and hypokalaemia which are resistant to calcium and potassium supplementation respectively

Normal plasma levels range from 0.7–1.0mmol/L; severe symptoms do not usually occur until levels drop below 0.5mmol/L.

Management

- Where possible, identify and treat the cause
- For severe, symptomatic hypomagnesaemia, 10mmol of magnesium sulphate can be given IV over 3–5min. This can be repeated once or twice as necessary.
- In less acute situations or for asymptomatic hypomagnesaemia, 10–20mmol $MgSO_4$ solution can be given over 1–2h and repeated as necessary or according to repeat plasma levels.
- A continuous IV infusion (e.g. 3–5mmol $MgSO_4$ solution/h) can be given however this is usually reserved for therapeutic indications where supranormal plasma levels (1.5–2mmol/L) of magnesium are sought, e.g. treatment of supraventricular and ventricular arrhythmias, pre-eclampsia and eclampsia, bronchospasm, post-myocardial infarction.
- Oral magnesium sulphate has a laxative effect and may cause severe diarrhoea.
- High plasma levels of magnesium may develop in renal failure; caution should be applied when administering iv magnesium.

Hypercalcaemia

Causes
- malignancy (e.g. myeloma, bony metastatic disease, hyper-nephroma)
- hyperparathyroidism
- sarcoidosis
- excess intake of calcium, Vitamin A or D
- drugs, e.g. thiazides, lithium
- immobilisation
- rarely, thyrotoxicosis, Addison's disease

Clinical features
Usually become apparent when total (ionised and unionised) plasma levels >3.5 mmol/L (normal range 2.2–2.6mmol/L). Symptoms depend on the patient's age, the duration and rate of increase of plasma calcium, and the presence of concurrent medical conditions.
- nausea, vomiting, weight loss, pruritus
- muscle weakness, fatigue, lethargy,
- depression, mania, psychosis
- drowsiness, coma
- abdominal pain, constipation
- acute pancreatitis
- peptic ulceration
- polyuria, renal calculi, renal failure
- arrhythmias

Management
1 Identify and treat cause where possible.
2 Carefully monitor haemodynamic variables, urine output, and ECG morphology with frequent estimations of plasma Ca^{2+}, PO_4^{3-}, Mg^{2+}, Na^+ and K^+
3 Intravascular volume repletion—this inhibits proximal tubular reabsorption of calcium and often lowers the plasma calcium by 0.4–0.6mmol/L. It should precede diuretics or any other therapy. Either colloid or 0.9% saline should be used, depending on the presence of hypovolaemia-related features.
4 Calciuresis—after adequate intravascular volume repletion, a forced diuresis with frusemide plus 0.9% saline (6–8L/day) may be attempted. An effect is usually seen within 12h. Loop diuretics inhibit calcium reabsorption in the ascending limb of loop of Henle. More aggressive frusemide regimens can be attempted but can potentially result in complications. Thiazides should not be used as tubular reabsorption may be reduced with increased $[CA^{2+}]$.

5 Dialysis/haemofiltration—may be indicated at an early stage for established oligo-anuric renal failure $\pm$ fluid overload.
6 Steroids can be effective for hypercalcaemia related to haematological cancers (lymphoma, myeloma), Vitamin D overdose and sarcoidosis.
7 Calcitonin has the most rapid onset of action with a nadir often reached within 12–24h. Its action is usually short-lived and rebound hypercalcaemia may occur. It generally does not drop the plasma level more than 0.5mmol/L.
8 Diphosphonates (e.g. etridonate), mithramycin and IV phosphate should only be given after specialist advice is taken in view of their toxicity and potential complications.

Drug dosage

diuretics	frusemide 10–40mg IV 2–4h (may be increased to 80–100mg IV every 1–2h)
steroids	hydrocortisone 100mg qds IV or prednisolone 40–60mg PO for 3–5 days
etridonate	
mithramycin	25g/kg slow IV bolus
phosphate	
calcitonin	3–4U/kg IV followed by 4U/kg SC bd

See also:

Hypocalcaemia

Causes
- Associated with hyperphosphataemia:
  - Renal failure
  - Rhabdomyolysis
  - Hypoparathyroidism (including surgery), pseudohypoparathyroidism
- Associated with low/normal phosphate:
  - Critical illness including sepsis, burns
  - Hypomagnesaemia
  - Pancreatitis
  - Osteomalacia
  - Over-hydration
- Massive blood transfusion (citrate-binding)
- Hyperventilation and the resulting respiratory alkalosis may reduce the ionised plasma calcium fraction and induce clinical features of hypocalcaemia

Clinical features
These usually appear when total plasma calcium levels < 2mmol/L and the ionised fraction is < 0.8mmol/L.
- Tetany (including carpopedal spasm)
- Muscular weakness
- Hypotension
- Perioral and peripheral parasthesiae
- Chvostek & Trousseau's signs
- Prolonged QT interval
- Seizures

Management
1 If respiratory alkalosis is present, adjust ventilator settings or, if spontaneously hyperventilating and agitated, calm ± sedate. Rebreathing into a bag may be beneficial.
2 If symptomatic, give 5–10ml 10% calcium chloride solution over 2–5min. Repeat as necessary.
3 Correct hypomagnesaemia or hypokalaemia if present.
4 If asymptomatic and in renal failure or hypoparathyroid, consider enteral/parenteral calcium supplementation and Vitamin D analogues.
5 If hypotensive or cardiac output is decreased following administration of a calcium antagonist, give 5–10ml 10% calcium chloride solution over 2–5min.

Hypophosphataemia

Causes
- Critical illness
- Inadequate intake
- Loop diuretic therapy (including low dose dopamine).
- Parenteral nutrition—levels fall rapidly during high dose intravenous glucose therapy, especially with insulin
- Alcoholism
- Hyperparathyroidism

Clinical effects
The main clinical feature of hypophosphataemia is muscle weakness affecting cardiac and skeletal muscle. The associated depletion of ATP also affects white blood cell function adversely. Depletion of 2,3–diphosphoglycerate reduces the efficiency of red cell oxygen carriage.

Treatment
Phosphate supplements (5–10mmol) should be given by intravenous infusion over 6h and repeated according to the plasma phosphate level.

See also:
Enteral nutrition, 72; Parenteral nutrition, 74; Calcium, magnesium &
phosphate, 140; Diuretics, 200

General acid–base management

Increased intake, altered production or impaired/excessive excretion of acid or base leads to derangements in blood pH. Augmented renal excretion of H^+ ions may result from hypokalaemia. With time, respiratory and renal adjustments correct the pH towards normality by altering the plasma level of PCO_2 or HCO_3^-.

Increased intake
- Acid: aspirin overdose
- Base: $NaHCO_3$ administration, antacid abuse, buffered replacement fluid (haemofiltration)

Altered production
- Increased acid production: Lactic acidosis (usually 2° to hypoperfusion), diabetic ketoacidosis
- Increased base production: Chronic hypercapnic respiratory failure, permissive hypercapnia.
- Decreased base production: Chronic hyperventilation

Altered excretion
- Increased acid loss: Vomiting, large gastric aspirates, diuretics (Cl^-), hyperaldosteronism, corticosteroids
- Increased base loss: Diarrhoea, small bowel fistula, urethroenterostomy, proximal renal tubular acidosis,
- Decreased acid loss: Renal failure, distal renal tubular acidosis, acetazolamide
- Decreased base loss: Chronic hypercapnic respiratory failure, permissive hypercapnia.

Principles of management

1 Correct (where possible) the abnormality, e.g. hypoperfusion
2 Consider addition of 'substrate' and physiological corrective functions
3 NaCl infusion for vomiting-induced alkalosis; insulin, Na^+ and K^+ in diabetic ketoacidosis
4 Correct pH in specific circumstances only, e.g. $NaHCO_3$ in renal failure

See also:
Haemo(dia)filtration 1, 54; Haemo(dia)filtration 2, 56; Peritoneal dialysis, 58;
Blood gas analysis, 94; Crystalloids, 166; Vomiting / gastric stasis, 326; Acute
renal failure—management, 322; Metabolic acidosis, 420; Metabolic alkalosis,
422

Metabolic acidosis

A subnormal arterial blood pH with a base deficit > 2mmol/L. Outcome in critically ill patients has been linked to the severity and duration of metabolic acidosis and hyperlactataemia.

Causes

- Tissue hypoperfusion, e.g. heart failure, hypovolaemia, sepsis. The anion gap is related to production of lactic and other organic acids. Although anaerobic metabolism contributes in part to this metabolic acidosis, other cellular mechanisms are involved though remain to be clearly defined
- Tissue necrosis, e.g. bowel, muscle
- Ketoacidosis—high levels of β-hydroxybutyrate and acetoacetate related to uncontrolled diabetes mellitus, starvation and alcoholism
- Renal failure—accumulation of organic acids, e.g. sulphuric.
- Drugs—in particular, aspirin (salicylic acid) overdose, acetazolamide (carbonic anhydrase inhibition), ammonium chloride. Vasopressor agents may be implicated, possibly by inducing regional ischaemia.
- Ingestion of poisons—e.g. paraldehyde, ethylene glycol, methanol
- Bicarbonate loss, e.g. severe diarrhoea, small bowel fistulae, large ileostomy losses
- Type B lactic acidosis (rare)—i.e. no evidence of tissue hypoperfusion.

Clinical features

- Dyspnoea
- Haemodynamic instability
- A rapidly increasing metabolic acidosis (over minutes to hours) is not due to renal failure. Other causes, particularly severe tissue hypoperfusion, sepsis or tissue necrosis should be suspected when there is associated systemic deterioration.

Management

1 The underlying cause should be identified and treated where possible rather than administering alkali or manipulating minute volume to normalise the arterial pH.
2 Urgent haemo(dia)filtration may be necessary if oligo-anuria persists.
3 Reversal of the metabolic acidosis is generally an indication of successful therapy. An increasing base deficit suggests that the therapeutic manoeuvres in operation are either inadequate or wrong.
4 The benefits of buffers such as Carbicarb and THAM (trishydroxy-methyl-aminomethane) remain unproved.

Causes of type B lactic acidosis

Acute infection
Diabetes mellitus
Drugs, e.g. phenformin, metformin, alcohols
Glucose-6-Phosphatase deficiency
Haematological malignancy
Hepatic failure
Pancreatitis
Renal failure
Short bowel syndrome (d-lactate)
Thiamine deficiency

421

See also:
  Haemo(dia)filtration 1, 54; Haemo(dia)filtration 2, 56; Peritoneal dialysis, 58; Blood gas analysis, 94; Lactate, 160; Sodium bicarbonate, 168; Inotropes, 184; Vasopressors, 188; Basic resuscitation, 258; Cardiac arrest, 260; Fluid challenge, 262; Dyspnoea, 266; Hypotension, 300; Heart failure—assessment, 312; Heart failure—management, 314; Acute renal failure—diagnosis, 320; Acute renal failure—management, 322; Abdominal sepsis, 340; Pancreatitis, 342; General acid–base management, 418; Diabetic ketoacidosis, 428; Salicylate poisoning, 440; Inhaled poisons, 450; Methanol and ethylene glycol, 454; Sepsis / infection, 490

Metabolic alkalosis

- A supranormal arterial blood pH with a base excess > 2mmol/L caused either by loss of (non-carbonic) acid or gain of base. As the kidney is usually efficient at excreting large quantities of bicarbonate, persistence of a metabolic alkalosis usually depends on either chronic renal failure or a diminished extracellular fluid volume with severe depletion of K^+.
- The patient is usually asymptomatic though, if spontaneously breathing, will hypoventilate.
- A metabolic alkalosis will cause a left shift of the oxyhaemoglobin curve, reducing oxygen availability to the tissues.

Causes

- Loss of total body fluid, Na^+, Cl^+, K^+ usually due to:
  - diuretics
  - large nasogastric aspirates, vomiting
  - secondary hyperaldosteronism with potassium depletion
- Use of haemofiltration replacement fluid containing excess buffer (e.g. lactate)
- Renal compensation for chronic hypercapnia. This can develop within 1–2 weeks. Although more apparent when the patient hyperventilates, or is hyperventilated to normocapnia, an over-compensated metabolic alkalosis can occasionally be seen in the chronic state (i.e. a raised pH in an otherwise stable long-term hypercapnic patient)
- Excess administration of bicarbonate
- Excess administration of citrate (large blood transfusion)
- Drugs, including laxative abuse, corticosteroids
- Rarely, Cushing's, Conn's, Bartter's syndrome

Management

1 Replacement of fluid, sodium, chloride (i.e. give 0.9% saline) and potassium losses are often sufficient to restore acid–base balance.
2 With distal renal causes related to hyperaldosteronism, addition of spironolactone (or potassium canrenoate) can be considered.
3 Active treatment is rarely necessary. If so, give ammonium chloride 5g tds PO. Hydrochloric acid has been used on occasion for severe metabolic alkalosis (pH > 7.7). It should be given via a central vein in a concentration of 1mmol HCl per ml water at a rate not exceeding 1mmol/kg/h.
4 Compensation for a long-standing respiratory acidosis, followed by correction of that acidosis, e.g. with mechanical ventilation, will lead to an uncompensated metabolic alkalosis. This usually corrects with time though treatments such as acetazolamide can be considered. Mechanical 'hypoventilation', i.e. maintaining hypercapnia, can also be considered.

See also:
   Haemo(dia)filtration 1, 54; Haemo(dia)filtration 2, 56; Blood gas analysis, 94;
Sodium bicarbonate, 168; Blood transfusion, 172; Acute renal failure—diagnosis
320; Acute renal failure—management, 322; Vomiting / gastric stasis, 326;
Hypokalaemia, 408; General acid–base management, 418

Hypoglycaemia

Causes

- Inadequate intake of carbohydrate
- Excess insulin or sulphonylurea
- Liver failure with depletion of glycogen stores
- Alcohol
- Hypoadrenalism (including Addison's disease), hypopituitarism
- Quinine, aspirin

Clinical features

- Nausea, vomiting
- Increased sympathetic activity, e.g. sweating, tachycardia,
- Altered behaviour and conscious level
- Seizures, focal neurological signs

Management

1 Monitor carefully with regular bedside estimations. The frequency should be increased in conditions known to precipitate hypoglycaemia, e.g. insulin infusion, liver failure, quinine treatment of malaria
2 Administer 25ml 50% glucose solution if the blood glucose is:
   - ≤3mmol/L or
   - ≤4mmol/L and the patient is symptomatic or
   - within the normal range but the patient is symptomatic (usually long-standing poorly-controlled diabetics)

   Repeat as necessary every few minutes until symptoms abate and the blood glucose level has normalised.
3 If the blood glucose is 3–4mmol/L and the patient is non-symptomatic, either reduce the rate of insulin infusion (if present), or increase calorie intake (enterally or parenterally). In insulin dependent diabetes mellitus, the insulin should continue with adequate glucose intake.
4 A continuous parenteral infusion of 10%, 20% or 50% glucose solution varying from 10–100ml/h may be required, depending on the degree of continuing hypoglycaemia and the patient's fluid balance/urine output. 5% glucose solution only contains 20Cal/100ml and should not be used to prevent or treat hypoglycaemia.
5 In the rare instance of no venous access, hypoglycaemia may be temporarily reversed by glucagon 1mg given either IM or SC.
6 Continuing hypoglycaemia in the face of adequate treatment and lack of symptoms should be confirmed with a formal laboratory blood sugar estimation to exclude malfunctioning of the bedside testing equipment.

Hyperglycaemia

Causes
- A common occurrence in critically ill patients due to a combination of impaired glucose tolerance, high circulating levels of endogenous catecholamines and corticosteroids, and regular administration of such drugs which antagonise the effect of insulin.
- Pancreatitis resulting in islet cell damage

Clinical features
None in the short-term other than polyuria from the osmotic diuresis. The patient may complain of thirst or show signs of hypovolaemia if fluid balance is allowed to become too negative.

Metabolic effects
Relative lack of insulin prevents cellular glucose uptake and utilisation resulting in:
- Increased lipolysis
- Altered cellular metabolism
- Increased risk of infection (decreased neutrophil action)

Management
1 Treatment should be given if blood glucose estimations persist > 10mmol/L.
2 A short-acting insulin infusion (e.g. actrapid) should be used and titrated to maintain normoglycaemia (4–8mmol/L). Usually 1–4 units/h are required though may need to be much higher in diabetics who become critically ill. Regular bedside monitoring of blood sugar should be performed; this should be hourly if unstable.
3 Oral hypoglycaemic agents should be generally avoided in the ICU patient because of their prolonged duration of action and unpredictable absorption.

Diabetic ketoacidosis

This may occur *de novo* in a previously undiagnosed diabetic or follow an acute insult (e.g. infection) in an otherwise controlled diabetic patient.

Monitoring

Adequate invasive monitoring is essential, particularly if the patient has circulatory instability or cardiac dysfunction. Urine output, blood gases and plasma electrolytes should also be monitored frequently.

Fluid and electrolyte management

1 Fluid and electrolyte repletion should not follow a strict regimen but must be tailored to individual needs.
2 If the patient shows signs of tissue hypoperfusion and haemodynamic instability, colloid solutions should be given by repeated fluid challenges to restore the circulating blood volume.
3 Otherwise or thereafter, fluid replacement with 0.9% saline should be given at a rate of 200ml/h until the salt and water debt has been replenished. Caution should be exercised to prevent sodium overload.
4 Hypotonic (0.45%) saline resuscitation may be appropriate in the non-shocked patient, especially if the plasma sodium is rising rapidly. This often occurs during treatment due to a shift of water into the cells and a shift of sodium from the cells in exchange for potassium.
5 Traditional regimens of rapid fluid replacement (e.g. 3–4 litres within the first 3–4h) are no longer encouraged because of the higher risk of cerebral oedema and of compromising cardiac or renal function.
6 Substitute 5% glucose solution (100–200ml/h) after replacing the sodium debt; this is usually when the blood sugar falls < 10mmol/L.

Electrolyte replacement

1 Carefully monitor K^+ replacement. Both acidosis and excessive K^+ administration cause hyperkalaemia while fluid and insulin will produce hypokalaemia. Check levels frequently, initially hourly, to maintain normokalemia. Infusion rates of 10–40mmol/h KCl will be needed.
2 Magnesium replacement—3–5mmol/h $MgSO_4$ is usually sufficient but should be confirmed by frequent laboratory estimations.

Hyperglycaemia

Correct slowly at a rate of 2–4mmol/h by adjusting the short-acting insulin infusion (usually 1–5U/h). Monitor blood glucose hourly. Continue IV insulin even after achieving normoglycaemia, until heavy ketonuria has disappeared and the base deficit has normalised. A glucose infusion may be needed to maintain normoglycaemia.

Other aspects of managing ketoacidosis

1 Seek a precipitating cause and treat as indicated. Approximately 50% are related to underlying disease, e.g. sepsis, myocardial infarction, stroke, infective gastroenteritis.
2 Only give antibiotics for proved or highly suspected infection.
3 Abdominal pain should not be dismissed as part of the syndrome.
4 A nasogastric tube should be inserted as gastric emptying is often delayed and acute gastric dilatation is common.
5 Avoid bicarbonate, even for severe acidosis (pH < 7.0). It causes an increased intracellular acidosis and depressed respiration due to a relative CSF alkalosis. Sodium overload may also occur.
6 Heparin 5000U SC bd is indicated in immobile or comatose patients.

Clinical features

These relate to:
- Excess fat metabolism to fatty acids with ketone production
- An osmotic diuresis with large losses of fluid (up to 6–10L), sodium (400–800mmol), potassium (250–800mmol) and magnesium

Symptoms are those resulting from hypovolaemia, metabolic acidosis and electrolyte imbalance with polyuria. Hyperventilation is a prominent feature.

Coma need not necessarily be present for life to be threatened.

Plasma amylase commonly exceeds 1000U/L but does not indicate pancreatitis. If suspected, perform an abdominal ultrasound.

Hyperosmolar diabetic emergencies

This is more common in elderly, non-insulin dependent diabetics though can present *de novo* in young adults.
Precipitating factors are similar to ketoacidosis, e.g. sepsis, myocardial infarction

Clinical features

- Fluid depletion is greater, blood glucose levels often higher, coma more frequent and mortality much higher than in diabetic ketoacidosis.
- Confusion, agitation and drowsiness which may persist for 1–2 weeks.
- A metabolic acidosis may be present but is not usually profound; ketoacidosis is not a feature.
- Hyperosmolality may predispose to thrombotic events; this is the major cause of mortality. Severe hyperosmolality does not always occur.
- Focal neurological signs and disseminated intravascular coagulation are occasionally recognised.

Management

As for diabetic ketoacidosis however:
1 Unless the patient shows signs of hypovolaemia and tissue hypoperfusion, in which case colloid challenges should be given for prompt resuscitation, fluid replacement should be more gradual as the risk of cerebral oedema is higher. This can be with either 0.9% saline or, if the plasma sodium is high, 0.45% saline at a rate of 100–200ml/h.
2 The plasma sodium rises with treatment, even with 0.45% saline, and can often increase in the first few days to 160–170mmol/L before gradually declining thereafter. Aim to correct slowly.
3 Serum phosphate and magnesium levels fall rapidly with this condition; replacement may be needed as guided by frequently taken plasma levels.
4 Patients may be hypersensitive to insulin and often require lower doses.
5 Unless otherwise contraindicated, these patients should be fully heparinised until full recovery (which may take ⩾5 days).

See also:
Electrolytes (Na^+, K^+, Cl^-, HCO_3^-), 138; Bacteriology, 148; Urinalysis, 156;
Crystalloids, 166; Fluid challenge, 262; Anticoagulants, 236; Antimicrobials, 248;
Acute myocardial infarction, 308; Oliguria, 318; Vomiting / gastric stasis, 326;
Abdominal sepsis, 340; Hyperkalaemia, 406; Hypokalaemia, 408;
Hypomagnesaemia, 410; Hypophosphataemia, 416; Hyperglycaemia, 426;
Diabetic ketoacidosis, 428; Sepsis / infection, 490

Thyroid emergencies

Thyrotoxic crisis

Presents as an exacerbation of the clinical features of hyperthyroidism (e.g. pyrexia, hyperdynamic circulation, heart failure, confusion). There is usually a precipitating factor such as infection, surgery, ketoacidosis, myocardial infarction or childbirth. It may present with exhaustion in the elderly with few features of hyperthyroidism. The diagnosis is confirmed by standard thyroid function tests.

Management
- Pyrexia should be controlled by surface cooling (avoid aspirin which displaces thyroxine from plasma proteins).
- Catecholamine effects should be reduced by β blockade (propranolol 1–5mg IV then 20–80mg qds PO) unless there is acute heart failure.
- Blockade of thyroxine synthesis is achieved by potassium iodide 200–600mg IV over 2h then 2g/day PO and carbimazole 60–120mg/day PO.
- Blockade of peripheral T4 to T3 conversion is achieved by dexamethasone 2mg qds IV.
- Careful fluid and electrolyte management is essential.

Myxoedema coma

Presents as an exacerbation of the features of hypothyroidism (e.g. hypothermia, coma, bradycardia, metabolic and respiratory acidosis, anaemia). There may be a precipitating factor (e.g. cold, infection, surgery, myocardial infarction, CVA, central nervous system depressant drugs). Diagnosis is confirmed by thyroid function tests.

Management
- Treatment of the complications of severe hypothyroidism (e.g. hypotension, heart failure, hypothermia, bradycardia, seizures) is more important than thyroid hormone replacement.
- Thyroxine replacement should be with low doses (0.1–0.2mg PO or PR unless ischaemic heart disease is possible, then start at 0.25mg).
- There are no definite advantages to using T3 replacement, high dose replacement regimens or intravenous treatment.
- Steroids (hydrocortisone 100mg qds IV) should be given since coexisting hypoadrenalism is masked by myxoedema.

Hypoadrenal crisis

Clinical features

Primary hypoadrenalism
- Glucocorticoid deficiency (e.g. weakness, vomiting, diarrhoea, abdominal pain, hypoglycaemia)
- Mineralocorticoid deficiency (e.g. dehydration, hyponatraemia, weight loss, postural hypotension, hyperkalaemia)
- Skin pigmentation due to ACTH excess.

Secondary hypoadrenalism
- May be due to steroid withdrawal after 2 weeks' treatment or hypopituitarism
- No skin pigmentation
- Features of mineralocorticoid deficiency may be absent.

Diagnosis

Diagnosis is confirmed by plasma cortisol and ACTH levels or a Synacthen test although treatment should begin on clinical suspicion. Synacthen is an ACTH analogue; 250µg given IM should produce a rise in plasma cortisol to >600nmol/L. A negative response is consistent with primary hypoadrenalism. Dexamethasone may be used for steroid replacement for 48h before a Synacthen test is performed since other steroid treatment may be detected in the plasma cortisol assay.

Management

- Salt and water deficiency should be corrected urgently. Initial fluid replacement should be with colloid if there is hypotension or evidence of poor tissue perfusion. Otherwise, 4–5L/day 0.9% saline will be needed for several days.
- Fluid management should be carefully monitored to ensure adequate replacement without fluid overload.
- Glucocorticoid replacement should be with hydrocortisone 50–100mg tds IV on day 1 then 20–50mg tds on days 2–3). Hydrocortisone may be changed to equivalent doses of dexamethasone when a Synacthen test is performed.

435

Poisoning

Poisoning—general principles

Poisoning should be considered in patients presenting with altered consciousness, respiratory or cardiovascular depression, vomiting, hypothermia or seizures. The history usually makes diagnosis obvious although clinical signs may be confused due to ingestion of multiple poisons or absent if effects are delayed. It should be remembered that poisons may enter the body via routes other than ingestion, e.g. inhalation or transdermally. Salicylate and paracetamol are extremely common agents in self poisoning and patients often present with no alteration of consciousness.

Investigation

All patients require urea and electrolyte, blood glucose and blood gas estimations. Urine samples and gastric aspirate should be saved for possible later toxicology analysis. Salicylate and paracetamol levels are necessary due to the common lack of early signs and to allow specific early treatment. Other drug levels may help in diagnosis but treatment is often supportive. Early support from the local Poisons Information Service should be solicited.

Supportive treatment

Treatment of cardiovascular and respiratory compromise and neurological disturbance should be by standard intensive care methods outlined elsewhere in the book. In the unconscious patient opiates and benzodiazepines may be reversed temporarily to allow assessment of the underlying status.

Gastric elimination

Gastric emptying should be considered if the poison is not a corrosive or hydrocarbon and has been ingested < 4h previously. If salicylates or tricyclics have been ingested gastric emptying is useful for 12h after ingestion. There are no clear advantages for forced emesis (ipecacuanaha 30ml in 200ml water) or gastric lavage. Forced emesis may be delayed for 30min and then may be intractable. Aspiration is a serious risk with either form of gastric emptying therapy; the patient should be intubated for airway protection if consciousness is at all impaired.

Activated charcoal

Activated charcoal is probably more effective than gastric emptying to prevent drug absorption. A charcoal:poison weight ratio of 10:1 is required. Poisons may be eliminated after absorption via the small bowel with activated charcoal 50–100g followed by 12.5g hourly NG. Activated charcoal is particularly useful for benzodiazepines, anticonvulsants, tricyclics, theophylline, phenothiazines and antihistamines.

Forced diuresis and dialysis

Forced diuresis with appropriate urinary acidification or alkalinisation (see table) is useful for water soluble poisons which are distributed predominantly extracellularly. Forced diuresis should not be used if renal function is abnormal. Small molecules may also be removed by haemodialysis (e.g. ethylene glycol, methanol, oxalic acid, formic acid).

Forced alkaline diuresis

- Used for soluble acidic drugs (e.g. salicylates)
- Frusemide or mannitol to maintain urine output > 200ml/h
- Intravenous crystalloid to prevent hypovolaemia
- Avoid excessive positive fluid balance
- Use 1.26% bicarbonate to maintain urinary pH > 7
- Stop bicarbonate if arterial pH > 7.5 and use 0.9% saline
- Alternate bicarbonate/saline with 5% glucose
- Monitor and replace potassium and magnesium carefully

Forced acid diuresis

- Used for soluble basic drugs (e.g. amphetamines, quinine, phencyclidine)
- Frusemide or mannitol to maintain urine output > 200ml/h
- Intravenous crystalloid to prevent hypovolaemia
- Avoid excessive positive fluid balance
- Use 750g NH_4Cl in each 500ml 5% glucose to maintain urinary pH < 7.0
- Alternate 0.9%saline with 5% glucose
- Monitor and replace potassium and magnesium carefully

See also:

Salicylate poisoning

Serious, life-threatening toxicity is likely after ingestion of > 7.5g salicylate.

Aspirin is the most common form ingested but salicylic acid and methylsalicylate are occasionally implicated.

Loss of consciousness is rare but metabolic derangements are complex (e.g. respiratory alkalosis due to stimulation of the respiratory centre, dehydration due to salt and water loss, renal bicarbonate excretion and hyperthermia, hypokalaemia, metabolic acidosis due to interference with carbohydrate, lipid and amino acid metabolism, hyperthermia due to uncoupling of oxidative phosphorylation and increased metabolic rate).

There may also be pulmonary oedema due to capillary leak, and bleeding due to reduced prothrombin levels.

Although gastric erosions are common with aspirin treatment, bleeding from this source is rare in acute poisoning.

Management

Gastric elimination
Due to delayed gastric emptying gastric elimination is worthwhile for up to 24h after ingestion. Activated charcoal (12.5g/h) should be given NG to adsorb salicylate remaining in the bowel and adsorb any salicylate back-diffusing across the bowel mucosa. Insoluble aspirin may form a gastric mass that is difficult to remove by gastric lavage.

Salicylate levels
Repeated levels should be taken since levels may continue to rise as absorption continues. Levels taken after 12h may underestimate the degree of toxicity due to tissue binding. If salicylate levels are < 3.1mmol/L after 1h of ingestion and there is no metabolic derangement observation, fluids and repeat levels are all that is required. Alkaline diuresis is required if levels > 3.1mmol/L or there is metabolic derangement but no renal failure. Levels > 6.2mmol/L (or > 3.1mmol/L with renal failure) require haemodialysis.

Alkaline diuresis
If urine flow cannot be maintained alkaline diuresis should be abandoned in favour of haemodialysis, although it is the alkalinisation rather than the diuresis which is more important for salicylate excretion. Urinary pH must be > 7.0 without arterial alkalosis (pH < 7.5). Potassium loss will occur with the bicarbonate infusion, due to the diuresis and as a toxic effect of the salicylate. Potassium levels must be monitored and corrected in a high dependency environment. Alkaline diuresis, if successful, should continue until salicylate levels < 3.1mmol/L. If alkaline diuresis continues for > 6h calcium supplements should be given.

Haemodialysis
Indications include salicylate levels > 6.2mmol/L or renal failure.

See also:
Toxicology, 14; Hypokalaemia, 408; Poisoning—general principles, 438

Paracetamol poisoning

Serious, life-threatening toxicity is likely after ingestion of > 15g.

Paracetamol is rapidly absorbed from the stomach and upper small bowel and is metabolised by conjugation in the liver.

Hepatic necrosis occurs due to the toxicity of an alkylating metabolite which is normally removed by conjugation with glutathione; glutathione is rapidly depleted with overdose.

Toxicity is usually asymptomatic for 1–2 days although laboratory assessment of liver function may become abnormal after 18h.

Hepatic failure, if manifest, develops after 2–7 days, an earlier onset being associated with more severe toxicity.

Management

If ingestion has occurred < 4h previously, gastric elimination techniques should be employed. Paracetamol levels may be taken to confirm ingestion but should not be interpreted for toxicity until after 4h from ingestion. The mainstay of treatment is to restore hepatic glutathione levels with its precursor, N-acetylcysteine.

N-acetylcysteine

Treatment is most effective if started within 10h of ingestion but is currently advised for up to 36h after ingestion. Treatment is required if the paracetamol levels are in the toxic range (see figure) or > 15g paracetamol has been ingested. It should be continued until paracetamol is not detected in the blood. N-acetylcysteine is given by continuous IV infusion (150mg/kg over 15min, 50mg/kg in 500ml 5% glucose over 4h then 50mg/kg in 500ml 5% glucose 8hrly).

Management of hepatic failure

- Early referral to a specialist hepatology centre is necessary since patients with established hepatic failure do not travel well. A rise in prothrombin time or bilirubin are early warning signs of significant hepatic damage.
- Encephalopathy requires airway protection, careful fluid and electrolyte management and prevention of intracranial hypertension.
- The high risk of infection requires prophylactic antibiotics and antifungals.
- Absorption of excessive gastrointestinal protein is managed by cathartics (e.g. lactulose 30ml PO or NG, magnesium sulphate enemas).
- Circulatory management requires avoidance of hypovolaemia while preventing fluid excess if there is cerebral oedema and arrhythmia control (especially those associated with hypokalaemia).
- Renal failure is commonly associated with paracetamol induced hepatic failure and should be managed with early haemofiltration to ensure stability of fluid management.

Graph for predicting treatment requirement

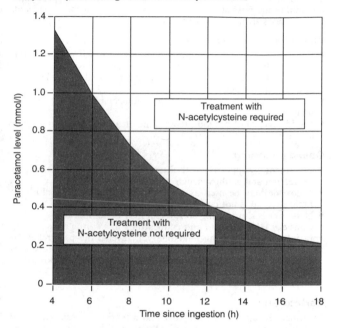

Treatment is required at lower levels if the patient is a known alcoholic or is taking enzyme inducing drugs, e.g. phenytoin.

443

Sedative poisoning

Patients present with alteration of consciousness, respiratory failure and, in some cases, cardiovascular disturbance. After prolonged immobility the possibility of rhabdomyolysis should be considered. In most cases treatment is supportive.

Benzodiazepine poisoning

- Benzodiazepines are common agents used for self poisoning but severe features are uncommon, except at extremes of age.
- Flumazenil may be used as a specific antidote (0.2–1.0mg IV given in 0.1mg increments).
- Flumazenil is short acting so benzodiazepine reversal may be temporary.
- Rapid reversal of benzodiazepines may lead to anxiety attacks or seizures.

Opioid poisoning

- Treatment is supportive with attention particularly to respiratory depression and cardiovascular disturbance.
- Naloxone may be used as an antidote (0.2–0.4mg IV) although rapid reversal is not desired in abusers.
- Naloxone is short acting so reversal may be temporary.
- Consider HIV infection and endocarditis in IV drug abusers.
- In iatrogenic poisoning naloxone will reverse the pain relief for which opioids were given. In these cases respiratory depression is better reversed by the non-specific respiratory stimulant doxapram (1.0–1.5mg/kg over 30sec intravenously followed by 1.5–4.0mg/min).

Barbiturates

Treatment is supportive with particular attention to respiratory and cardiovascular depression. Vasodilatation may be extreme requiring fluid support and, in some cases, inotropic support. Phenobarbitone may be eliminated by forced alkaline diuresis.

Tricyclic antidepressant poisoning

Tricyclic antidepressants are prescribed to patients who are at greatest risk of a suicide attempt. They are rapidly absorbed from the gastrointestinal tract, although gastric emptying is delayed.

Clinical features

- Anticholinergic effects (dilated pupils, dry mouth, ileus, retention of urine)
- Arrhythmias (particularly associated with prolonged QT interval and QRS waves.
- Hyperreflexia with extensor plantars, visual hallucinations and seizures. Drug levels do not correlate with severity.
- Metabolism is usually rapid and improvement can be expected within 24h.

Management

1 There is no specific treatment for tricyclic antidepressant poisoning.
2 Patients require ECG monitoring during the first 24h and until ECG changes have disappeared for 12h.
3 Gastric elimination is worthwhile for 24h after ingestion since tricyclics slow gastric emptying.
4 Activated charcoal via a nasogastric tube will adsorb tricyclics remaining in the bowel.
5 Cardiac arrhythmias are more common if there is acidosis. Bicarbonate should be used urgently to achieve an arterial pH of 7.5. If arrhythmias occur with no acidosis and fail to respond to conventional treatment bicarbonate (25–50ml 8.4% IV) may still be useful.
6 Seizures are best managed with diazepam.

See also:
Ventilatory support—indications, 4; Blood gas analysis, 94; ECG monitoring, 102; Blood pressure monitoring, 104; Toxicology, 152; Sodium bicarbonate, 168; Basic resuscitation, 258; Tachyarrhythmias, 304; Generalised seizures, 360; Poisoning—general principles, 438

Amphetamines including Ecstasy

Amphetamines, including 3,4methylenedioxymethamphetamine (MDMA, 'Ecstasy') and 3,4methylenedioxyethamphetamine ('Eve'), are stimulants taken predominantly for recreational use, or as appetite suppressants. These drugs are hallucinogenic at higher doses. MDMA has been shown to cause rapid decreases in central nervous system 5–hydroxytryptamine and 5–hydroxyindole-3–acetic acid levels and increases in dopamine release.

Clinical features of overdose

Agitation, hyperactivity, hypertension, hallucinations, paranoia followed by exhaustion, coma, convulsions and hyperthermia.

Idiosyncratic responses to Ecstasy and Eve are more common with numerous reports of mortality and major morbidity following ingestion of just 1–2 tablets. These appear related to ingestion in hot environments, e.g. nightclubs, and concurrent dehydration. Features include profound hyperthermia (> 40°C), agitation, seizures, muscle rigidity, hypertension, tachycardia, sweating, coma, liver failure, disseminated intravascular coagulation and rhabdomyolysis. These complications lead to hypovolaemia, electrolyte imbalance (particularly hyperkalaemia) and a metabolic acidosis.

Some patients taking Ecstasy or Eve have been admitted with water intoxication and acute hyponatraemia following ingestion of large amounts of water.

Management

1 Supportive care including airway protection, fluid resuscitation, electrolyte correction and, if needed, mechanical ventilation.
2 Early stages of amphetamine poisoning can be often controlled with tepid sponging, chlorpromazine, β-blockade. Forced acid diuresis to increase urinary excretion is rarely needed.
3 Severe complications should be managed as they arise, e.g. rapid cooling for hyperpyrexia, anticonvulsants for seizures, forced alkaline diuresis ± fasciotomies for rhabdomyolysis, platelet and fresh frozen plasma infusions for coagulopathy.
4 Dantrolene may be given to treat the hyperpyrexia at a dose of 1mg/kg IV, repeated to a cumulative maximum dose of 10mg/kg, particularly if the temperature is > 40°C.

449

Inhaled poisons

Carbon monoxide

Carbon monoxide poisoning should be considered in anyone found in a smoke filled, enclosed space. Carbon monoxide displaces oxygen from haemoglobin, to which it has 200 times greater affinity and thus prevents oxygen carriage. There is also a direct toxic myocardial effect and inhibition of mitochondrial oxidative phosphorylation.

Clinical features
- A cherry red appearance of the skin and mucosae are classical but not common.
- PaO_2 will be normal unless there is respiratory depression and pulse oximetry is misleading.
- The half life of carboxyhaemoglobin is 4h when breathing room air and 50min when breathing 100% oxygen.

Management
- Carboxyhaemoglobin levels should be measured by a co-oximeter and treatment started immediately with oxygen at the maximum concentration that can be delivered (FiO_2 1.0 if ventilated and 0.6–1.0 if self ventilating).
- If carboxyhaemoglobin levels >25% or carbon monoxide poisoning is associated with mental disturbance the optimal treatment is hyperbaric oxygen at 3 atmospheres for 30min, repeated 6hrly if levels remain >25%. Death is likely with carboxyhaemoglobin levels >60%.
- High concentration oxygen treatment should continue until carboxyhaemoglobin levels <10%.

Cyanide

- Severe cyanide poisoning has an extremely rapid onset and occurs in some cases of smoke inhalation. Survival may be associated with anoxic brain damage.
- Diagnosis must be made clinically since a blood cyanide level takes 3h to perform.

Clinical features
Clinical features include anxiety, headache, loss of consciousness and vomiting. The skin remains pink and hypotension may be severe. An unexplained metabolic acidosis is suggestive.

Management
- High concentration oxygen should be given.
- Sodium thiosulphate (150mg/kg intravenously followed by 30–60mg/kg/h) converts cyanide to thiocyanate and should be used if there is unconsciousness. In milder cases rapid, natural detoxification reduces cyanide levels by 50% within 1h allowing supportive therapy only.
- Dicobalt edetate (300mg IV) is the specific antidote to cyanide but is severely toxic in the absence of cyanide. It is therefore best avoided.

See also:
Oxygen therapy, 2; Ventilatory support—indications, 4; Blood gas analysis, 94; ECG monitoring, 102; Blood pressure monitoring, 104; Toxicology, 152; Basic resuscitation, 258; Inhalation injury, 294; Metabolic acidosis, 420; Poisoning—general principles, 438

Household chemicals

Corrosives

Strong acids and alkalis are increasingly available in the household and ingestion may lead to shock and bowel perforation. Gastric elimination techniques must be avoided since aspiration of corrosives may cause severe lung damage. Early surgical repair of perforation may be necessary.

Petroleum

Although not strictly a household chemical, access to petroleum in the home is easy.

Clinical features
Gastrointestinal ingestion and absorption gives clinical features similar to those of alcohol intoxication with more severe central nervous system depression.

Management
- Gastric elimination techniques must be avoided since a few drops of petroleum spilling into the lungs can lead to a severe pneumonitis. This is due to the low surface tension and vapour pressure of petroleum allowing rapid spread through the lungs.
- Treatment involves supportive therapy and 250ml liquid paraffin orally.

Paraquat

Paraquat is widely available as a selective weedkiller which is inactivated on contact with the soil. A dose of 2–3g is usually fatal (equivalent to 80–120g of granules or 10–15ml of industrial liquid concentrate).

Clinical features
- Very little of the ingested paraquat is absorbed from the gut but a large dose will lead rapidly to shock with widespread tissue necrosis.
- A burning sensation in the mouth and abdomen is more common in poisoning, as is the development of painful mouth ulcers and, after several days, a relentless, proliferative alveolitis causing death by pulmonary fibrosis.

Management
- Treatment should begin on clinical grounds in view of the severity of toxicity and the time taken for laboratory confirmation.
- Urgent gastric emptying is required with instillation of 500ml water containing 150g Fuller's earth and 25g magnesium sulphate afterwards.
- Severe diarrhoea may ensue requiring careful fluid management.
- If paraquat poisoning is confirmed 200–500ml of 30% Fuller's earth is given 2hrly for 24h via a nasogastric tube.
- A forced diuresis should be started to encourage renal excretion.
- Pulmonary fibrosis is more severe when breathing high oxygen concentrations; if oxygen is required the lowest concentration possible should be given accepting a low PaO_2. Liposomal superoxide dismutase and glutathione peroxidase have been used experimentally.

See also:
Toxicology, 152; Poisoning—general principles, 438

Methanol and ethylene glycol

Methanol

Toxicity mainly arises due to oxidation of methanol to formic acid and formaldehyde. The oxidative pathway is an enzymatic process involving alcohol dehydrogenase but proceeds at 20% of the rate of ethanol oxidation.

Clinical features
Clinical features of poisoning include blindness (due to concentration of methanol in the vitreous humour), severe metabolic acidosis, headache, nausea, vomiting and abdominal pain.

Management
- Metabolism of methanol is slow so treatment will need to be prolonged (several days).
- Treatment includes gastric emptying (within 4h of ingestion), sodium bicarbonate titrated to correct arterial pH and ethanol to saturate the oxidative pathway.
- On presentation 1ml/kg ethanol (50%) is given orally followed by 0.5ml/kg 2hrly for 5 days.
- If methanol levels are > 1000mg/L haemodialysis is used until levels are < 250mg/L.

Ethylene glycol

Ethylene glycol is partially metabolised to oxalic acid which is responsible for a severe metabolic acidosis, renal failure and seizures.

Clinical features
Clinical suspicion is aroused by odourless drunkenness, oxalate crystals in the urine or blood and the severe acidosis. As little as 50ml can be fatal.

Management
Treatment is as for methanol.

Trauma and Burns

Multiple trauma 1

Such patients are admitted either after surgery or for close observation and medical management. The principles of management are to:
- maintain or quickly restore adequate tissue perfusion and gas exchange
- control pain
- secure haemostasis and correct any coagulopathy
- provide adequate nutrition
- monitor closely and deal promptly with any complications

Circulatory management
- Patients are often cold and vasoconstricted on admission. This serves to camouflage concurrent hypovolaemia and compromise tissue perfusion.
- Adequate monitoring must be instituted at an early stage.
- Development of a persisting tissue oxygen debt has been shown to lead to subsequent multiple organ dysfunction which may not become clinically apparent for 3–7 days. Therefore, adequate perfusion must be restored promptly by repeated fluid challenges. Addition of a vasodilating agent, e.g. glyceryl trinitrate, may be beneficial.
- An increasing metabolic acidosis should prompt suspicion of inadequate resuscitation, covert haemorrhage or tissue necrosis. Myocardial depression or failure may also be implicated.

Respiratory management
- If ventilated, ensure haemodynamic stability, removal of any metabolic acidosis, adequate rewarming and satisfactory gas exchange before attempting to wean. If the patient remains unstable, it is advisable to delay extubation in case urgent surgery is required.
- If spontaneously breathing, give supplemental oxygen to provide adequate arterial oxygenation, encourage deep breathing to prevent atelectasis and secondary infection, and ensure sufficient analgesia albeit not too much to suppress ventilatory drive.

Haematological management
- Maintain haemoglobin >9–10g/dL to assist oxygen transport. Cross-matched blood should be readily available for secondary haemorrhage.
- Correct any coagulopathy with fresh frozen plasma, ± platelets, and, occasionally, other blood products, e.g. cryoprecipitate.

Peripheries
Injury to the limb may result in nerve injuries, obstruction of the vascular supply, or muscle damage which may lead to compartment syndrome and rhabdomyolysis. A high level of suspicion should be held and corrective surgery undertaken promptly if necessary.

See also:
Ventilatory support—indications, 4; Chest drain insertion, 34; Nutrition—use and indications, 70; Blood gas analysis, 94; Blood pressure monitoring, 104; Central venous catheter—use, 108; Central venous catheter—insertion, 110; Full blood count, 144; Coagulation monitoring, 146; Lactate, 160; Colloids, 170; Blood transfusion, 172; Coagulants & antifibrinolytics, 242; Basic resuscitation, 258; Fluid challenge, 262; Pneumothorax, 288; Haemothorax, 290; Hypotension, 300; Anaemia, 386; General acid–base management, 418; Metabolic acidosis, 420; Multiple trauma 2, 460; Head injury 1, 462; Head injury 2, 464; Sepsis / infection, 490; Pain, 496; Rhabdomyolysis, 504

Multiple trauma 2

Analgesia

- Adequate analgesia is imperative to avoid circulatory instability and decreased chest wall excursion, especially following chest, abdominal or spinal trauma.
- Initially, analgesia is usually given IV or IM. Increased use of regional techniques (depending on absence of infection and coagulopathy) and patient-controlled analgesia has facilitated pain relief and weaning.
- Opiates are recommended for initial analgesia. Non-steroidals are particularly effective for bony pain though may occasionally precipitate coagulopathies, stress ulceration and renal failure.
- Agitation may be due to causes other than pain, e.g. infection, intracranial lesion.

Nutrition

Early nutrition has been shown to reduce post-operative complications. This should ideally be enteral, an approach which has been demonstrated as safe even after abdominal laparotomy for trauma.

Infection

- Depending on the site of trauma, the type of wound (open/closed, clean/dirty), and the need for surgery, prophylactic antibiotic cover varying from 3 doses to 1–2 weeks may be needed.
- The trauma patient is at high risk of developing secondary infection, in particular chest, wound sites, intravascular catheter insertion sites and, post-abdominal trauma, intra-abdominal abscesses. Preventive measures and strict infection control should be undertaken.
- Intravascular catheters inserted during emergency resuscitation under non-sterile conditions should be replaced.

Prophylaxis

- Attention should be paid to pressure areas; this may involve the use of specialised mattresses or support beds.
- Clear instructions should be obtained from the surgeon regarding care of the wound and drain sites.
- Especially after orthopaedic procedures on the pelvis and lower limb, or if the patient will remain immobilised, heparin prophylaxis against deep venous thrombosis should be instituted.

Review

- Regular review of the patient is necessary to ensure complications are detected and dealt with promptly. This may require repeat laparotomy, ultrasound or CT scanning.
- Later complications include pancreatitis, acalculous cholecystitis, and multiple organ dysfunction (including ARDS).

Head injury 1

The head may be injured with or without significant trauma to other parts of the body. Priority in management of the multiply injured patient must be placed on securing adequate gas exchange and circulatory resuscitation, and dealing with any life-threatening injury, e.g. an arterial injury, before definitive treatment for head injury.

The patient will usually be admitted to the ICU after CT scanning has identified the extent of injury. The neck should also be imaged by CT, particularly if the patient is ventilated. It is also likely that surgery will have been undertaken for any significant space-occupying lesion or for elevation of a depressed fracture.

General management

- An unstable neck fracture should be assumed until excluded by an expert opinion and appropriate investigations.
- Most head injury patients admitted to non-neurosurgical ICUs will have diffuse or local brain injury for which a non-operative approach has been adopted. The Regional Neurosurgery Centre should be contacted if raised intracranial pressure is present as local policy may encourage early bone flap decompression or referral for invasive monitoring (e.g. intracranial pressure, jugular venous bulb O_2 saturation).
- If a basal skull fracture is suspected (e.g. X-rays, rhinorrhoea, otorrhoea), avoid nasal insertion of feeding or endotracheal tubes.
- Deterioration in conscious level, developing neurological deficits or focal signs (e.g. unilateral pupillary dilatation) should prompt urgent repeat CT scanning for late complications, e.g. subdural haematoma.

Complications

- Actively manage raised intracranial pressure.
- Actively treat seizures with anticonvulsants to prevent further hypoxaemic cerebral damage, reduce cerebral oxygen requirements and ICP. The patient should be loaded with IV phenytoin as prophylaxis against further fits. Consider causes such as hypoglycaemia, development of a new space-occupying lesion and infection.
- Diabetes insipidus suggests hypothalamic injury and carries a poor prognosis. Desmopressin 1–4µg IV should be given daily to maintain urine outputs of 100–150ml/h.

Indications for consideration of intracranial pressure monitoring

1 Indications
- Glasgow coma score $\leqslant 8$ and any abnormality on CT scan
- GCS $\leqslant 8$ and a normal CT scan but any two of the following:
- Age > 40 years
- Hypotension
- Decerebrate posturing
- GCS > 8 but:

Requiring general anaesthesia for treatment of other injuries

Requiring treatment likely to increase ICP, e.g. high levels of PEEP

2 Contraindications
- coagulopathy

3 ICP monitoring should be continued:
- as long as the ICP is elevated
- during active management of ICP
- for up to 3 days in the absence of significant elevation

463

See also:
Ventilatory support—indications, 4; Endotracheal intubation, 28; Intracranial pressure monitoring, 126; Jugular venous bulb saturation, 128; Anticonvulsants, 230; Neuroprotective agents, 232; Generalised seizures, 360; Intracranial haemorrhage, 364; Raised intracranial pressure, 368; Multiple trauma 1, 458; Multiple trauma 2, 460; Head injury 2, 464; Spinal cord injury, 466

Head injury 2

Analgesia

- Adequate analgesia (usually opiates) must be given to the head-injured patient as pain and agitation will increase intracranial pressure, thereby causing a secondary insult.
- Short-acting sedation and muscle relaxation are useful for rapid assessment of the underlying conscious level and any focal neurological deficit.

Respiratory management

- Aggressive hyperventilation is no longer recommended apart from short-term management of raised intracranial pressure. If ventilated, maintain the $PaCO_2$ at 3.5–4kPa.
- Face or neck injuries may have required emergency cricothyroidotomy or tracheostomy to obtain a patent airway. If orotracheally intubated, ensure local swelling has subsided (nasendoscopy, air leak around deflated cuff) before extubation.
- Severe agitation and confusion may last for several weeks; this will often delay weaning and extubation. Judicious sedation, e.g. with chlorpromazine, may be necessary.

Circulatory management

- Hypotension should be avoided with adequate fluid resuscitation ± vasopressor therapy.
- Elevated blood pressures may be tolerated unless excessive.
- β-blockers may be useful in reducing the myocardial effects of excessive catecholamine levels.

Other drug therapy

- Antibiotic prophylaxis is not routinely recommended.
- High-dose steroid therapy has not been shown to be beneficial.
- Trials of neuroprotective agents e.g. free oxygen radical scavengers, are currently in progress. At present, no drug therapy is of proved benefit.

See also:
   Blood pressure monitoring, 104; Hypotensive agents, 190; Opioid analgesics, 222; Anticonvulsants, 230; Antimicrobials, 248; Neuroprotective agents, 232; Fluid challenge, 262; Hypotension, 300; Hypertension, 302; Generalised seizures, 360; Multiple trauma 1, 458; Multiple trauma 2, 460; Head injury 1, 462

Spinal cord injury

Spinal injury, with or without damage to the cord, may be apparent soon after admission to hospital however deterioration may occur, requiring a high index of suspicion and careful monitoring.

Immobilisation

- The spine should be immobilised until a senior surgical / orthopaedic opinion has confirmed that no unstable fracture is present.
- Place a hard cervical collar if a neck fracture is possible. This does not stabilise the spine; either skull traction or operative stabilisation will be needed for an unstable fracture.
- Move the patient by 'log-rolling' or straight-lifting, using at least four staff members. Exercise care with neck manipulation; intubation should be performed by an experienced operator.

Circulatory instability

- So-called 'spinal shock' may occur with marked hypotension due to sympathetic outflow disturbance. Hypovolaemia should be excluded first. Consider damage to other organs / vessels, e.g. spleen, aorta.
- Vasopressor therapy may be necessary if evidence of tissue hypoperfusion persists, e.g. oliguria, metabolic acidosis.
- Postural hypotension and circulatory instability (including symptomatic bradycardia) is commonplace for the first few weeks. Autonomic dysfunction affects 50% of cervical and high thoracic cord injuries.

Respiratory management

- High cervical cord injury above C5 results in loss of diaphragmatic function whereas above C8 can result in loss of intercostal function. This may compromise or prevent breathing and weaning from IPPV.
- When able, the patient should be managed in an upright posture
- Atelectasis is common and requires regular physiotherapy.
- Early tracheostomy may be indicated to facilitate support and comfort.

General measures

- Carefully monitor neurological function to enable early detection of spinal cord compression and referral for urgent remedial surgery.
- Give heparin 5000U bd SC for prophylaxis against thromboembolism.
- The incidence of stress ulceration is high. Ideally, enteral nutrition should be instituted at an early stage though this may prove unsuccessful. Drug therapy, e.g. sucralfate, H_2-blockers may be needed.
- Enteral feeding may be difficult to institute initially as there is a high incidence of gastric distension and paralytic ileus following spinal cord injury. A nasogastric tube should be inserted for gastric decompression. An enterostomy may eventually be required to enable long-term feeding.
- Bowel and bladder function may be deranged. Long-term silastic bladder catheters and regular laxative and enema therapy should be instituted at an early stage.
- Special care is needed to prevent pressure sores.
- Institute regular exercises to prevent contractures.
- Psychological support for patient and family is crucial, particularly if long-term disability is likely.
- High-dose steroid therapy may be beneficial if started within 8h.
- Hyperbaric oxygen therapy is of unproved benefit.
- After spinal injury, muscle relaxants may cause severe hyperkalaemia.

See also:

Burns—fluid management

Major thermal injuries (i.e. > 20% body surface area) are admitted to an intensive care unit, usually specialised in the management of burns, in view of the need for meticulous attention to fluid resuscitation, prevention of infection, and the frequent need for mechanical ventilation.

Monitoring

- The fluid loss from major burns requires careful assessment of intravascular volume status. The traditional markers of fluid resuscitation in burns of central venous pressure, urine output and haematocrit are inadequate.
- Either invasive or non-invasive cardiac output monitoring is needed for accurate titration of fluid. This is particularly applicable in the presence of a hyperdynamic, vasodilated circulation which often commences within 1–2 days. Although infection is not necessarily present, vasopressor therapy may be needed to maintain adequate systemic blood pressures.
- Pulmonary artery and central venous catheters should not be inserted through affected skin areas if at all possible.
- Insertion of intravascular catheters, urinary catheters and nasogastric tubes should be carried out soon after admission as rapid onset swelling within a few hours may make these procedures impossible.

Fluid management

- The extent of injury will have been estimated by the plastic surgeons who will also determine the proportion of full thickness dermal injury. This is used to calculate the degree of fluid resuscitation required.
- Fluid resuscitation in the UK commonly follows the Mount Vernon (albumin-based) formula whereas the Parkland (crystalloid-based) formula is frequently used in the US. Colloids may reduce oedema at non-burn sites and restore blood volume more quickly than crystalloids.
- These formulae only provide an approximate guide and frequently underestimate losses both into the interstitial spaces and through the lost skin barrier. Evaporative losses are approximately 2ml/kg/h. Water losses may be increased if wounds are not covered. Losses increase further with inhalation injury.
- Overzealous fluid infusion should be avoided to minimise oedema.
- The increased permeability and fluid leak phase lasts approximately 1–2 days. After 2–5 days, a diuretic phase usually commences during which time excess tissue fluid is lost and the body swelling reduces.

- Electrolyte levels (in particular potassium and magnesium) can fluctuate widely in both periods and require careful monitoring and replacement as necessary.
- Though some haemolysis may occur, blood transfusion requirements are usually low. However, debridement will result in major blood loss often requiring major transfusion (> 8–10Units). A coagulopathy will occur, in part due to a dilutional effect of massive albumin infusion.

Fluid resuscitation regimen (adapted from Mount Vernon formula)

Note: this regimen should be used as a guide only.

1 Divide first 36h from the time of burn into six consecutive periods of 4, 4, 4, 6, 6 and 12h. For each period give 0.5ml 4.5–5% albumin × body wt [kg] × %burn
2 Give blood as necessary to maintain haemoglobin > 10g/dL.
3 Commence enteral nutrition as soon as possible
4 Give 1.5–2ml/kg/h 5% glucose
5 Reassess cardiorespiratory variables and urine output at frequent intervals to determine whether volume replacement is inadequate or excessive. Adjust fluid input as necessary.

469

See also:
Blood pressure monitoring, 104; Central venous catheter—use, 108; Central venous catheter—insertion, 110; Pulmonary artery catheter—use, 112; Pulmonary artery catheter—insertion, 114; Colloid osmotic pressure, 162; Crystalloids, 166; Colloids, 170; Fluid challenge, 262; Hypotension, 300; Oliguria, 318; Burns—general management, 470

Burns—general management

Surgery

- Escharotomy may be needed on hospital admission to affected limbs, as well as the neck and/or chest if a circumferential burn is present.
- Debridement of necrotic tissue is often begun within the first few days as early grafting is associated with improved outcome. Coverage is obtained using either split skin grafts from the patient's own unaffected skin, donor skin grafts or even experimental 'skin'. Blood loss may be rapid and massive, e.g. 100ml per 1% of body surface grafted.

Wound care

- Early application of dressings and Flamazine (silver sulphadiazine) cream which has anti-bacterial properties against Gram negative bacteria may usefully prevent secondary infection.
- Early grafting often takes place within the first 2–3 days to provide a skin protective barrier.

Nutrition

- Enteral nutrition should be commenced soon after admission as studies have shown that early enteral nutrition improves outcome.
- Target intake is protein of 1g/kg + 2g/%burn and a calorie intake of 20Cal/kg + 50Cal/%burn.

Infection

- Prophylactic antibiotics are often not given to burn patients.
- Body temperature rises on Day 1–2 as high as 40°C, may persist for several days and does not indicate secondary infection.
- Likely infecting agents include streptococci, staphylococci and Gram negative bacteria such as pseudomonas. Appropriate antibiotic treatment should be given as indicated.

Other considerations

- Any suspected inhalation injury should be diagnosed and treated.
- Ensure adequate analgesia (opiates). Ketamine is a useful anaesthetic as it has analgesic properties in addition.
- tetanus toxoid should be given soon after hospital admission.
- Reduce heat & fluid losses by placing the patient on a heated air fluidised bed and by early coverage of burnt skin through application of occlusive dressings and placement of affected limbs in transparent plastic bags.
- Stress ulceration can usually be avoided through prompt resuscitation and early enteral nutrition.
- Pressure sores and contractures should be prevented by careful nursing and physiotherapy.
- Suxamethonium should be avoided from 5–150 days post-burn because of the risk of rapid and severe hyperkalaemia.
- Increasing resistance to non-depolarising muscle relaxants may be seen.

See also:
Enteral nutrition, 72; Infection control, 78; Special support surfaces, 82; Non-opioid analgesics, 224; Opioid analgesics, 222; Muscle relaxants, 228; Antimicrobials, 248; Hyperkalaemia, 406; Burns—fluid management, 468; Sepsis / infection, 490; Pyrexia, 500; Rhabdomyolysis, 504

Electrocution

The effects of electrocution are due to the effects of the current and the conversion of electrical energy to heat energy on passage through the tissues. Important factors are:

- Energy delivered—heat = amperage^2 × resistance × time, i.e. the amperage is the most important determinant of heat production.
- Resistance to current flow—tissues are resistant to current flow in the following decreasing order: bone, fat, tendon, skin, muscle, blood vessels, nerves. A high skin resistance and short duration of contact concentrate the effects locally. However, skin contaminants, moisture and burning reduce resistance.
- Type of current—Alternating current is more dangerous than direct current. Tetanic muscle contractions may prevent the victim from releasing the current source whereas the single, strong muscle contraction with direct current often throws the victim clear. Alternating current is more likely to reach central tissues with consequent sustained apnoea and ventricular fibrillation (with as little as 50–100mA for 1–10msec).
- Current pathway—cardiorespiratory arrest is more likely the closer the contact is with the chest and heart.

Lightening strike differs from contact electrocution in that high intensity, ultra-short duration of current may produce cardiac arrest with little tissue destruction.

Clinical features

- Tachyarrhythmias—including ventricular tachycardia and fibrillation.
- Asystole—more likely with high current (> 10 A).
- Myocardial injury—heat injury, coronary artery spasm, arrhythmias, myocardial spasm.
- Respiratory arrest—tetanic contraction of the diaphragm, arrhythmias, cerebral medullary dysfunction.
- Trauma—tetanic muscle contraction, falling or being thrown clear.
- Burns—to skin and internal tissues

Management

Most severe electrical injuries require urgent field treatment prior to hospital admission.

1 The first priority is to ensure that the source of the electrical injury is not a hazard to rescuers.
2 Management of cardiorespiratory arrest.
3 Prevention of further injury, e.g. spinal protection, removal of smouldering clothes

After hospital admission and restoration of the circulation management is directed towards the complications.

1 Maintain ventilatory support.
2 Management of hypovolaemia associated with burn injury. Fluid requirements are usually greater than for victims of thermal burns and require close monitoring.
3 Check cardiac enzymes for degree of myocardial injury. Treat heart failure and / or arrhythmias as indicated.
4 Management of rhabdomyolysis and covert compartment syndrome.
5 Surgical debridement of necrotic tissue and fixation of bony injury.

See also:
Ventilatory support—indications, 4; Blood pressure monitoring, 104; Opioid analgesics, 222; Antimicrobials, 248; Basic resuscitation, 258; Cardiac arrest, 260; Fluid challenge, 262; Hypotension, 300; Multiple trauma 1, 458; Multiple trauma 2, 460; Multiple trauma 2, 460; Head injury 1, 462; Head injury 2, 464; Burns—fluid management, 468; Burns—general management, 470; Metabolic acidosis, 420; Rhabdomyolysis, 504

Near-drowning

Following near-drowning the major complications are lung injury, hypothermia and the effects of prolonged hypoxia. Although hypothermia bestows protective effects against organ damage, rewarming carries particular hazards.

Pathophysiology

Prolonged immersion usually results in inhalation of fluid however 10–20% of patients develop intense laryngospasm leading to so-called 'dry drowning'. Traditionally, fresh water drowning was considered to lead to rapid absorption of water into the circulation with haemolysis, hypo-osmolality and possible electrolyte disturbance whereas inhalation of hypertonic fluid from sea water drowning produced a marked flux of fluid into the alveoli. In practice, there seems to be little distinction between fresh and sea water as both cause loss of surfactant and severe inflammatory disruption of the alveolar-capillary membrane leading to an ARDS-type picture. Initially, haemodynamic instability is often minor. A similar picture often develops after 'dry drowning' and subsequent endotracheal intubation. Acute hypothermia often accompanies near-drowning with loss of consciousness and haemodynamic alterations.

Management

1 Oxygen—FIO_2 0.6–1should be given, either by face mask if the patient is spontaneously breathing or via mechanical ventilation. Comatose patients should be intubated. Early CPAP or PEEP may be useful.
2 Bronchospasm is often present and may require nebulised β_2 agonists, IV aminophylline and either nebulised or adrenaline.
3 Fluid replacement should be directed by appropriate monitoring. Inotrope therapy may be necessary if hypoperfusion persists after adequate fluid resuscitation. Intravascular fluid overload is uncommon and the role of early diuretic therapy with a view to lowering intracranial pressure is controversial. Haemolysis may require blood transfusion to maintain haemoglobin > 10g/dL.
4 Arrhythmias may arise secondary to myocardial hypoxia, hypothermia and electrolyte abnormalities. These should be treated conventionally.
5 Metabolic acidosis may be profound however sodium bicarbonate therapy is rarely indicated as the acidosis will usually correct on restoration of adequate tissue perfusion.
6 Rewarming follows conventional practice; cardiopulmonary bypass may be considered if core temperature is < 30°C. Resuscitation including cardiac massage should be continued until normothermia is achieved.
7 Cerebral protection usually follows raised intracranial pressure protocols though, as mentioned above, the role of diuretic therapy and fluid restriction is controversial. Signs of brain damage such as seizures may become apparent and should be treated as they arise.
8 Antibiotic therapy (e.g. clindamycin, or cefuroxime plus metronidazole) should be given if strong evidence of aspiration exists. Otherwise, take specimens for culture and treat as indicated.
9 Decompress the stomach using a nasogastric tube to lessen any risk of aspiration. Enteral feeding can be initiated afterwards.

See also:
   Ventilatory support—indications, 4; Positive end expiratory pressure, 20;
Continuous positive airway pressure, 22; Bronchodilators, 176; Antiarrhythmics,
192; Antimicrobials, 248; Adult respiratory distress syndrome 1, 280; Adult
respiratory distress syndrome 2, 282; Metabolic acidosis, 420; Hypothermia, 498

Obstetric Emergencies

Pre-eclampsia & eclampsia

The hallmark of pre-eclampsia is hypertension with proteinuria. It is considered mild if proteinuria is 0.25–2g/L and severe if >2g/L. Eclampsia is the same condition associated with seizures. They are associated with cerebral oedema and, in some cases, haemorrhage. A reduced plasma volume, raised peripheral resistance and disseminated intravascular coagulation all impair tissue perfusion, with possible renal and hepatic failure. Pulmonary oedema may occur secondary to increased peripheral resistance and low colloid osmotic pressure.

Management

Hypertensive crises and convulsions may continue for 48h postpartum, during which time close monitoring in a high dependency or intensive care area is essential.

Circulatory management
- High blood pressure is due to arteriolar vasospasm so controlled plasma volume expansion is essential as the first line treatment.
- A standard fluid challenge regimen may be used in the intensive care area with little risk of fluid overload.
- Oliguria may coexist with reduced plasma volume; controlled plasma volume expansion is usually more appropriate than diuretic therapy.
- If plasma volume expansion fails to control hypertension antihypertensives such as labetalol, nifedipine or hydralazine may be used.

Convulsions
- Convulsions are best avoided by good blood pressure control.
- Initial seizure control may be achieved with small doses of benzodiazepines or chlormethiazole.
- Prophylactic anticonvulsants therapy with phenytoin may be considered in pre-eclampsia.
- Excess sedation should be avoided due to the risk of aspiration although continued seizures may require elective intubation, mechanical hyperventilation and further anticonvulsant therapy.
- Magnesium sulphate is an effective treatment for eclamptic convulsions. Magnesium levels should be monitored and kept between 2.5–3.75mmol/L. Above 3.75mmol/L toxicity with possible cardiorespiratory arrest may be seen.

Early fetal delivery
The definitive treatment for eclampsia is fetal delivery but the needs of the fetus must be balanced against those of the mother. If fetal maturity has been reached immediate delivery after control of seizures and hypertension is necessary.

Drug dosages

Labetalol	start at 2mg/min IV or quicker if a rapid response is required. Labetalol is usually effective once 200mg has been given after which a maintenance infusion of 5–50mg/h may be continued.
Nifedipine	10mg SL is an often effective alternative, given every 20min if necessary.
Hydralazine	5–10mg by slow IV bolus, repeat after 20–30min. Alternatively, by infusion starting at 200–300µg/min and reducing to 50–150µg/min.
Magnesium	4g over 20min followed by 1–1.5g/h by intravenous infusion until seizures have stopped for 24h.

See also:
Ventilatory support—indications, 4; Blood pressure monitoring, 104; Central venous catheter—use, 108; Central venous catheter—insertion, 110; EEG / CFM monitoring, 130; Coagulation monitoring, 146; Colloid osmotic pressure, 162; Colloids, 170; Hypotensive agents, 190; Anticonvulsants, 230; Fluid challenge, 262; Hypertension, 302; Generalised seizures, 360

HELLP syndrome

HELLP syndrome is a pregnancy related disorder associated with haemolysis, elevated liver function tests and low platelets. Criteria used for the diagnosis of HELLP are shown opposite.
- Microangiopathic haemolysis results from destruction of red cells as they pass through damaged small vessels.
- Hepatic dysfunction is characterised by periportal necrosis and hyaline deposits in the sinusoids. In some cases hepatic necrosis may proceed to hepatic haemorrhage or rupture.
- Thrombocytopenia results from increased platelet consumption, although prothrombin time and activated partial thromboplastin time are normal, unlike DIC.

Clinical features
- Epigastric or right upper quadrant pain with malaise.
- Nausea and vomiting.
- Generalised oedema is usual but hypertension is less common. Presentation may occur post-partum.

Management
- Priorities for management include basic resuscitation and exclusion of hepatic haemorrhage or ruptured liver. In the latter case an early Caesarean section and definitive surgical repair are urgent.
- Microangiopathic haemolysis and thrombocytopenia may respond to plasma exchange and fresh frozen plasma infusion.
- Platelet transfusions should be avoided unless there is active bleeding.

Criteria for diagnosis of HELLP syndrome

Haemolysis	Abnormal blood film
	Hyperbilirubinaemia
	LDH $>600U/L$
Elevated liver enzymes	AST $>70U/L$
Thrombocytopenia	Platelets $<100 \times 10^9/L$

See also:
   Plasma exchange, 60; Liver function tests, 142; Full blood count, 144;
Coagulation monitoring, 146; Blood products, 240; Basic resuscitation, 258;
Vomiting / gastric stasis, 326; Haemolysis, 390; Platelet disorders, 392

Post-partum haemorrhage

Usually due to incomplete uterine contraction after delivery but may be due to retained products. The magnitude of haemorrhage may be severe and life- threatening.

Resuscitation

The principles of resuscitation are the same of those applying to any haemorrhagic condition. Blood transfusion requirements may be massive and there may therefore be a need to replace coagulation factors. There may be significant retroplacental bleeding which may lead to underestimation of blood volume loss. It is safer to manage fluid and blood replacement with haemodynamic monitoring.

Aortic compression

Temporary reduction of haemorrhage may be achieved by compressing the aorta with a fist pushed firmly above the umbilicus, using the pressure between the fist and vertebral column to achieve compression. This manoeuvre may buy time while definitive surgical repair is organised.

Stimulated uterine contraction

Prostaglandin F2α injected locally into the uterus or IM is an effective method of stimulating uterine contraction and may avoid the need for surgery.

Arterial occlusion

Angiographic embolisation or internal iliac artery ligation may avoid the need for hysterectomy in some cases. The disadvantages of these procedures include a significant delay in organisation and, in the latter case, the high failure rate.

483

See also:
   Blood pressure monitoring, 104; Central venous catheter—use, 108; Central
venous catheter—insertion, 110; Full blood count, 144; Coagulation monitoring,
146; Blood transfusion, 172

Amniotic fluid embolus

- An uncommon but dangerous complication of childbirth.
- There is a high early mortality associated with acute pulmonary hypertension.
- The initial response of the pulmonary vasculature to the presence of amniotic fluid is intense vasospasm resulting in severe pulmonary hypertension and hypoxaemia.
- Right heart function is initially compromised severely but returns to normal with a secondary phase during which there is severe left heart failure and pulmonary oedema.
- Amniotic fluid contains lipid-rich particulate material which stimulates a systemic inflammatory reaction. In this respect the progress of the condition is similar to other causes of multiple organ failure with associated capillary leak and disseminated intravascular coagulation.
- Diagnosis is supported by amniotic fluid and fetal cells in pulmonary artery blood and urine.

Management

Management is entirely supportive, requiring invasive monitoring with pulmonary artery catheterisation. If amniotic fluid embolism occurs prior to delivery urgent Caesarean section must be performed to prevent further embolisation.

Respiratory support
Oxygen (FIO_2 0.6–1.0) must be provided. In many cases CPAP or mechanical ventilation will be required.

Cardiovascular support
Standard resuscitation principles apply with controlled fluid loading and inotropic support being started as required. Isoprenaline has the advantage of providing pulmonary dilatation.

Haematological management
Management of the coagulopathy requires blood product therapy guided by laboratory assessment of coagulation times. In addition, some cases improve after treatment with cryoprecipitate, possible due to the effects of fibronectin replacement.

See also:
   Ventilatory support—indications, 4; Continuous positive airway pressure, 22;
Pulmonary artery catheter—use, 112; Pulmonary artery catheter—insertion, 114;
Fluid challenge, 262; Pulmonary embolus, 296; Heart failure—assessment, 312;
Heart failure—management, 314; Systemic inflammatory response, 488

Inflammation

Systemic inflammatory response

Exposure to an exogenous insult can result in an exaggerated, generalised and inappropriate inflammatory response. Stimulation of inflammatory pathways leads to activation of macrophages, endothelium, neutrophils, platelets, coagulation, fibrinolytic and contact systems with release of inflammatory mediators and effectors (e.g. cytokines, prostanoids, free oxygen radicals, proteases, nitric oxide, endothelin). This results in microvascular obstruction and occlusion, blood flow redistribution, interstitial oedema and fibrosis, and cellular mitochondrial dysfunction. The consequences of this may be organ dysfunction, varying from 'mild' to severe, and single to multiple organ (i.e. MODS), including cardiovascular collapse, renal failure, disseminated intravascular coagulation and thrombocytopenia. Adult respiratory distress syndrome (ARDS) is the respiratory component of this pathophysiological response.

Causes include:

- Infection
- Trauma, burns
- Pancreatitis
- Inhalation injuries
- Massive blood loss/ transfusion
- Miscellaneous including drug-related (including overdose), myocardial infarction, drowning, hyperthermia, pulmonary embolus

Treatment

Largely supportive though the cause should be removed/treated if at all possible. Treatment includes antibiotics, drainage of pus, fixation of femoral / pelvic fractures and debridement of necrotic tissue.

An important facet of organ support is to minimise iatrogenic trauma. It is sufficient to maintain survival with relative homeostasis until recovery takes place rather than attempting to achieve normal physiological or biochemical target values. An example of this is permissive hypercapnia.

Specific treatment regimens remain contentious and largely based on anecdote. Multicentre studies have to date shown little overall benefit (see Immunotherapy) though it is generally agreed that rapid resucitation and restoration of oxygen delivery, and prompt removal of any treatable cause is desirable in preventing the onset of SIRS.

Because of non-standardisation of definitions, outcome data are conflicting though single organ 'failure' carries a 30–50% mortality rate while $\geqslant 3$ organ 'failures' lasting $\geqslant 3$ days carries a mortality in excess of 80%. Recovery is usually complete in survivors, though, in rare cases, symptomatic renal or respiratory sequelae may persist.

Definitions (AACP/SCCM Guidelines—Crit Care Med 1992; 20: 864–74)

Systemic inflammatory response syndrome (SIRS)
Two or more of:
- Temperature $> 38°C$ or $< 36°C$
- Heart rate > 90 bpm
- Respiratory rate > 20 breaths/min or $PaCO_2 < 32mmHg$ (4.3kPa)
- WBC $> 12\,000$ cells/mm^3, < 4000/mm^3, or $> 10\%$ immature forms

Multi-organ dysfunction syndrome (MODS)
Presence of altered organ function in an acutely ill patient such that homeostasis cannot be maintained without intervention.

Multiple organ failure (MOF) is the extreme of MODS but has not achieved worldwide uniformity of definition.

Current UCL Hospitals principles of management

Respiratory	$SaO_2 > 90$–95% (may have to settle for lower) Permissive hypercapnia
Cardiovascular	Maintain cardiac output/oxygen delivery and blood pressure compatible with adequate organ perfusion (e.g. no metabolic acidosis)
Renal	Maintain adequate metabolic and fluid homeostasis by intravascular filling, diuretics, vasoactive agents, and/or renal replacement techniques
Haematological	Maintain haemoglobin > 9–10g/dl, platelets > 20–40×10^9/L, INR < 1.5–2.5
Gastrointestinal	Stress ulcer treatment (prophylaxis generally by enteral nutrition), observe for pancreatitis and acalculous cholecystitis
Infection	Antibiotics, pus drainage, careful infection control
Nutrition	Preferably early and by enteral route
Pressure area/ mouth/joint care	
Psychological support	To both patient and family

See also:
Ventilatory support—indications, 4; Infection control, 78; Blood pressure monitoring, 104; Bacteriology, 148; Antimicrobials, 248; Adult respiratory distress syndrome 1, 280; Adult respiratory distress syndrome 2, 282; Inhalation injury, 294; Hypotension, 300; Acute myocardial infarction, 300; Abdominal sepsis, 340; Pancreatitis, 342; Multiple trauma 1, 458; Multiple trauma 2, 460; Burns—fluid management, 468; Burns—general management, 470; Poisoning—general principles, 438; Sepsis / infection, 490; Pyrexia, 500

Sepsis / infection

Sepsis is defined as the systemic response to a insult of proven or high likelihood of infection. Whereas infection can be applied to a localised phenomenon, sepsis initiates a systemic inflammatory response thereby affecting distant organs.

Sites of infection before and after admission to an ICU

Organ	Primary site of infection necessitating admission to ICU	Secondary site of infection while in ICU
Brain	Relatively uncommon	Rare
Sinuses	Rare	Relatively uncommon
Cannula sites	Rare	Very common
Chest	Common	Very common
Urine	Relatively uncommon	More common
Abdomen	Common	Uncommon
Bone	Rare	Rare
Heart valves	Relatively uncommon	Relatively uncommon

Treatment

- Drain pus
- Change cannula sites if necessary
- Appropriate antibiotic therapy after laboratory specimens taken.

A high degree of input from microbiological ± infectious disease specialists is recommended to advise on best options for empiric therapy and for possible modifications based on early communication of positive laboratory results (including antibiotic sensitivity patterns).

Empiric antibiotic therapy is guided on the severity of illness of the patient, likely site of infection and likely infecting organism(s), whether the infection is community-acquired or nosocomial (including ICU-acquired), patient immunosuppression, and known antibiotic resistance patterns of hospital and local community organisms. In general, critically ill patients should receive parenteral antibiotics at appropriate dosage, taking into account any impaired hepatic or renal clearance, or concurrent haemofiltration therapy.

The duration of treatment remains highly contentious. Apart from specific conditions such as endocarditis, tuberculosis and meningitis where prolonged therapy is advisable, it may be sufficient to stop within 3–5 days provided the patient has shown adequate signs of recovery. Alternatively, patients not responding or deteriorating should be considered to be either treatment failures or inappropriately treated (i.e. no infection was present in the first place). The presence of pyrexia, neutrophilia, chest X-ray changes, pyuria, purulent sputum and other commonly accepted markers of infection are poorly specific in the intensive care patient. Indeed, a pyrexia may settle on stopping antibiotic treatment. Anecdotally, we find a falling platelet count to be a good marker of sepsis while a rise in levels is seen during recovery. Cessation or change of antibiotic therapy must be considered on individual merits according to the patient's condition and any subsequent laboratory results. An advantage of ceasing therapy is the ability to take further specimens for culture in an antibiotic-free environment.

Definitions (AACP/SCCM Guidelines—Crit Care Med 1992; 20: 864–74)

Infection
Microbial phenomenon characterised by an inflammatory response to the presence of micro-organisms or the invasion of normally sterile host tissue by those organisms

Bacteraemia
The presence of viable bacteria in the blood.

Sepsis
The systemic response to infection. Definition as for SIRS but as a result of infection.

Severe sepsis
Sepsis associated with organ dysfunction, hypoperfusion or hypotension. These may include, but are not limited to, lactic acidosis, oliguria or an acute alteration in mental status.

Septic shock
Sepsis with hypotension, despite adequate fluid resuscitation, plus presence of perfusion abnormalities.

Specimen antibiotic regimens (organism unknown)

Sepsis of unknown origin	Quinolone OR 2nd/3rd generation cephalosporin OR carbapenem + aminoglycoside + metronidazole
Pneumonia—community acquired	2nd/3rd generation cephalosporin + erythromycin
Pneumonia—nosocomial	Quinolone OR 3rd generation cephalosporin OR carbapenem ± teicoplanin, vancomycin or gentamicin
Abdominal	Quinolone OR 2nd/3rd generation cephalosporin OR carbapenem ± aminoglycoside + metronidazole
Gynaecological	Quinolone OR 2nd/3rd generation cephalosporin OR carbapenem ± aminoglycoside + metronidazole
Nephro-urological	Quinolone OR 2nd/3rd generation cephalosporin OR carbapenem ± aminoglycoside
Meningitis	Cefotaxime

491

See also:
Infection control, 70; Blood pressure monitoring, 104; Bacteriology, 148; Antimicrobials, 248; Acute chest infection 1, 276; Acute chest infection 2, 278; Hypotension, 300; Abdominal sepsis, 340; Meningitis, 362; Systemic inflammatory response, 488; Pyrexia, 500

Anaphylactoid reactions

Minor reactions to allergens (itching, urticaria) are common before a severe reaction occurs; any such history should be taken seriously and potential allergens avoided. Most reactions are acute in onset and clearly related to the causative allergen. However, some complement mediated reactions may take longer to develop.

Clinical features

- Respiratory—laryngeal oedema, bronchospasm, pulmonary oedema, pulmonary hypertension
- Cardiovascular—hypotension, tachycardia, generalised oedema
- Other—urticaria, angio-oedema, abdominal cramps, rigors

Management

1 Stop all infusions and blood transfusions and withhold any potential drug or food allergen. Blood and blood products should be returned to the laboratory for analysis.
2 Start oxygen (FIO_2 0.6–1.0). If there is evidence of persistent hypoxaemia consider urgent intubation and mechanical ventilation.
3 If there is laryngeal obstruction, bronchospasm or facial oedema give IM or nebulised adrenaline and IV hydrocortisone. If there is not rapid relief of airway obstruction, consider urgent intubation or, in extremis, emergency cricothyroidotomy or tracheostomy. Persistent bronchospasm may require an adrenaline infusion, aminophylline infusion or assisted expiration (manual chest compression).
4 Hypotension should be treated with adrenaline IV/IM and rapid colloid infusion. Large volumes of colloid may be required to replace the plasma volume deficit in severe anaphylaxis.
   - Severe oedema may coexist with hypovolaemia.
   - Plasma volume has not been adequately replaced if the haemoglobin is higher than normal.
   - Hetastarch is the most appropriate fluid for colloid resuscitation unless the reaction is due to a hydroxyethyl starch.
5 Persistent hypotension should be treated with further adrenaline, hydrocortisone and colloid infusion guided by central venous pressure ± pulmonary artery catheter monitoring. An adrenaline infusion may be required to overcome myocardial depression. The use of military anti-shock trousers or noradrenaline should be considered to divert blood centrally and increase peripheral resistance.
6 Urticaria requires chlorpheniramine IV or PO depending on the severity of the reaction.
7 After control of the anaphylactoid reaction advice should be sought from the immunology laboratory and appropriate samples taken for confirmation.
8 Reactions to long-acting drugs or fluids will require continued support (perhaps for many hours).

Drug dosages

Laryngeal oedema and bronchospasm

	Initial dose	*Continued treatment*
Adrenaline	0.3–0.5mg IM or 0.5mg nebulised	start at 0.05µg/kg/min
Hydrocortisone	200mg IV	
Aminophylline	6mg/kg IV over 15min	0.5mg/kg/h adjusted according to levels

Hypotension

	Initial dose	*Continued treatment*
Adrenaline	0.5–1.0mg IM or 0.05–0.2mg IV	start at 0.05µg/kg/min
Hetastarch 6%	500ml	according to response
Hydrocortisone	200mg IV	200mg IV qds
Chlorpheniramine		10mg IV tds

Urticaria

Chlorpheniramine	10mg IV tds or 4mg PO tds
Hydrocortisone	50–100mg IV tds
Prednisolone	20mg PO daily

493

See also:
Ventilatory support—indications, 4; Endotracheal intubation, 28; Tracheostomy, 30; Central venous catheter—use, 108; Central venous catheter—insertion, 110; Colloids, 170; Blood transfusion, 172; Inotropes, 184; Blood products, 240; Steroids, 250; Basic resuscitation, 258; Fluid challenge, 262

Miscellaneous Disorders

Pain

Pain results from many insults, e.g. trauma, invasive procedures, specific organ disease and inflammatory processes. Pain relief is necessary for physiological and psychological reasons:

- Anxiety and lack of sleep
- Increased sympathetic activity contributing to an increased metabolic demand.
- The capacity of the circulation and respiratory system to meet the demands of metabolising tissues may not be adequate.
- Myocardial ischaemia is a significant risk.
- The endocrine response to injury is exaggerated with consequent salt and water retention.
- Physiological attempts to limit pain may include immobility and muscle splinting and consequent reductions in ventilatory function and cough.

Pain perception

The degree of tissue damage is related to the magnitude of the pain stimulus. The site of injury is also important; thoracic and upper abdominal injury is more painful than injury elsewhere. However, the perception of pain is dependent on other factors, e.g. simultaneous sensory input, personality, cultural background and previous experiences of pain.

Management of pain

Systemic analgesia

- Opioid analgesics form the mainstay of analgesic drug treatment in intensive care.
- Small, frequent IV doses or a continuous infusion provide the most stable blood levels. Since the degree of analgesia is dependent on blood levels it is important that they are maintained.
- Higher doses are required to treat rather than prevent pain.
- The dose of drug required for a particular individual depends on their perception of pain and whether tolerance has built up to previous analgesic use.
- The use of non-opioid drugs may avoid the need for or reduce the dose required of opioid drugs.

Regional analgesia

- Regional techniques reduce respiratory depression but require experience to ensure procedures are performed safely.
- Epidural analgesia may be achieved with local anaesthetic agents or opioids.
- Opioids avoid the vasodilatation and hypotension associated with local anaesthetic agents but do not produce as profound analgesia.
- The combination of opioid and local anaesthetic is synergistic.
- Intravenous opioids should be avoided or close monitoring should continue for 24h after cessation of epidural opioids due to the potential for late respiratory failure.
- Local anaesthetic agents may be used to block superficial nerves, e.g. intercostal nerve block with 3–5ml 0.5% bupivicaine plus adrenaline.

Non-pharmacological techniques

Adequate explanation, positioning and physical techniques may all reduce drug requirements.

Regimens for epidural analgesia

Lumbar LA	10–15ml 0.5% bupivicaine followed by an infusion of 5–20ml/h 0.125% bupivicaine
Thoracic LA	4–6ml 0.5% bupivicaine followed by an infusion of 6–10ml/h 0.125% bupivicaine
Opioid	5mg morphine gives up to 12h analgesia
Combined	An infusion of 3–4ml/h 0.125% bupivicaine with 0.3–0.4mg/h morphine or 25–50µg/h fentanyl

See also:

Opioid analgesics, 222; Non-opioid analgesics, 224; Multiple trauma 1, 458; Multiple trauma 2, 460; Head injury 1, 462; Head injury 2, 464; Burns—general management, 470; Post-operative intensive care, 510

Hypothermia

Clinical features

- Above 33°C—shivering is usually marked in an attempt to correct body temperature.
- Below 33°C—neurological signs of dysarthria and slowness appear.
- Below 31°C—hypertonicity and sluggish reflexes with cardiovascular dysfunction become life threatening.
- Below 28°C—arterial pulses often become impalpable . Hypothermic rigidity is difficult to distinguish from death.
- Prognosis depends on the degree and duration of hypothermia.

ECG changes

Sinus bradycardia is followed by atrial flutter and fibrillation with ventricular ectopics. The PR interval, QRS complex and QT interval are prolonged. Atrial activity eventually ceases. The 'J' wave is most often seen < 31°C and ventricular fibrillation is common < 30°C giving way to asystole < 28°C.

Complications

Hypoxaemia is common due to hypoventilation and ventilation perfusion mismatch. Hypovolaemia and metabolic acidosis are common. Renal tubular damage may result from renal blood flow reduction. Acute pancreatitis, rhabdomyolysis and gastric erosions are common.

Management

1 Oxygen (FIO$_2$ 0.6–1.0).
2 Fluid replacement with careful monitoring.
3 Rewarming—All hypothermic patients with no evidence of other fatal disease should be assumed fully recoverable. In the event of cardiac arrest full resuscitation should continue until the patient is normothermic (ventricular fibrillation is resistant to defibrillation between 28–30°C). The technique used for rewarming depends on the core temperature (measured with a low reading rectal thermometer and the clinical circumstance.

Rapid central rewarming
In cases where the temperature is < 28°C (< 33°C with acute exposure hypothermia), or where there is cardiac arrest, rapid rewarming may be achieved by peritoneal dialysis, gastric or bladder lavage with warmed fluids. These techniques may achieve rewarming rates of 1–5°C/h. Active surface rewarming with a heated blanket can achieve rates of 1–7°C/h and is less invasive. Haemodynamic changes may be dramatic during active rewarming requiring careful monitoring and support. If extracorporeal rewarming is available rates of 3–15°C/h may be achieved with the addition of cardiovascular support.

Spontaneous rewarming
Spontaneous rewarming proceeds at a rate inversely proportional to the duration of hypothermia. With good insulation (space blanket) rewarming rates of 0.1–0.7°C/h can be achieved. Core temperature may fall during spontaneous rewarming as cold blood is returned from the periphery to the central circulation.

Causes of hypothermia

- Coma and immobility
- Cold water immersion
- Exposure
- Hypothyroidism,
- Hypopituitarism
- Sepsis
- Erythroderma

See also:

Pyrexia

Causes

Infection
The commonest cause in the ICU patient, though probably over diagnosed. Main sites are chest and intravascular cannula sites. Urinary tract infections are difficult to diagnose in the presence of a urethral catheter. Similarly, the respiratory tract is routinely colonised with bacteria within a few days of ICU admission; differentiation between colonising and pathogenic bacteria is difficult. Seek malaria in patients having visited endemic areas. Antibiotic therapy may itself be a cause of pyrexia.

Inflammation
Inflammation unrelated to infection will usually generate a pyrexic response, e.g. systemic inflammatory response syndrome, post-cardiac surgery, post-burns, post-myocardial infarction, vasculitis, glomerulonephritis, hepatitis, acalculous cholecystitis. Other than specific therapy, e.g. immnosuppression for vasculitis, management is generally symptom-orientated to include cooling.

Adverse drug reaction
Numerous drugs may induce an idiosyncratic pyrexia, including antibiotics, sedative and paralysing agents, and amphetamines. Usually removal of the offending drug is sufficient but, occasionally, more active measures have to be taken, including active cooling and dantrolene.

Ambient heating
Excessive heating or prevention of heat loss may result in pyrexia. Attention should be paid to strong sunlight, excess temperature control settings on specialised beds or mattresses, and heat-retaining bed clothing.

Miscellaneous
Miscellaneous causes of pyrexia include neoplasm and post-cerebral insult

Principles of management

1 Cooling aids symptomatic recovery, reduces metabolic rate and lowers pressor requirements.
   - Increase evaporative losses, e.g. tepid sponging, wet sheets, ice packs
   - Increase convective losses, e.g. fanning to improve air circulation
   - Antipyretics e.g. paracetamol, aspirin, chlorpromazine
   - More aggressive cooling if temperature > 40°C
2 For suspected infection:
   - Clinical examination, seeking localising signs.
   - Further investigations as appropriate: (i) microbiological, e.g. blood, sputum, wound sites, (ii) haematological, e.g. neutrophilia, platelet count, (iii) radiological, e.g. chest X-ray, abdominal ultrasound, CT
   - Specific treatments, e.g. change catheters, drain pus.
   - Commence or alter antibiotic therapy if patient is symptomatic and new infection suspected or patient not responding to current regimen. Modify in light of patient response and laboratory results.

See also:
   Bacteriology, 148; Virology, serology & assays, 150; Blood transfusion, 172;
Antimicrobials, 248; Acute chest infection 1, 276; Acute chest infection 2, 278;
Acute myocardial infarction, 308; Abdominal sepsis, 340; Burns—general
management, 470; Sepsis / infection, 490; Hyperthermia, 502; Post-operative
intensive care, 510; Vasculitides, 508; Malaria, 514

Hyperthermia

Hyperthermia is defined as a core temperature above 41°C.

Clinical features

- Delirium and seizures are associated with temperatures of 40–42°C
- Coma is associated with temperatures above 42°C.
- Tachycardia
- Tachypnoea
- Salt water depletion
- Rhabdomyolysis
- Disseminated intravascular coagulation
- Heart failure with ST depression and 'T' wave flattening.

Causes

- Hyperthermia may be an extreme form of pyrogen induced fever associated with infection, inflammation, neoplasm or cerebro-vascular accident.
- Heat stroke is associated with severe exercise in high environmental temperatures and humidity. there may be excess clothing or hypo-volaemia reducing the body's ability to dissipate heat production.
- Malignant hyperthermia is a drug induced myopathy associated with a hereditary calcium transfer defect in patients receiving volatile anaesthetics, muscle relaxants, antidepressants, alcohol or Ecstasy. Heat production is increased by muscle catabolism, spasm and peripheral vasoconstriction.
- The neuroleptic malignant syndrome is a drug induced hyperther-mic syndrome secondary to phenothiazines or butyrophenones. It is associated with muscle rigidity, akinesia, impaired consciousness and autonomic dysfunction and continues for 1–2 weeks.

Management

1 Rapid cooling should be instituted for patients with temperatures >41°C.
2 Supportive treatment includes fluid replacement and seizure con-trol.
3 Clothing should be removed and patients should be nursed in a cool environment.
4 Surface cooling may be achieved with a fan, tepid sponging, wet sheets, ice packs or a cool bath.
5 Handling should be minimised and active cooling measures should be stopped when the core temperature is <39°C.
6 Internal cooling may be considered by gastric lavage or peritoneal lavage using cooled fluids.
7 Phenothiazines may be used to reduce temperature and prevent shivering (not in neuroleptic malignant syndrome)
8 Muscle relaxants should be used if the patient is ventilated.
9 For malignant hyperthermia the offending drug should be stopped and dantrolene 1mg/kg given IV every 5min to a max-imum dose of 10mg/kg.
10 Mechanical ventilation with high FiO_2 and treatment of hyper-kalaemia are required.
11 The neuroleptic malignant syndrome is treated by stopping the offending drug, giving dantrolene as above and dopamine ago-nists (e.g. L-dopa or bromocriptine).

Rhabdomyolysis

Breakdown of striated muscle which may result in compartment syndrome, acute renal failure and electrolyte abnormalities (hyperkalaemia, hypocalcaemia, hyperphosphataemia).

Causes
- Trauma, especially crush injury
- Prolonged immobilisation, e.g. after fall, drug overdose
- Drugs, e.g. opiates, Ecstasy
- Hyperpyrexia
- Vascular occlusion (including lengthy vascular surgery)
- Infection
- Burns/electrocution
- Congenital myopathy (rare)

Diagnosis
- Suggested by disproportionately high serum creatinine compared to urea (usual ratio is approximately 10:1)
- Raised creatine kinase (usually $> 2000IU/L$)
- Myoglobinuria (this produces a positive urine dipstick to blood; laboratory analysis is required to confirm myoglobin rather than blood or haemoglobin. The urine is usually red or black but may appear clear despite significant rhabdomyolysis.

General management
- Prompt fluid resuscitation
- Hypocalcaemia should not be treated unless the patient is symptomatic; administered calcium may form crystals with the high circulating phosphate
- Hyperkalaemia may be resistant to medical management and require urgent haemodialysis or haemodiafiltration.

Compartment syndrome
- Suspect if limb is tender or painful and peripheries are cool. Loss of peripheral pulses and tense muscles are late signs
- Manometry (muscle compartments pressures > 20–$25mmHg$).
- Arm, legs and buttock compartments may be affected.
- Management involves either prophylactic fasciotomies if at high risk or close monitoring (including regular manometry) with decompression if pressures exceed 20–$25mmHg$.
- Fasciotomies may result in major blood loss.

Renal failure
- Renal failure is produced by a combination of hypovolaemia, hypotension and myoglobin blocking the renal tubules.
- Renal failure may be prevented by prompt rehydration and a forced alkaline diuresis with 0.9% saline 6–10L/day for 3–5 days, aiming to produce an equivalent amount of urine. The urinary pH should be maintained $\geqslant 6$ and blood pH < 7.5 using up to 500ml/h 1.24% sodium bicarbonate solution to increase urinary excretion of myoglobin. Frusemide and/or mannitol may be needed to avoid fluid overload and potassium, sodium, calcium and magnesium levels regularly monitored and managed as appropriate.
- If renal failure is established, dialysis or filtration techniques will be required, usually for a period of 6–8 weeks.

Rheumatic disorders

Rheumatoid arthritis

A debilitating arthritis that may present to intensive care through pulmonary involvement or through complications of treatment (e.g. renal failure, immunosuppression, bleeding disorders). Pleuro-pulmonary involvement may precede the arthritic symptoms and is more common in those with active rheumatoid disease and middle aged men. Care is required when intubating patients with rheumatoid arthritis since the neck joints may sublux.

Rheumatoid pleurisy
Rheumatoid pleurisy, often with effusion, is most common and is usually asymptomatic. However, effusions may be recurrent or chronic and may impede respiratory function. The effusion is an exudate, low in glucose and often high in cholesterol.

Rheumatoid lung
Rheumatoid lung is a diffuse interstitial pneumonitis with bi-basal fibrotic changes on the chest X-ray. The condition may be difficult to distinguish from idiopathic pulmonary fibrosis and produces a restrictive pulmonary defect. The mainstay of treatment is early systemic steroid therapy, although chronic cases do not respond.

Systemic lupus erythematosis (SLE)

A non-organ specific autoimmune disease characterised by anti-nuclear antibodies with high titres of anti-double stranded DNA antibodies. A vasculitis is prominent although cutaneous and central nervous system involvement are not vasculitic. SLE may present to intensive care through pulmonary, renal or central nervous system involvement.

Renal failure
Renal failure is vasculitic in origin and may progress to end stage renal failure requiring long term dialysis. Early treatment with systemic steroids and immunosuppressives may halt the disease progress.

Lupus pleurisy and pericarditis
Unlike rheumatoid pleurisy the pleural involvement in SLE is often painful and associated with large pleural effusions.

Pulmonary haemorrhage
Pulmonary haemorrhage is associated with renal failure and may be life threatening. Plasma exchange may be helpful.

Interstitial pneumonitis
Interstitial pneumonitis is uncommon in SLE. It is more likely that parenchymal infiltrates are infective in origin secondary to immuno-suppressive therapy.

Pulmonary thromboembolic disease
Patients typically have a prolonged activated partial thromboplastin time due to circulating lupus anticoagulant. but are more prone to thrombotic episodes. Lupus anticoagulant is associated with antic-ardiolipin antibodies and a false positive VDRL. Recurrent pulmon-ary emboli may be associated with chronic pulmonary hypertension. Treatment is long term anticoagulation.

See also:

Vasculitides

Vasculitis should be suspected in any patient with multi-system disease especially involving the lungs and kidneys.

Wegener's granulomatosis

A systemic vasculitis characterised by necrotising granulomas of the upper and lower respiratory tract, glomerulonephritis and small vessel vasculitis. Wegener's granulomatosis is associated with positive core antineutrophil cytoplasmic antibodies (c-ANCA), particularly granular with central attenuation on immunofluorescence. Intensive care admission is usually through renal and pulmonary involvement.

Renal failure
Focal necrotising glomerulonephritis leads to progressive renal failure. Treatment with steroids and cyclophosphamide may give complete remission.

Upper airway disease
Most patients will have nasal symptoms including epistaxis, nasal discharge and septal perforation. Intensive care admission may be required rarely for severe epistaxis. Ulcerating lesions of the larynx and trachea may cause subglottic stenosis. This is usually insidious but may present problems on attempted intubation.

Pulmonary involvement
Usually associated with haemoptysis, dyspnoea and cough with rounded opacities on the chest X-ray. There may be cavitation. Nodules may be solitary. Alveolar haemorrhage may be life threatening. The mainstay of treatment is steroids and cyclophosphamide which may produce complete remission. Plasma exchange may be helpful.

Polyarteritis nodosa (PAN)

PAN is a necrotising vasculitis affecting small and medium sized muscular arteries. Intensive care admission may be provoked by renal failure, ischaemic heart disease, hypertensive crisis and bronchospasm although true pulmonary involvement is uncommon. Diagnosis may be confirmed by mesenteric angiography or renal biopsy. Treatment involves renal replacement therapy, high dose steroids and cyclophosphamide.

Goodpasture's syndrome

Anti-glomerular basement membrane (anti-GBM) antibodies bind at the glomerulus and alveolus. Patients present with a proliferative glomerulonephritis and haemoptysis. Diagnosis is confirmed by positive anti-GBM antibodies and renal biopsy. Treatment is with immunosuppressive therapy and plasma exchange.

See also:
Plasma exchange, 60; Airway obstruction, 268; Steroids, 250; Haemoptysis, 292; Acute renal failure—diagnosis, 320; Acute renal failure—management, 322; Rheumatic disorders, 506

Post-operative intensive care

Patients may be admitted to the ICU after surgery, either electively (table opposite) or after unexpected peri-operative complications.

General care
- Ensure surgical and anaesthetic plan has been agreed, e.g. overnight ventilation, special precautions (wire cutters if mandible wired, patient movement, haemodynamic targets).
- Provide adequate analgesia.
- Ensure adequate rewarming (may require vasodilators).
- Provide appropriate thrombosis prophylaxis.
- Blood gas, electrolyte and haemoglobin monitoring.

Post-operative respiratory problems
Most common in those with pre-existing respiratory disease, especially those associated with a reduced vital capacity or peak expiratory flow rate. Problems include:
- Exacerbation of chronic bronchitis
- Retained secretions
- Basal atelectasis
- Pneumonia

Anaesthesia and surgery (especially upper abdominal surgery) reduce functional residual capacity , thoracic compliance and cough. There is also reduced macrophage function and systemic inflammatory activation with infection and acute lung injury as consequences.

Therapeutic aims
Pre-operative preparation may help avoid some of the problems:
- Cessation of smoking for > 1 week
- Bronchodilatation
- Respiratory muscle training
- Chest physiotherapy
- Avoidance of hypovolaemia in the nil-by-mouth period

Post-operatively, the clearance of secretions and maintenance of basal expansion are very important. These require the provision of effective analgesia and chest physiotherapy ± intermittent positive pressure breathing (in the co-operative patient). Post-operative mechanical ventilation ensures basal expansion and secretion clearance where anaesthetic recovery is expected to be prolonged or surgery ± pre-existing disease increase the risk of secretion retention and atelectasis.

Post-operative circulatory problems
- Prevention of hypovolaemia is crucial in avoiding inflammatory activation and, therefore, many post-operative complications.
- Haemorrhage is usually obvious and managed by resuscitation, correction of coagulation disturbance and surgery.
- Sub-clinical hypovolaemia is common after anaesthesia and surgery. Hypothermia and high catecholamine levels help to maintain central venous pressure and blood pressure despite continuing hypovolaemia. Avoidance of reductions in stroke volume or tissue acidosis are the best indicators of adequate resuscitation.
- Post-operative fluid management requires a high degree of suspicion of hypovolaemia; fluid challenges with colloid should be used to confirm and treat hypovolaemia where there is any circulatory disturbance, metabolic acidosis or oliguria.

Reasons for elective ICU admission

- Airway monitoring: e.g. major oral, head and neck surgery
- Respiratory monitoring: e.g. cardiothoracic surgery, upper abdominal surgery, prolonged anaesthesia, previous respiratory disease
- Cardiovascular monitoring: e.g. cardiac surgery, vascular surgery, major abdominal surgery, prolonged anaesthesia, previous cardiovascular disease
- Neurological monitoring: e.g. neurosurgery, cardiac surgery with circulatory arrest,
- Elective ventilation: e.g. cardiac surgery, major abdominal surgery, prolonged anaesthesia, previous respiratory or cardiac disease

See also:

HIV related disease

Patients with HIV related diseases may present to intensive care electively after surgical procedures, particularly diagnostic biopsies of brain or lung, but also in all circumstances where elective ventilation would be offered after major surgical procedures. Other cases present with complications of HIV related disease, especially pulmonary infection (e.g. *Pneumocystis carinii*, CMV) or seizures (e.g. cerebral lymphoma, cerebral abscess, meningitis). HIV related diseases are now considered to be chronic manageable conditions with an often good short-term prognosis. It is therefore reasonable that intensive care facilities should be offered.

Infection control

The protection of staff from transmission of HIV follows basic measures. Body fluids should not be handled (wear gloves) and the face and eyes should be protected where there is a risk of splash contamination.

Needles should be disposed of in appropriate burn bins without re-sheathing and any fluid spillages should be cleaned up immediately. Robust procedures are usually adhered to where a patient is known to be HIV positive; the real risk is in the patient of unknown HIV status. It should be remembered that patients presenting to intensive care with non-HIV related illness may be unknown positives. It follows therefore that precautions should be taken for all patients.

Pneumocystis carinii pneumonia

- This is the commonest respiratory disorder affecting HIV positive patients. The majority survive their first attack but prognosis is not as good in those requiring mechanical ventilation. Intensive, early support with CPAP and appropriate chemotherapy may avert the need for ventilatory support.
- Diagnosis is usually made clinically without waiting for laboratory confirmation.
- First line drug treatment is with high dose co-trimoxazole or pentamidine with adjuvant high dose steroids. Co-trimoxazole has advantages over pentamidine since its onset of effect is quicker and it has a broader spectrum of antibacterial activity covering the common secondary pathogens. Pentamidine is usually used where co-trimoxazole fails or where patients cannot take co-trimoxazole.
- Methylprednisolone is used to suppress peribronchial fibrosis and alveolar infiltrate. It is usual for there to be an initial deterioration on treatment lasting several days.
- Respiratory support is provided with CPAP (5–10cmH$_2$O) or BiPAP if hypoxaemic despite high FIO$_2$. Lower CPAP pressures should be used where possible since patients with *Pneumocystis carinii* pneumonia have a considerable risk of pneumothorax.
- Mechanical ventilation is reserved for those who have a rising with deteriorating gas exchange and fatigue despite CPAP or BiPAP.
- Chest X-ray changes respond very slowly.

512 IV drug abusers

As a group, IV drug abusers are at high risk for HIV related disease. However, they tend to present to intensive care more commonly as a result of the drug abuse (e.g. drug withdrawal syndromes, overdose, sepsis, endocarditis, hepatitis B or C, rhabdomyolysis).

Drug Dosages

Co-trimoxazole	120mg/kg/day in divided doses IV for 10–14 days then PO to complete 21 days
Pentamidine	4mg/kg/day IV
Methylprednisolone	1g/day for 3 days

See also:
Ventilatory support—indications, 4; Endotracheal intubation, 28; Continuous positive airway pressure, 22; Infection control, 78; Bacteriology, 148; Virology, serology & assays, 150; Antimicrobials, 248; Steroids, 250; Acute chest infection 1, 276; Acute chest infection 2, 278; Pneumothorax, 288

Malaria

Malaria should be suspected in any patient returning from endemic areas with a febrile illness which may have cerebral, abdominal, lung or renal features. Rarely, people living near airports may be bitten by a transported Anopheles mosquito. There may be considerable delay (weeks to months) between the mosquito bite and signs of infection. It is caused by protozoal infection with the Plasmodium genus. The most severe form is *P. falciparum* which causes malignant, tertian malaria. Other forms (*P. malariae, P. vivax, P. ovale*) rarely cause significant life-threatening disease and will not be discussed further.

Pathophysiology

P. falciparum invades erythrocytes regardless of age. High levels of parasitaemia > 5% are considered severe in non-immune travellers. The cells may haemolyse or be destroyed in liver or spleen. Anaemia may be severe. Increased vascular permeability, cytokine release, red cell agglutination and intravascular coagulation (DIC) may occur.

Clinical features

- Symptoms include headache, fever with rigors, myalgia, abdominal pain, vomiting and diarrhoea. Signs include splenomegaly, jaundice, tender hepatomegaly and anaemia. Low $[Na^+]$ is common.
- Only a minority of patients with *P. falciparum* have paroxysms of fever with 'cold' and 'hot' stages.

If > 5% parasitaemia, features include:

- Cerebral malaria, causing coma, delirium, seizures or focal deficits.
- Cough and haemoptysis or acute respiratory distress
- Blackwater fever is associated with massive intravascular haemolysis, jaundice, haemoglobinuria, collapse, and acute renal failure
- Acute renal dysfunction occurs in a third of adult patients
- Acute cardiovascular collapse ('algid malaria') and metabolic acidosis
- Thrombocytopenia, DIC and spontaneous bleeding

Diagnosis

- Plasmodia seen in RBC in thick or thin smears of peripheral blood. The parasitaemia intensity may vary from hour to hour and may be scanty in number. The smear should be carefully scrutinised and repeated if doubt persists.
- Leucocytosis is not a feature of malaria
- Splenomegaly is almost invariable during the second week of illness

Treatment

1 Early IV quinine infusion is the mainstay of treatment of severe malaria. Levels should be monitored daily and dosage adjusted as appropriate. Complications include hypoglycaemia and tinnitus.
2 A 2–3Litre exchange transfusion should be considered if the patient is severely ill or if parasitaemia levels > 10%.
3 Careful attention must be paid to fluid and electrolyte balance, prevention of fluid overload, and management of renal failure.
4 Treatment of hypoglycaemia, renal failure, coagulopathy, metabolic acidosis, seizures, ARDS, anaemia and hyperpyrexia follow conventional lines
5 Steroids are not recommended for cerebral oedema.
6 Suspect coincident Gram negative infection if stocked.

Drug dosage

Quinine	20mg quinine salt/kg IV over 4h, then 10mg/kg infusion over 4h, repeated 8hrly until the patient can swallow, then tablets (10mg quinine salt/kg 8hrly) to complete 7 days' treatment. Halve maintenance dose to 5mg salt/kg 8hrly if continuing parenteral therapy for >48h.
Tetracycline	Add 250mg qds PO if malaria acquired in quinine-resistant area, e.g. Thailand

See also:

Brainstem death

The correct diagnosis of brainstem death is a medical emergency since it allows discontinuation of pointless ventilation and retrieval of organs for donation. The diagnosis of brainstem death is usually followed by asystole within a few days. There are a number of requirements before brainstem function testing can be performed to confirm the diagnosis. The patient must have an underlying diagnosis that is compatible with brainstem death. Patients must have been in a coma for at least 6h and there should be a minimum of 2h following a cardiac arrest. There must be no hypothermia (temperature > 35°C) and there must be no evidence or suspicion of depressant drugs, urea, electrolyte or glucose abnormality or muscle relaxant effect. The performance of brain stem death tests should not proceed until relatives and all medical and nursing staff involved with the patient have had a chance to take part in discussions although the test itself does not require consent. Cessation of mechanical ventilation is seen by many lay people as the final point of death. Clearly, this final step is easier if all are aware that it is to happen. If organ donation is considered, the transplant coordinator should be involved early.

Brain stem death testing

Procedures vary internationally. In the UK clinical assessment of brain stem reflexes must be performed by 2 doctors who have been registered for > 5 years. In addition an EEG is commonly required in other countries.

Pupillary light reflex
Pupils should appear fixed in size and fail to respond to a light stimulus.

Corneal reflexes
These should be absent bilaterally

Pain response
There should be no cranial response to supraorbital pain.

Vestibulo-ocular reflexes
After confirming that the tympanic membranes are clear and unobstructed 20ml iced water is syringed into the ear. The eyes would normally deviate toward the opposite direction. Absence of movement to bilateral cold stimulation confirms an absent reflex.

Oculo-cephalic reflexes
Also called 'doll's eye' reflexes. With the eyelids held open brisk lateral rotation of the head normally produces opposite rotation of the eyeball as if to fix the gaze on an object. This rotation is lost in brain stem death.

Gag reflex
The gag reflex is absent in brain stem death. However, the gag reflex is often lost in patients who are intubated.

Apnoea test
While the reflex assessments are being performed the patient should be pre-oxygenated with 100% oxygen. The ventilator is disconnected and 6L/min oxygen is passed into the trachea via a catheter. Apnoeic oxygenation can sustain SaO_2 for prolonged periods but there is an inevitable rise in $PaCO_2$ which should stimulate respiratory effort. After 3–15min disconnection blood gas analyses are performed until $PaCO_2 > 8kPa$. Any respiratory effort negates the diagnosis of brain stem death.

Care of the potential organ donor

Patients with suspected brainstem death should be considered candidates for organ donation unless there is evidence of:
- Cancer (except primary central nervous system
- HIV or hepatitis surface antigen positive
- High risk for HIV
- Uncontrolled sepsis
- Significant systemic disease
- Slow virus infection.

The transplant co-ordinator should be contacted early (before the family are approached) to confirm likely suitability. If the family are amenable, the transplant co-ordinator will then initiate organ donation procedures. Do not reject those brain dead potential donors who, for example, have fully treated infections or acute renal failure without consultation with the transplant co-ordinator.

Management

1 Confirm brainstem death with appropriate testing.
2 Laboratory tests for blood group, HIV and hepatitis status and electrolytes.
3 Confirm organ donation is permissible by the coroner (or equivalent)
4 Maintain optimal cardiorespiratory status with fluid ± inotropes, optimal ventilation and physiotherapy. Diabetes insipidus should be treated with DDAVP.
5 Contact surgical and anaesthetic teams.

Organ suitability

- Kidneys—Age 4–70, acceptable U & E and Creatinine
- Heart—Age 0–50, acceptable CXR and ECG
- Lungs—Age 0–50, acceptable CXR and Blood gases
- Liver—Age 0–55, no alcohol or drug abuse, acceptable LFTs
- Corneas—Age 0–100, no previous intraocular surgery

The transplant co-ordinator will advise on other organ and tissue suitability, e.g. pancreas, trachea, bowel, skin.

See also:
Urea & creatinine, 136; Electrolytes (Na$^+$, K$^+$, Cl$^-$, HCO$_3^-$), 138; Virology, serology & assays, 150; Fluid challenge, 262; Inotropes, 184; Brain stem death, 516

ICU Organisation

ICU layout

The intensive care unit should be easily accessible by departments from which patients are admitted and close to departments which share engineering services. It is desirable that critically ill patients are separated from those requiring coronary care or high dependency care where a quieter environment is often needed. It is possible to provide intensive care and high dependency care in the same unit so long as patients can be separated within the unit. However, the differing requirements of these patients may limit such flexibility. The floor sizes given below represent a minimum guide.

Size

Intensive care bed requirements depend on the activity of the hospital with additional beds required for regional specialties such as cardiothoracic surgery or neurosurgery. Small (< 6 beds) or very large (> 14 beds) units may be difficult to manage although larger units may be divided operationally and allow better concentration of resources.

Patient areas

- Patient areas must provide unobstructed passage around the bed with a floor space of $20m^2$ per bed. Curtains or screens are required for privacy.
- Floors and ceilings must be constructed to support heavy equipment (some may weigh 1000 kg).
- Doors must allow for passage of bulky equipment as well as wide beds.
- Every bed should have access to a wash hand basin.
- The specification should include at least 1 cubicle per 6 beds with $30m^2$ floor area for isolation. Air conditioning should allow for positive and negative pressure control in cubicles, temperature and humidity control.
- Services must include adequate electricity supply (at least 20 sockets per bed) with emergency back-up supply. Oxygen (3), medical air (2) and suction (2) outlets must be available for every bed.
- The bed areas should have natural daylight and patients and staff should ideally have an outside view.
- Communications systems include an adequate number of telephones to avoid all telephones being in use at once, intercom systems to allow bed to bed communication and a system to control entry to the department.
- Computer networks should enable communication with central hospital administration and laboratory systems.

Other areas

Other areas include storage space ($12m^2$ per bed), dirty utility ($20m^2$), clean utility ($10m^2$), offices ($45m^2$), doctor's bedroom ($15m^2$), laboratory ($15m^2$), seminar room ($30m^2$), cleaner's room ($10m^2$), staff rest room, locker room, toilets, relatives' area, bedroom and interview room.

ICU staffing (medical)

Intensive care has evolved from the early success in simple mechanical ventilation of the lungs of polio victims to the present day where patients admitted to intensive care will usually have failure or dysfunction of one or more organ systems requiring mechanical support and monitoring. The intensive care unit should have dedicated consultant sessions allocated with additional allocation for management and audit activities. These sessions should be divided between several intensive care specialists. In addition, the intensive care specialist should be supported by junior doctors in training who can provide 24h per day cover on a rota which provides for adequate rest.

Required skills of intensive care medical staff

Management
Senior intensive care medical staff, together with their senior nursing colleagues, command the primary responsibility for the financial management of the intensive care unit. It is through their actions that treatment of the critically ill is initiated and perpetuated; they are ultimately responsible for the activity of the unit and patient outcome.

Decision making
In the ICU most decisions are ultimately made by team consensus. Clinical decisions in the intensive care unit can be thought of under three categories: (i) decisions relating to common or routine problems for which a unit policy exists; (ii) decisions relating to uncommon problems requiring discussion with all ICU and non-ICU staff currently involved and (iii) decisions of an urgent nature taken by intensive care staff without delay.

Practical skills
Expertise in the management of complex equipment, monitoring procedures and performance of invasive procedures are required.

Clinical experience
Medical staff require experience in the recognition, prevention and management of critical illness, infection control, anaesthesia and organ support.

Technical knowledge
The intensive care specialist has an important role in the choice of equipment used in the intensive care unit.

Pharmacological knowledge
Drug therapy regimens are clearly open to the problems of drug interactions and, in addition, pharmacokinetics are often severely altered by the effects of major organ system dysfunction, particularly involving the liver and kidneys.

Teaching and training
The modern intensive care specialist has acquired a number of skills that cannot be gained outside the intensive care unit. It is therefore necessary to be able to provide this education to junior doctors in training for intensive care.

ICU staffing (nursing)

Critically ill patients require close nursing supervision. Many will require 1:1 nursing throughout a 24h period while others are of a lower dependency and can share nurses. A few patients are so ill with the need for multiple interventions that their real nursing requirement is > 1:1. In addition to the bedside nurses, the department needs additional staff to manage the day to day operation of the unit, to assist in lifting and handling of patients, to relieve bedside nurses for rest periods and to collect drugs and equipment. These additional nurses can be termed the 'fixed nursing establishment' and the nature of their duties is such that they will usually be higher grade nurses. The bedside nurses are a 'variable establishment' and their numbers are dependent on activity such that more patients require higher numbers. Most departments fix their variable establishment by assuming an average activity.

Fixed establishment

In the UK providing 1 nurse per shift for 24h per day 7 days per week requires 4.5 nurses. In addition, staff handover, annual leave, study leave and sickness are usually calculated at 22% such that 1 additional nurse is required. Thus the provision of 1 nurse in charge of each shift and 1 nurse to support the bedside nurses requires 11 additional nurses. In larger units there may be a need for additional support nurses and less in smaller units.

Variable establishment

The same principles apply for the provision of bedside nurses. Thus, to provide 1:1 nursing for a bed requires 5.5 nurses and to provide 1:2 nursing requires 2.75 nurses. The total number required depends on the occupancy and the nurse to patient ratio for each occupied bed. One of the difficulties in staffing an intensive care unit relates to the variable dependency and occupancy. An average dependency weighted occupancy (average occupancy × average nurse to patient ratio) should be used to set the establishment of bedside nurses with additional nurses being drafted in from a bank or agency to cover peak demands.

Skill Mix

Nursing skill mix is the subject of much controversy as the need for economy is balanced against the need for quality. As stated above the fixed nursing will usually be of higher grade since the role incorporates the administration of the unit and supervisory nursing. The bedside nurses will be made up of those who have received post-qualification training in intensive care and those who have not. The ratio of trained to untrained intensive care nurses should be of the order of 3:1 to facilitate in-service teaching.

Fire safety

Fires affecting the ICU are rare but are particularly difficult in that patients are not easily evacuated, yet their lives depend on services which fire may disrupt. Smoke, while dangerous to staff and the less critically ill patients who may be breathing spontaneously, is less of a problem to those on mechanical ventilation since their fresh gas supply is from outside the affected environment. It therefore follows that, in the event of fire, the priority is to ensure safety and means of escape for the staff first.

Control of smoke

Smoke and toxic gases are a common association with fire and may, in themselves, be flammable, particularly in association with high concentrations of oxygen. The main techniques for control of smoke include containment (e.g. fire resisting walls, doors and seals) and dispersal (e.g. positive pressure air conditioning); the latter being used in patient areas. The possibility of flammable or toxic fumes should be considered when equipping and furnishing the intensive care unit.

Escape from fire

- Escape routes should be well marked and unobstructed.
- The nature of critical illness is such that not all patients can be evacuated.
- The staff should escape first by proceeding to the nearest exit away from the fire.
- Patients should be evacuated in the order of the least sick first.
- Evacuation of patients should be managed by someone trained in the use of breathing apparatus; in most cases this will be the fire brigade.
- If patients are to be evacuated they should be moved to a place of safety on the same floor as the intensive care unit. Patients should not be moved downstairs.
- In the majority of fires containment will reduce the need for full evacuation.

Preventing fire

- Automatic smoke or heat alarms should be provided in all areas.
- Cooking areas and laboratory areas must be separated from patient areas by fire doors.
- Fire doors are provided to protect staff and patients and should not be wedged open.
- If a closed door would compromise the care given to patients but is essential to separate fire compartments then an electro-mechanical device should hold the door open and be disabled by the fire alarm.
- Fire extinguishers of the appropriate types should be readily available and staff should be properly trained in their use.

Communication

Good communication is essential to the smooth running of the ICU. This includes communication between the ICU staff, patient, visiting professionals and relatives.

Patient communication

Critically ill patients may still be able to hear conversation despite sedation or apparent unconsciousness. Bedside discussions should take this into account and all procedures should be explained to the patient in simple terms before starting. The patient who is not competent to consent to treatment may appreciate verbal discussion or explanation.

Doctor—nurse communication

It is essential that the multidisciplinary approach to intensive care involves medical and nursing staff in decision making. Ward rounds are a forum for such interdisciplinary communication and the consultant leading the round should ensure that all present are truly involved. The plan for the day can be set on the ward round but is more likely to succeed if all involved in effecting the plan are involved in setting it. Similarly, all changes from the plan, whether due to unforeseen emergencies or due to failure of the patient to respond, should be fully discussed.

Communication with visiting teams

The intensive care staff should be responsible for the day to day care of critically ill patients, including coordinating the input from various non-ICU professionals involved in the management of patients and effecting the treatment plan. The admitting team should be involved in major decisions. Visiting medical staff should not see patients without being accompanied by a member of the intensive care medical staff.

Communication with relatives

Relatives are often overwhelmed by the environment of an intensive care unit, are worried about the patient and are easily confused by the information they are given about critically ill patients. Most communication should be face to face, avoiding lengthy discussions on the telephone. Where several people are imparting information, differences in emphasis or content destroy any chance of effective communication. It is essential that the bedside nurse is present when relatives are spoken to since there are often questions and concerns which crop up later and are directed to the nurse; it is worth remembering that the relatives have greater contact with the nurses and often build up a relationship with them. Where admitting teams need to communicate with relatives about a specific aspect of the illness the bedside nurse and, ideally, a member of the intensive care medical staff, should be present. Most interviews with relatives should be away from the bedside although it is often helpful to impart simple information at the bedside, particularly to demonstrate particular issues. Again it must be remembered that the patient may hear the conversation. While it is helpful to interview all relatives together this is not always practical, either because they cannot all be present at once or because they do not relate to each other. Information often changes when delivered second hand so it is better to communicate directly with various relatives separately in these circumstances.

Medicolegal aspects

The intensive care unit is a source of many medicolegal problems. Patients are often not competent to consent to treatment. They may be admitted following trauma, violence or poisoning, all of which may involve a legal process. Admission may also follow complications of treatment or medical mishaps occurring elsewhere in the hospital. The nature of critical illness is such that complications are common and litigation may follow.

Consent

Many procedures in intensive care are invasive or involve significant risk. The patient is often not competent to consent for such treatment such that the next of kin must be involved. It is essential that the risks and benefits are explained to the person giving assent and a chance is given for the patients wishes to be taken into account. It is all too easy to achieve assent from a relative without giving adequate explanation of the options. Research presents consent problems in the critically ill and requires close ethical committee supervision.

Note-keeping

It is impossible to record everything that happens in intensive care in the patients' notes. The 24h observation chart provides the most detailed record of what has happened but summary notes are essential. Such notes must be factual without unsubstantiated opinions about the patient or about previous treatment. All entries must be timed and signed. Records of ward rounds must record the name of the consultant leading the round. it must be remembered that the notes may be used later in legal proceedings. They may be used against you but if well kept will usually form the best defence. In the event of a medical mishap the episode should be clearly documented after witnessed explanation to relatives.

Dealing with the police

Most police enquiries relate to patients who are admitted after suspicious circumstances. While there is a duty to patient confidentiality it may be in the patient's interests to impart information about them. This may be with the consent of the patient or the next of kin. Written statements or verbal information may be requested. Any information given should avoid opinion and stick to facts.

Dealing with the coroner

The Coroner must be informed of any death where a death certificate cannot be issued. Death certificates can be issued where the death is due to a natural cause and the patient has been seen professionally by the doctor within 14 days prior to death. The table documents the conditions requiring the Coroner to be informed. Where there is any doubt the Coroner should be informed.

Deaths which must be informed to the Coroner

Unidentified body
No doctor attending within prior 14 days
Death without recovery from anaesthesia
Sudden or unexplained death
Medical mishap
Industrial accident or disease
Violence, accident or misadventure
Suspicious circumstances
Alcoholism
Poisoning
Death in custody

Audit

Audit has become an essential part of medical practice. The main purpose is to improve quality of care which, in the intensive care unit, must involve all members of the multidisciplinary team. Change in practice in one discipline will inevitably have a knock-on effect in others. Audit may involve a review of activity, performance against pre-determined indicators or cost-effectiveness. Audit may focus on specific topics or may encompass the performance of several intensive care units. Successful audit requires commitment from senior staff to ensure practice is defined, data are collected and change is effected where necessary. Where change is suggested by audit a further review is required to ensure that such change has occurred. Intensive care is a small specialty which may create difficulties for individual hospitals to carry out successful audit alone. In these circumstances it is better that several intensive care units group together for the purposes of audit.

Data collection

Ideally, a basic data set should be common to all intensive care units nationally to allow meaningful comparisons to be made. This requires the data set to be detailed enough to answer questions posed but not so detailed that collection becomes unsustainable. Resources must be provided in terms of computer databases and staff to collect and analyse data. Those collecting the data should be provided with regular summary reviews to ensure that enthusiasm continues. and quality control is maintained. Methods of data entry should consider the time involved and the fact that most of those collecting data are not keyboard experts. Typographical mistakes destroy the value of collected data such that error trapping and data validation must form part of the housekeeping in any database used. Some audit topics require data collection that is not part of the basic data set. Collecting appropriate data requires clarity in setting the question to be answered and care in choosing data items that will truly answer the question.

Audit meetings

Regular audit meetings should follow a pre-defined timetable. This helps to ensure maximum staff attendance and also sets target dates for data collection and analysis. Audit meetings should be chaired and have defined aims. Discussion of the topic being audited must lead to recommended changes in practice and these must be followed through after the meeting. It is clear that all staff cannot attend all meetings. Dissemination of information prior to implementing proposed changes is necessary to stand some chance of carrying them through.

ICU scoring systems

Various ICU scoring systems have evolved to provide:
- An index of disease severity, e.g. APACHE, SAPS.
- An index of workload and consumption of resources, e.g. TISS.
- A means of comparison for
  (i) auditing performance—either in the same ICU or between ICUs.
  (ii) research, e.g. evaluation of new products or treatment regimens.
- Patient management objectives, e.g. sedation, pressure area care.

Other than the Glasgow Coma Score, there is no universal system practised by every ICU. While APACHE is the predominant system used in the USA and UK for scoring disease severity, SAPS is more popular in mainland Europe. Interpretation of the same system can also be highly variable.

TISS (Therapeutic Intervention Scoring System)
- This system attaches a score to procedures and techniques performed on an individual patient (e.g. use and number of vasoactive drug infusions, renal replacement therapy, administration of enteral nutrition).
- It has been used by some ICUs to develop a means of costing individual patients by attaching a monetary value to each TISS point scored.
- It is also used as an index of workload activity.
- A discharge TISS score can be used to estimate the amount of nursing interventions required for a patient in step-down facilities (e.g. a High Dependency Unit) or on the general ward.
- TISS does not accurately measure nursing workload activity as it fails to cater for tasks and duties such as coping with the irritable or confused patient, dealing with grieving relatives, etc...

Glasgow Coma Scale
First described by Teasdale and Jennett in 1974, it utilises eye opening, best motor response and best verbal response to categorise neurological status. It is the only system used universally in ICUs though limitations exist in mechanically ventilated, sedated patients. It can be used for prognostication and is also frequently used for therapeutic decision making, e.g. elective ventilation in patients presenting with a GCS < 8.

Sedation
A variety of systems gauge and record the level of sedation in a mechanically ventilated patient. This assists the staff to titrate the dose of sedative agents to avoid either over- or under-sedation. The forerunner developed in 1974 was the Ramsay Sedation Score which consists of a 6–point scoring system separated into 3 awake and 3 asleep levels where the patient responds to a tap or loud auditory stimulus with either brisk, sluggish or no response at all. The main problem lies in achieving reproducibility of the tap or loud auditory stimulus. We currently use an in-house 8–point system.

Glasgow coma scale

Score	Eyes open	Best motor response	Best verbal response
6	—	obeys commands	—
5	—	localises pain	orientated
4	spontaneously	flexion withdrawal	confused
3	to speech	decerebrate flexion	inappropriate words
2	to pain	decerebrate extension	incomprehensible sounds
1	never	no response	silent

UCLH Sedation Score

3	Agitated and restless
2	Awake and uncomfortable
1	Aware but calm
0	Roused by voice, remains calm
-1	Roused by movement
-2	Roused by noxious or painful stimuli
-3	Unrousable
A	Natural sleep

ICU scoring systems—APACHE II

APACHE (Acute Physiology And Chronic Health Evaluation)

- Devised by Knaus *et al.*, this system utilises a point score derived from the degree of abnormality of readily obtainable physiological and laboratory variables in the first 24h of ICU admission, plus extra points for age and chronic ill health.
- The summated score provides a measure of severity while the percentage risk of subsequent death can be computed from specific coefficients applied to a wide range of admission disorders (excluding burns and cardiac surgery).
- APACHE I, first described in 1981, utilised 34 physiological and biochemical variables.
- A simplified version (APACHE II) utilising just 12 variables was published in 1985 and extensively validated in a number of countries.
- A further refinement published in 1990, APACHE III, claims to improve upon the statistical predictive power by;
  1 Adding five new physiological variables (albumin, bilirubin, glucose, urea, urine output)
  2 Changing thresholds and weighting of existing variables
  3 Comparing both admission and 24h scores
  4 Incorporating the admission source (e.g. A&E, ward, operating theatre)
  5 Reassessing effects of age, chronic health and specific disease category.
- Wide acceptance of APACHE III may be limited as its risk stratification system is proprietary and has to be purchased.

APACHE II score (Crit Care Med 1985; 13: 818–829)

Acute physiology score

	+4	+3	+2	+1	0	+1	+2	+3	+4
Core temperature (°C)									
	˜ 41	39–40.9		38.2–38.9	36–38.4	34–35.9	32–33.9	30–31.9	¶ 29.9
Mean BP (mmHg)									
	˜ 160	130–159	110–129		70–109		50–69		¶ 49
Heart rate (/min)									
	˜ 180	140–179	110–139		70–109		55–69	40–54	¶ 39
Respiratory rate (/min)									
	˜ 50	35–49		25–34	12–24	10–11	6–9		¶ 5
If FIO_2 ˜0.5: A-aDO_2 (mmHg)									
	˜ 500	350–499	200–349		< 200				
If FIO_2 <0.5: PO_2 (mmHg)									
					> 70	61–70		55–60	¶ 55
Arterial pH									
	˜ 7.7	7.6–7.69		7.5–7.59	7.33–7.49		7.25–7.32	7.15–7.24	¶ 7.15
Serum Na^+ (mmol/L)									
	˜ 180	160–179	155–159	150–154	130–149		120–129	111–119	¶ 110
Serum K^+ (mmol/L)									
	˜ 7	6–6.9		5.5–5.9	3.5–5.4	3–3.4	2.5–2.9		< 2.5
Serum creatinine (μmol/L) NB double points score if acute renal failure									
	˜ 300	171–299	121–170		50–120		< 50		
Haematocrit (%)									
	˜ 60		50–59.9	46–49.9	30–45.9		20–29.9		< 20
Leukocytes (/mm^3)									
	˜ 40		20–39.9	15–19.9	3–14.9		1–2.9		< 1
Neurological points = 15 – Glasgow Coma Score									

Age points:

Years	≤44	45–54	55–64	65–74	≥75
Points	0	2	3	5	6

Chronic health points

2 points for elective post-operative admission or 5 points if emergency operation or non-operative admission, if patient has either:

- Biopsy proven cirrhosis, portal hypertension or previous hepatic failure
- Chronic heart failure (NYHA Grade 4),
- Chronic hypoxia, hypercapnia, severe exercise limitation, 2° polycythaemia or pulmonary hypertension
- Dialysis-dependent renal disease
- Immunosuppression by disease or drugs

ICU scoring systems—SAPS II

- Has a similar role to APACHE II, but more widely utilised in mainland Europe, the Simplified Acute Physiology Score (SAPS) was devised by LeGall et al in 1984 (SAPS I) and modified by the same group in 1993 (SAPS II).
- As for APACHE II, burns and cardiac surgical patients are excluded from analysis.
- The original version used 14 readily measured clinical and bio-chemical variables while the updated version, SAPS II, comprises 12 physiology variables, age, type of admission (medical, scheduled or unscheduled surgical) and three underlying disease variables.
- A point score is based on the degree and prognostic importance of derangement of these variables in the first 24h following ICU admission. The point scoring was assigned following logistic regression modelling of data obtained from 8369 patients in 137 adult ICUs in both Europe and North America and validated in a further 4628 patients.
- The claimed advantage of this system is that it estimates the risk of death without having to specify a primary diagnosis.

(JAMA 1993; 270: 2957–2963)

Point score in brackets

Age	< 40 (0); 40–59 (7); 60–69 (12); 70–74 (15); 75–79 (16); ⩾ 80 (18)
Heart rate (bpm)	< 40 (11); 40–69 (2); 70–119 (0); 120–159 (4); ⩾ 160 (7)
Systolic BP (mmHg)	< 70 (13); 70–99 (5); 100–199 (0); ⩾ 200 (2)
Body temp (°C)	< 39 (0); ⩾ 39 (3)
PaO_2/FIO_2 (kPa) only if ventilated or on CPAP	< 13.3 (11); 13.3–26.5 (9); ⩾ 26.6 (6)
Urine output (lL/day)	< 0.5 (11); 0.5–0.999 (4); ⩾ 1 (0)
Serum urea (mmol/L)	< 10 (0); 10–29.9 (6); ⩾ 30 (10)
White cell count (/mm^3)	< 1 (12); 1–19.9 (0); ⩾ 20 (3)
Serum K^+ (mmol/L)	< 3 (3); 3–4.9 (0); ⩾ 5 (3)
Serum Na^+ (mmol/L)	< 125 (5); 125–144 (0); ⩾ 145 (1)
Serum HCO_3^- (mmol/L)	< 15 (6); 15–19 (3); ⩾ 20 (0)
Serum bilirubin (μmol/L)	< 68.4 (0); 68.4–102.5 (4); ⩾ 102.6 (9)
Glasgow coma score	< 6 (26); 6–8 (13); 9–10 (7); 11–13 (5); 14–15 (0)
Chronic disease	metastatic cancer (9), haematological malignancy (10), AIDS (17)
Type of admission	scheduled surgical (0); medical (6); unscheduled surgical (8)

ICU scoring systems—trauma

Scoring systems have been developed in trauma for:
- Rapid field triage to direct the patient to appropriate levels of care
- Quality assurance
- Developing and improving trauma care systems by categorising patients and identifying problems within the systems
- Making comparisons between groups from different hospitals, in the same hospital over time, and/or undergoing different treatments.

The Injury Severity Score (ISS) is a severity scoring system patients based on the anatomical injuries sustained. The Revised Trauma Score (RTS) utilises measures of physiological abnormality to predict survival. A combination of ISS and RTS—TRISS—was developed to overcome the shortcomings of anatomical or physiological scoring alone. The TRISS methodology uses ISS, RTS, patient age and whether the injury was blunt or penetrating to provide a measure of the probability of survival.

Injury Severity Score

1 Use AIS90 (Abbreviated Injury Score 1990) dictionary to score injury
2 Identify highest abbreviated injury scale score for each of the following:
- Head & neck
- Abdomen & pelvic contents
- Bony pelvis & limbs
- Face
- Chest
- Body surface
3 Add together the squares of the three highest area scores

Revised trauma score

	measure	coded value	× weighting	= score
Respiratory rate (breaths/min)	10–29	4		
	> 29	3		
	6–9	2	0.2908	
	1–5	1		
	0	0		
Systolic blood pressure (mmHg)	> 89	4		
	76–89	3		
	50–75	2	0.7326	
	1–49	1		
	0	0		
Glasgow coma scale	13–15	4		
	9–12	3		
	6–8	2	0.9368	
	4–5	1		
	3	0		

Total = revised trauma score

Index

.